Ultrasonography in Ophthalmology 14

Documenta Ophthalmologica Proceedings Series

VOLUME 58

The titles published in this series are listed at the end of this volume.

Ultrasonography in Ophthalmology 14

Proceedings of the
14th SIDUO Congress,
Tokyo, Japan 1992

Edited by
J.M. THIJSSEN
H.C. FLEDELIUS
S. TANE

SPRINGER-SCIENCE+BUSINESS MEDIA, B.V.

Library of Congress Cataloging-in-Publication Data
SIDUO Congress (14th   1992   Tokyo, Japan)
    Proceedings of the 14th SIDUO Congress, Tokyo, Japan, 1992 /
  edited by J.M. Thijssen and H.C. Fledelius and S. Tane.
        p.   cm. -- (Documenta ophthalmologica. Proceedings series , v.
  58)
    Includes index.
    ISBN 978-94-010-4015-0   ISBN 978-94-011-0025-0 (eBook)
    DOI 10.1007/978-94-011-0025-0
    1. Ultrasonics in ophthalmology--Congresses.   I. Thijssen, J. M.
  II. Fledelius, H.   III. Tane, S.   IV. Title.   V. Series.
    [DNLM 1. Eye Diseases--ultrasonography--congresses. 2. Eye--
  ultrasonography--congresses.   3. Ultrasonography--methods--
  congresses.   W3 D0637 v.58 1995 / WW 143 S569p 1995]
  RE79.U4S5   1992
  617.7'1543--dc20
  DNLM/DLC
  for Library of Congress   95-14247
ISBN 978-94-010-4015-0

Printed on acid-free paper

Table of Contents

PART THREE: DIAGNOSIS OF INTRAOCULAR DISEASES

Preface

The 14th Congress of SIDUO, held in Tokyo from October 26 to October 30, 1992, was the first congress meeting to be held in Asia in the 30-year history of SIDUO. The congress was organized by the Department of Ophthalmology, St. Marianna University School of Medicine, with the support of the Japanese Ophthalmological Society, the Japan Society of Ultrasonics in Medicine and the Japan Society of Ophthalmologists.

The organizing committee consisted of the following members.

Congress President:	Sadanao Tane, M.D. (Professor and Chairman, St. Marianna University School of Medicine)
Vice-presidents:	Atsushi Sawada, M.D. (Professor and Chairman, Miyazaki Medical College)
	Masayasu Ito, Ph.D. (Tokyo University of Agriculture and Technology)
Secretary General:	Yasuo Sugata, M.D. (Tokyo Metropolitan Komagome Hospital)
Finance Committee:	Koji Ohashi, M.D. (Assistant Professor, St. Marianna University School of Medicine)
	Akira Komatsu, M.D. (Assistant Professor, St. Marianna University School of Medicine)
	Toshio Kaneko, M.D. (Assistant Professor, St. Marianna University School of Medicine)
Publicity and Exhibition Committee:	
	Hideyuki Hayashi, M.D. (Assistant Professor, School of Medicine, Fukuoka University)
	Akihiro Kaneko, M.D. (National Cancer Center)

The Honorary Presidents were Yukio Yamamoto, M.D. (Tokyo Tama Geriatrics Hospital) and Yasuo Uemura, M.D. (Professor Emeritus, Keio University).

The opening ceremony began with the *Francois Memorial Lecture* given by Professor Peter Till (Standardized Echography: Quantitative Analysis of

Tissue Backscatter – A Major Source of Information for Tissue Diagnoses). Subsequently, Professor Pier-Enrico Gallenga gave the *Invited Lecture 1* (History of Ophthalmic Diagnostic Ultrasound), and Professor Karl C. Ossoinig gave the *Invited Lecture 2* (The Diagnosis and Differential Diagnosis of Neoplastic Lesions of the Extraocular Muscles with Standardized Echography).

These lecturers were followed by an awards ceremony, and the SIDUO Pioneer Award was bestowed upon Professor K.C. Ossoinig. Following Professor Gilbert Baum and Professor Arvo Oksala, Professor Ossoinig is the third recipient of this award, which is given to a member for prominent, unique achievements, and which expresses our appreciation and gratitude for important contributions to the development of ophthalmic ultrasonography.

This volume of the Documenta Ophthalmologica Proceedings Series of SIDUO-XIV carries 47 of the 89 scientific papers presented as general lectures at the congress. The topics of these papers have been compiled in the following sections: 1. Instrumentation and techniques; 2. Biometric ultrasound; 3. Diagnosis of intraocular diseases; 4. Diagnosis of orbital- and periorbital diseases.

The section on development of new techniques and equipment covers such issues as computer analysis of ultrasonic images, development of the digital color display, high-resolution and high-frequency imaging display, three-dimensional imaging display, application of the new annular array probe and fax network ultrasound diagnosis.

The section on ultrasonic biometry covers microbiometry of the depth of the retino-choroidal layer, determination of the external muscles in the orbit and of the optic nerve, and their clinical estimation, and finally, various problems associated with the determination of intraocular lens power.

The section on diagnosis of intraocular diseases discusses the use of standardized echography in routine examinations, and its effectiveness in the differential diagnosis of various inflammatory diseases and tumors, as well as the use of B-scan ultrasonography.

The section on the diagnosis of orbital and periorbital diseases reports that, in spite of the introduction of other imaging modalities such as CT and MRI, the simple, safe, quick method of echography has been the method of choice for screening examinations. In this section, Doppler echography of blood flow examination has been used for the practical diagnosis of various ophthalmological diseases and evaluation of their stage, following the rapid progress of technology and equipment.

Finally, our heartfelt gratitude is extended to Professor K.C. Ossoinig, who expressed kind consideration and provided instructions that assisted in our preparations for hosting the SIDUO-XIV Congress in Tokyo. We are also grateful to Professor, P.E. Gallenga, Professor P. Till, Professor G. Cennamo, Professor G. Hasenfratz, Dr. J.M. Thijssen, Dr. H.C. Fledelius and Dr. H.J. Shammas for their helpful advice.

We would also like to express our gratitude to Professor Emeritus Akira

Nakajima (Juntendo University, President of the International Council of Ophthalmology), and Professor Emeritus Toshio Wagai (Juntendo University, former President of the Japan Society of Ultrasonics in Medicine), and to the members of the Advisory Board, for their instructions and advice.

Sadanao Tane, M.D. President SIDUO 14

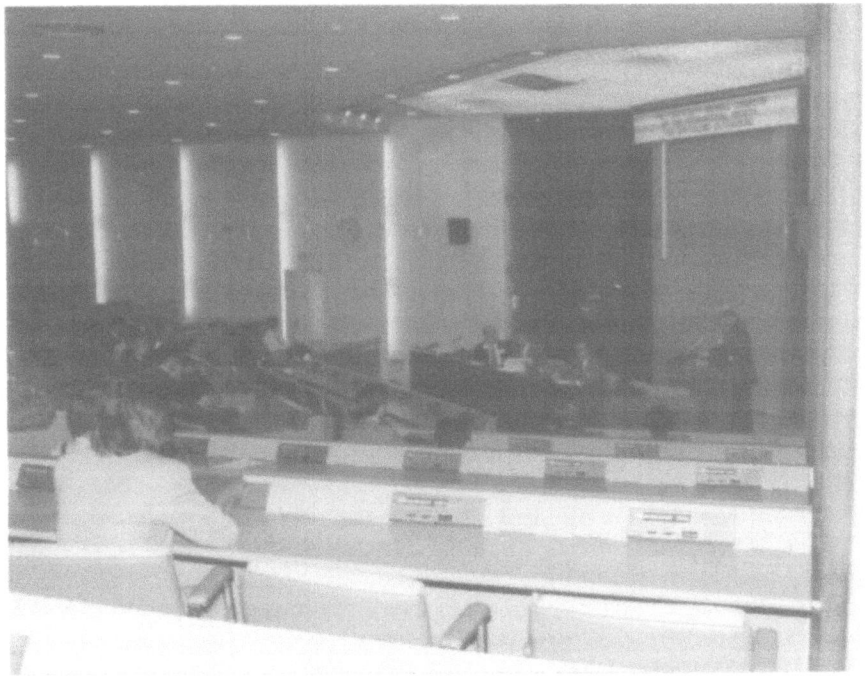

Professor Karl C. Ossoinig presenting his invited lecture. Lecture Hall of the National Cancer Center, Tokyo.

Message from Akira Nakajima, M.D.
President of the International Council of Ophthalmology.
Professor Emeritus, Juntendo University

Professor Tane, President of the 14th SIDUO Congress, participants of the congress, ladies and gentlemen, I am very glad to have the 14th SIDUO Congress here in Tokyo at last. I sincerely hope, and I am sure, that the congress, so well prepared by the local organizing committee, headed by Professor Tane, will be a great success. Our friends from abroad will play an essential role in the success of the meeting.

I attended the meetings of SIDUO, in particular the meetings in Muenster in 1966 and in Philadelphia were impressive to me. The topics of the congress were basic, technical and clinical, but few were clinical routine at that time. Now, in 1992, ultrasound is playing an indispensable role in ophthalmic practice. Ultrasonic phacoemulsification is a preferred method for cataract surgery. Axial length measurement by ultrasound is an indispensable preparatory step for insertion of IOLs. A- and B-mode are essential for ophthalmic diagnosis. The progress took place in the last two decades. I sincerely hope that the topics to be discussed during this congress will produce new and useful clinical armamentarium in the 21st century.

I wish that our friends from abroad will enjoy the beautiful autumn of Tokyo and will have a most pleasant stay in Japan. I wish all the best for the success of the 14th SIDUO Congress. Thank you for your attention.

Standardized Echography: Quantitative Analysis of Tissue Backscatter – A Major Source of Information for Tissue Diagnoses

2nd SIDUO Jules François Memorial Lecture

PETER TILL

(Vienna, Austria)

1. Introduction

Acoustic tissue signals are reliable and precise indicators of the tissues reflectivity under controlled and standardized conditions only. Specifically designed and standardized A-scan instrumentation and examinations techniques are absolutely required in order to obtain meaningful and diagnostic, both repeatable and comparable tissue signals. Both this special design and its standardization were developed by Ossoinig resulting in a series of so-called Standardized Echography Instruments [9, 16, 19, 20, 24, 32, 50]. The Mini-Scan A (Biophysic/Alcon; 1989) was the most precise digital instrument that became available for Standardized Echography. The Biovision S (BVI/Telsar; 1994) is the latest of these developments combining a fast digital Standardized A-scan with a high-resolution B-scan unit.

The first standardized A-scan was Ossoinig's Kretztechnik 7000. This instrument had been purchased by the 2nd Eye Department at the University of Vienna in 1963. It gradually was modified over a period of several years in cooperation with Kretztechnik in order to optimize its electronic design for tissue diagnosis. The modifications were based on the results of numerous clinical and experimental studies done in Vienna between 1963 and 1968 [1–3, 5, 7, 10–14, 17, 18, 21–23, 25–29]. This modified Kretztechnik 7000 instrument became the first prototype of Standardized A-scan.

The first commercially available instrument utilizing the Kretztechnik 7000 technology was the 7900 S. It combined the special A-scan design with a semi-automatic immersion B-scan unit (for both linear and compound scanning) and thus became also the first commercially available B-scan in ophthalmology [9, 13–17, 19–22]. It was produced in a small series only. Kretztechnik developed the 7900 S series with Ossoinig on the basis of his experience with the Kretz 7000 and used it as another more advanced prototype for the Kretztechnik 7200 MA which became available world-wide in 1971.

The Kretztechnik 7200 MA then was the gold standard of A-scan echography for the following decades [30–38, 40–44, 46, 48–50]. The Sonokretz-

J M Thijssen, H C Fledelius and S Tane (eds), Ultrasonography in Ophthalmology 14 xvii–xxxi
© 1995 Kluwer Academic Publishers, Dordrecht

Ocuscan (Sonometrics/Cilco), the Ophthascan S (Biophysic/Alcon), and finally the Mini-A-Scan (Biophysic/Alcon) were all the successors of the Kretz 7200 MA instrument utilizing the same principle but applying the greatly advanced electronic technologies of their time [50]. All of these Standardized A-scan units (combined with a real-time B-scan or as stand-alone units) were based entirely on the specifications laid down for the design of the Kretz 7200 MA.

2. Instrumentation

The specific design of a Standardized A-scan instrument [27, 28, 40–42] includes the design and function of the A-scan probe: it utilizes a plane transducer with a diameter of 5 mm, works with an effective frequency of 8 MHz ($\pm 5\%$) and emits a non-focused, parallel beam. Based on physical principles, it should be kept in mind that the effective sound beam width depends on the setting of the instrument sensitivity and on the reflectivity of the echo producing tissue structures under examination.

A narrow-band amplifier is used to optimize the instruments signal-to-noise ratio. A special low-pass filtering procedure is applied to optimize the visual signal evaluation on the instrument screen, the so-called visual pattern recognition. The filtering also serves the purpose of specific smoothing of the left ascending limbs of membrane spikes as obtained at Tissue Sensitivity of the Standardized A-scan instrument, and thus of differentiating smooth large interfaces (i.e., detached retina) from coarse large strongly reflecting surfaces (i.e., dense fibrovascular membranes) [48, 49]. Other very important designs of the signal processing applied in Standardized A-scans for the purpose of optimal display of significant acoustic information include a constant ratio between horizontal and vertical display dimensions and, in particular, a special **S-shaped amplifier characteristic curve**.

When signal intensities are plotted (in dB along the x-axis) against signal heights (in mm along the y-axis) this special amplifier produces a curve (amplifier characteristic curve) that has the shape of an asymmetric S: the central portion is steep, whereas the lower and, especially, the upper ends taper off (are compressed) [25, 28, 32, 34, 40–42, 44, 46, 48, 50]. The S-shaped amplifier characteristic curve is responsible for two very important acoustic properties of the instrument: (a) its relative sensitivity (acoustic acuity) and (b) its dynamic range (acoustic field of view).

The *relative sensitivity* is the capacity of the instrument to display different echo intensities as clearly different signal intensities (spike heights). A great relative sensitivity means that even minimal differences in echo intensities can be displayed as differently high spikes on the screen of the instrument. Poor relative sensitivity implies that echoes must differ greatly in intensity to be displayed as different signal heights. The *dynamic range* indicates the difference (in dB) between the weakest echo signal that is still displayed (in 5% of the display height) at a given instrument sensitivity setting and the strongest echo signal that – at the same instrument sensitivity setting – is displayed in 95% height of the display. The larger this total dynamic range is, the more echo signals can differ in intensity and still be displayed clearly (neither subthreshold, nor overloaded).

Relative sensitivity and dynamic range of an amplifier are principles in opposition to each other: the greater the relative sensitivity of an amplifier is, the smaller its dynamic range becomes, and vice versa. A **linear amplifier**, for instance, provides a great relative sensitivity, especially in its upper range of signal heights; a linear amplifier, however, is deficient in its dynamic range. In practice, a linear amplifier can display very small differences in tissue reflectivity, but can display only relatively thin layers of a tissue at any given instrument sensitivity setting. The stronger a tissue attenuates the ultrasound, the thinner is the tissue layer seen echographically at a given sensitivity setting. **Logarithmic amplifiers** can provide great dynamic range. The larger their dynamic range is, however, the poorer becomes their relative sensitivity. Thus neither linear nor logarithmic amplifiers are satisfactory for the echographic evaluation of tissues and for acoustic tissue diagnoses. These objectives require both a wide dynamic range (so that thick tissue layers may be evaluated at a single system sensitivity) and a great relative sensitivity (to be able to distinguish minor acoustic differences in tissue structures).

The **special S-shaped amplifier** developed by Ossoinig for Standardized Echography combines the advantages of both the linear and logarithmic amplifiers without introducing their disadvantages. The steeply rising central portion of the S-shaped amplifier curve provides great relative sensitivity (acoustic acuity) whereas the lower and upper (compressed) ends of the curve provide sufficient dynamic range (acoustic field). In order to explain the situation better to ophthalmologists, Ossoinig compared the functions of the special S-shaped as well as linear and logarithmic amplifiers with the function of normal vs. diseased human eyes: just as the normal human eye utilizes the great visual acuity of the macular region together with the wide visual field provided by the peripheral retina, so the S-shaped amplifier uses the central portion for achieving great acoustic acuity and the peripheral (lower and upper) ends of the curve for a wide acoustic field. The linear amplifier, though providing excellent acoustic acuity, lacks peripheral field (comparable to an eye with tube vision). The logarithmic amplifier, though providing excellent acoustic field (actually unnecessarily wide field), entirely lacks acoustic acuity (comparable to an eye with central scotoma) [44].

The special S-shaped amplifier is defined by a specific amount of total dynamic range (difference in dB between 5% and 95% high signals at a given system sensitivity). The simple fact that an A-scan instrument uses an S-shaped amplifier curve does not make this instrument standardized even when the total dynamic range is the required 33 dB. The distribution of this dynamic range along the curve is of crucial importance; it has been defined by Ossoinig [46] through a range of 16 dB between 1 and 30 mm of display height (2 to 57%). The more an S-shaped amplifier deviates from the standard first fully established in the Kretz technik 7200 MA instrument, the more the resulting tissue echograms may differ from the standard patterns and the less useful the resultant echograms will be for tissue diagnoses. The latter stems from the fact, that the standard curve was derived from years of experimentation and clinical examinations aimed at the purpose of achieving optimal results. Only A-scan instruments which are designed (though using different approaches in technical and electronic terms) to produce results in signal processing, which are identical to those of the Kretz technik 7200 MA, can be called standardized.

3. Examination Techniques

Instrument Settings
All instrument parameters which influence the appearance and diagnostic value of tissue echograms are designed optimally in a Standardized A-scan instrument. Some of these parameters such as the low-pass filtering and the amplification characteristics are fixed designs and cannot (and should not) be altered by the examiner. The examiner may change certain instrument parameters as needed during the examination. The extremely important instrument sensitivity settings are used here as an example. Two types of system sensitivity settings are predominantly used in Standardized Echography: (a) Tissue Sensitivity and (b) Measuring Sensitivity.

Tissue Sensitivity
Tissue Sensitivity is a high, defined system sensitivity of a Standardized A-scan unit which is the single most frequently used gain setting in Standardized Echography. It is determined for each instrument/probe combination with the help of a Tissue Model (see below). The detection of intraocular, orbital and periorbital lesions as well as their differentiation, and frequently even their measurement, are all performed at this instrument setting. Only few conditions or echographic objectives require an increase of the instrument gain above Tissue Sensitivity by 6 to 12 dB (e.g., early endophthalmitis) or a decrease below Tissue sensitivity (e.g., most precise measurements of thin tissue layers such as the retinochoroidal layer; see Measuring Sensitivity). Tissue Sensitivity is a constant setting for a given A-scan instrument/probe combination. Any repair of the instrument, but especially changes of the probe (including aging of the transducer), and at any rate an exchange of the probe, make it mandatory to check and, if changed, to correct the system sensitivity setting (in dB) that represents Tissue Sensitivity. It is recommended to check an instrument/probe combination in regular intervals for this sensitivity setting even if no such changes are known to have occurred.

Tissue Model
Tissue Sensitivity is determined for each instrument/probe combination with the help of a Tissue Model. Prototypes of the Tissue Model were developed

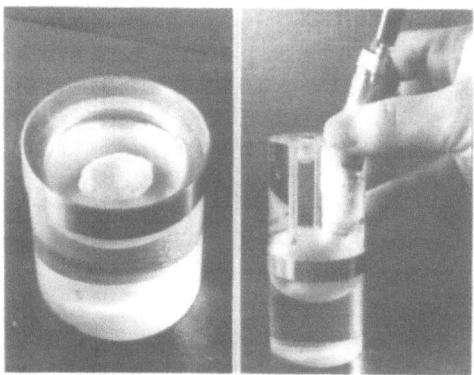

Figure 1 Tumor Model of the early 1960s designed by Ossoinig and Steiner *Left* open lower half of model showing a piece from a liver metastasis of a carcinoma of the pancreas *Right* Closed Tumor Model with hand-held probe in place for display of signals from the tumor

and tested by Ossoinig in the 1960s at the 2nd Eye Clinic in Vienna. They were first reported by him in 1964 at the first SIDUO Congress at the Charité University in Berlin [1]. At this meeting, Ossoinig reported special examination techniques for use in what later would be termed Standardized Echography: a topographic, kinetic and quantitative echography for the diagnosis of tumors in the eye and orbit using the 'time-amplitude method' – the 'A-scan'. Also at this meeting, he defined a certain optimal instrument sensitivity (the later Tissue Sensitivity), and suggested as test model a tumor phantom (Fig. 1). During the discussion he stressed that "it is of greatest importance to use a high, defined sensitivity to display a characteristic pattern from normal orbital tissues which is the key to differentiating them from pathological tissues [1].

Originally, a variety of reflectors such as large glass or steel surfaces in water or silicone oil were tested to find such an optimal sensitivity setting. In living tissues, however, echoes are primarily caused by scattering at small interfaces rather than by reflection at large mirror-like surfaces such as technological reflectors. It has been experimentally proven that scattering in tissues and reflection at such large targets are so different that their echoes are not comparable under practical circumstances [4]. It, therefore, became necessary to use scattering tissue models for setting a Standardized Instrument at Tissue Sensitivity.

A variety of human tissues obtained from surgery or autopsy (e.g., normal liver, liver metastases from carcinoma, etc.) were utilized by Ossoinig in 1964 (Fig. 1) [4]. In addition to the difficulty in obtaining such tissues, they rarely show uniform patterns and vary from case to case. The same is true for formalin-fixated tissues which exhibit continuing acoustic changes over a period of years. Suspensions of tumor cells obtained from rat or mouse ascites were also taken up. Unfortunately, it was impossible to get clean

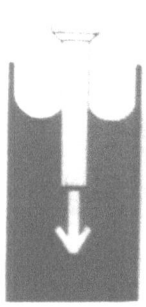 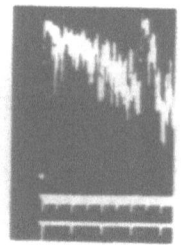 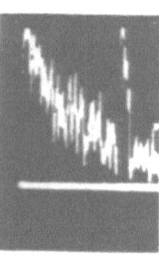

Figure 2. Schematic drawing (*left*) explains the immersion of the hand-held probe with tip at defined distance from the bottom of the Tissue Model (as determined from the microsecond scale on the screen of the Standardized A-scan instrument). *Center:* Echo pattern from Citrated Blood Model at higher than Tissue Sensitivity. *Right:* Echo pattern from the blood cells has medium height (signal-free zones above and below the chain of blood spikes are about equal in size) – indicating Tissue Sensitivity of the instrument/probe combination used.

populations of uniform cells. The suspensions were rather uncontrolled mixtures of living and dead tumor and blood cells, including necrotic debris. While cell cultures did produce more uniform tissue models, they failed to be useful mainly because of insufficient amounts of cells available at any one time. In order to use them as a tissue model, an amount of $20 \, mm^3$ was needed.

Finally **citrated human blood** of specific cell count and cell sedimentation rates of the donor turned out to be a very useful biological standard. Human blood cells are obtainable in sufficient amounts of one cell type and can easily be manipulated in terms of cell count and cell distribution. Citrated blood models were used since 1965 as the only useful standard for setting a Standardized A-scan Instrument at Tissue Sensitivity [8, 10, 11, 19, 25–28, 29, 30, 31, 33, 34, 38]. Each blood model consisting of a small glass container filled with citrated human blood of defined cell density had to be freshly prepared at the time of use. Before use, the blood was stirred with a glass rod and then left alone for 5 minutes. For the adjustment (or checking of) the Tissue Sensitivity, the probe was immersed into the citrated blood from above and held at a defined distance from the bottom of the glass container (Fig. 2). The instrument sensitivity was then adjusted in order to display the blood pattern in medium spike height.

The time-consuming preparation of such tissue models, their lack of durability and the limited accuracy inherent in any biological system such as this were significant disadvantages. For these reasons, standardization of A-scan Instruments remained difficult and restricted to a few major centers. Although citrated blood models allowed for a reliable standardization of A-scan instrumentation and techniques, the desire for a more simple and,

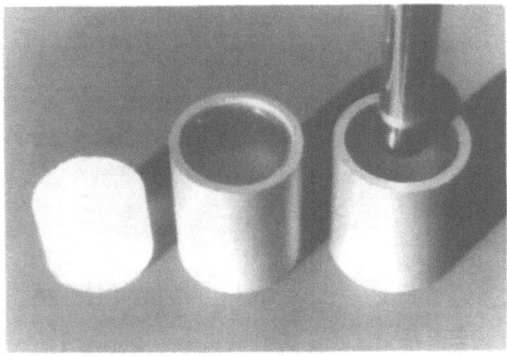

Figure 3. Plain substance of TM (*left*), its commercial form as contained in a metal shell (*center*), and the ultrasonic probe set on its top surface wetted with a liquid (*right*).

especially, durable model stimulated investigators to search for inorganic materials which could replace the blood model.

In 1975, I succeeded in finding an inorganic material, a silicon resin which was ideal in serving as matrix for a durable tissue model [39]. In this resin, a specified number of glass micro-beads of defined size and in equal and regular distribution (Fig. 3) provides the tissue model echoes. This solid Tissue Model (TM) replaced the citrated blood models which Ossoinig had developed as the standard for setting a Standardized A-scan Instrument at Tissue Sensitivity [43]. Since 1975 the TM is used for adjusting Tissue Sensitivity of each instrument/probe combination [44,45]. Every Standardized Instrument is equipped with a TM.

Figure 3 illustrates the TM with and without its metal shell. It also shows how the probe is placed on the top surface of the TM using a liquid (water, saline or methylcellulose) as contact agent. As in the citrated blood model (Fig. 2), the pattern obtained from within the TM (excluding the initial spike on the left and the maximized surface spike on the right) is utilized to adjust the Standardized A-scan instrument at Tissue Sensitivity. Tissue Sensitivity is obtained when the internal TM pattern is displayed in medium spike height (with the triangular signal-free zones above and below the spikes being of equal size). Figure 4 illustrates this procedure.

In blind studies, we examined the accuracy and reliability of these solid Tissue Models [47]. These blind studies were performed in the following manner: examiner A adjusted the Standardized A-scan instrument Kretz technik 7200 MA to Tissue Sensitivity by using the TM and by judging the echographic display without watching the dB dial of the instrument; examiner B recorded the dB setting in each adjustment without watching the echographic display. Each time, the probe was first completely removed from the TM and then re-applied to its surface; also, each time the dB control dial was reset at zero before proceeding with the next adjustment. The standard

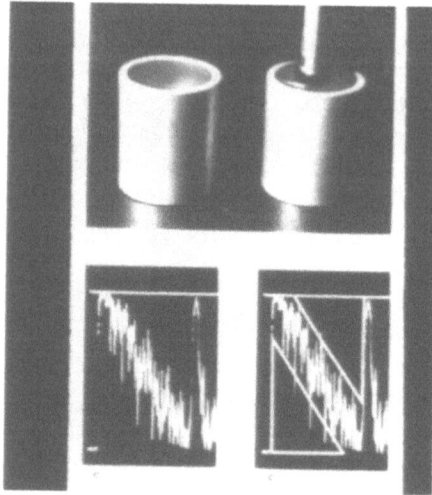

Figure 4. Top: TM with and without A-scan probe. *Bottom:* Echograms obtained at Tissue Sensitivity [T] (medium spike height; equal size of signal-free triangles above and below the TM spikes).

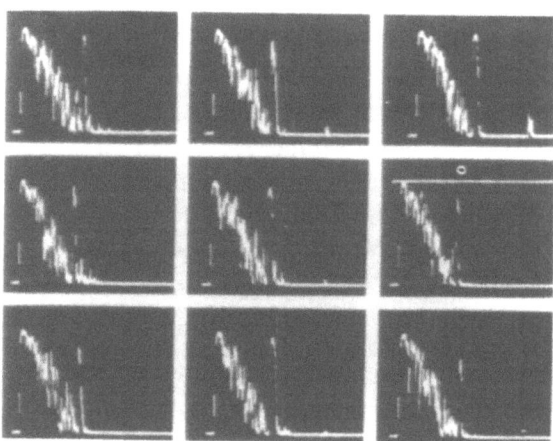

Figure 5. TM echograms in medium spike height as obtained in a blind-study setting from 9 different Tissue Models.

deviation found in a statistical evaluation of these Tissue Sensitivity settings was ±0.65 dB. Figure 5 shows echograms from different TMs. These echograms were obtained by adjusting the instrument to Tissue Sensitivity using each TM independently; the standard deviation in these settings was ±0.88 dB. Figure 6 demonstrates echograms obtained from a TM at temperatures of 16 degrees Celsius (left), 45 degrees Celsius (center) and 21 degrees

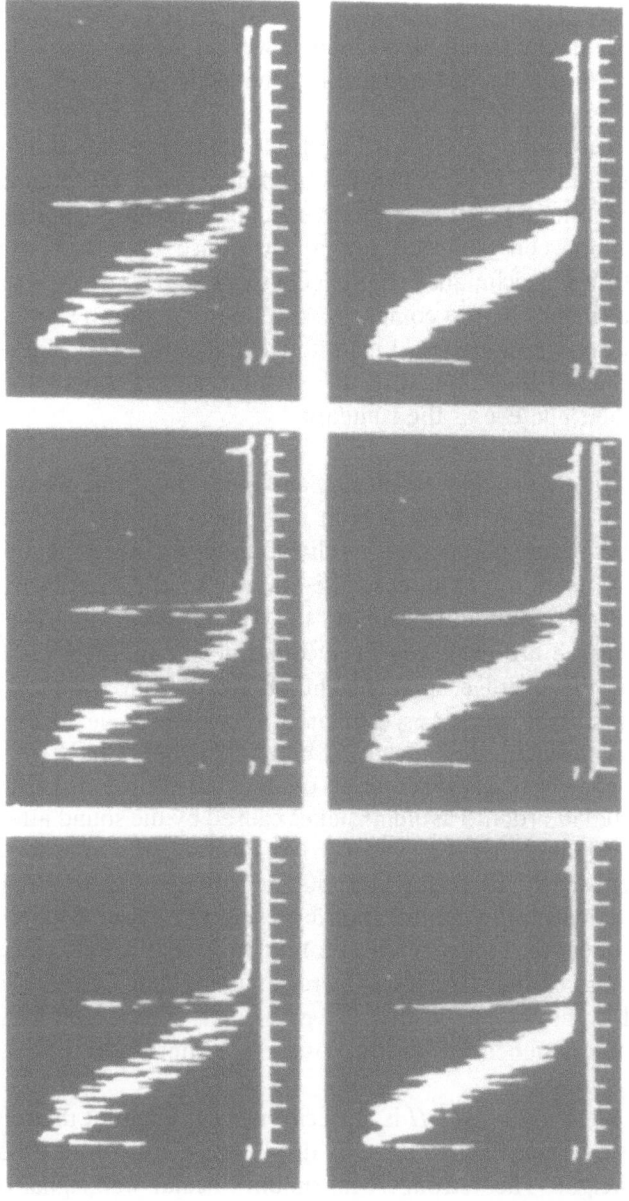

Figure 6 Echograms obtained from a single TM with the Standardized A-scan instrument Kretz 7200 MA set at Tissue Sensitivity with a fixed probe (*top* patterns) and a probe shifted along the TM surface back and forth (*bottom* patterns) The *left* 2 echograms were obtained at temperature (of TM and envirement) of 16° Celsius The *central* 2 echograms were obtained at a temperature of 45° Celsius, and the *right* 2 echograms were obtained at a temperature of 21° Celsius

Celsius (right) with the probe held fixed (top row) and with the probe being quickly shifted back and forth across the surface, in order to obtain an average pattern (bottom row). No significant differences can be noted. Since 1975, annual comparisons of the standard TM (serial #001) with freshly prepared and defined citrated blood models were done and showed that the acoustic parameter of this TM remained unchanged.

Quantitative Echography [3, 27, 34, 37, 38, 44] comprises two different methods: (a) Quantitative Echography I is used mainly for the differentiation of tissues (e.g., tumors). (b) Quantitative Echography II is applied for the differentiation between detached retina and dense fibrovascular vitreous membranes. In both techniques the reflectivity of the tissue under examination (tumor or membrane) is compared with that of a known standard. This comparison is done indirectly in Quantitative Echography I using a Tissue Model. The comparison is done directly in Quantitative Echography II using the sclera of the same eye as the standard.

Quantitative Echography Type I is an easy and quick procedure which necessitates the use of a Standardized A-scan instrument and the use of a TM. Quantitative Echography I provides a reliable though gross estimation of the reflectivity of a tissue, e.g., a tumor. The Standardized A-scan instrument is set at a defined high system sensitivity, the Tissue Sensitivity. The surface signals of the tissue are displayed in maximal height (perpendicular sound approach) and the average spike height obtained from within the tissue (excluding the surface spikes) is estimated as a percentage of the display height. In tissues which attenuate the sound beam significantly (medium to large angle kappa) only the first stretch of 10 microseconds of tissue signals is to be evaluated in order to avoid mistakes caused by the sound attenuation.

The key to Quantitative Echography I is the use of a constant, defined and high system sensitivity setting – Tissue Sensitivity. This sensitivity is set for each instrument/probe combination by using the Tissue Model (Fig. 3) by using reproduction as discribed before. Once it is known for a given instrument/probe combination, it can be re-set at any time by either choosing the known dB value of the instrument gain (e.g., Kretz 7200 MA) or by pushing a button designed for this purpose (e.g., Mini A-scan).

Quantitative Echography Type II is a precise measurement of the reflectivity of a single large surface. This is done by displaying the involved echo signals in maximum height. The "strongest maximum" ocular wall signal obtained in a transocular examination of the same eye (usually from the inferior periphery of the ocular wall) is used as standard to compare with. "Maximum" in this context means that the sound beam reaches the surface perpendicularly and thus produces the highest possible echo spike at this part of the large ocular wall surface; "strongest" in this context means the highest of all maximum signals achieved by aiming the beam perpendicularly at

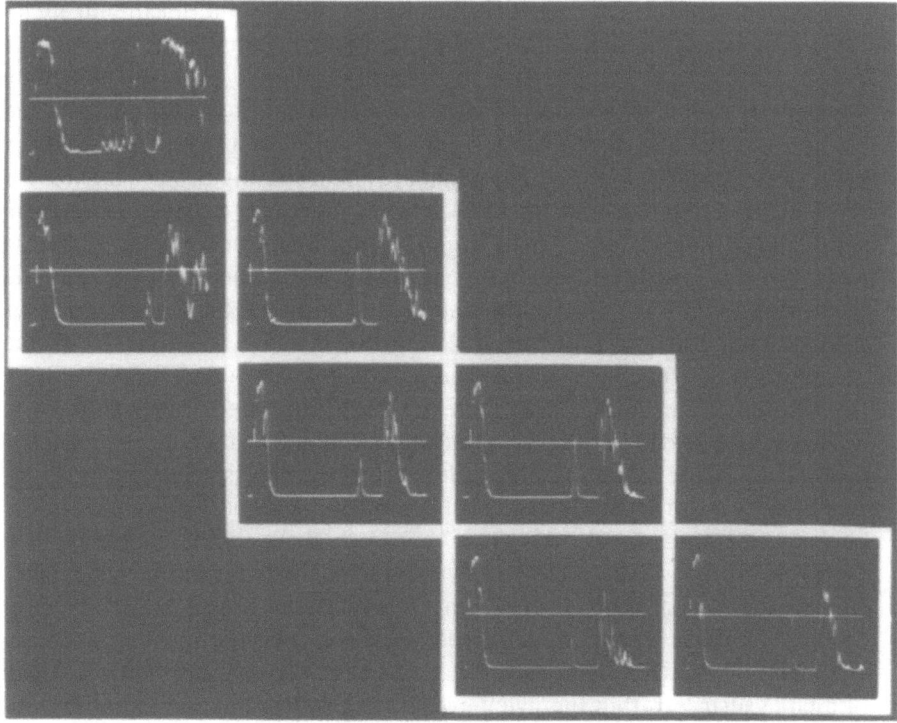

Figure 7. Series of Standardized A-scan echograms (Kretz 7200 MA) obtained from a fibrovascular membrane at Tissue Sensitivity (*top left*) and at continuously lower system sensitivity settings toward the bottom. The horizontally paired echograms were obtained at the same sensitivity setting but the right one was displayed with improved perpendicularity of the beam at the surface of the membrane. Hence the right echogram in each pair shows the high membrane signal. Whenever the maximum membrane spike rose beyond the horizontal marker line, the instrument setting was lowered (next echograms displayed at a lower level in the figure). The aim was to finally display the maximized membrane spike high enough that the peak temporarily just touched the marker line without ever rising higher beyond the line while the examiner tried to better maximize the spike by minimally angling and shifting the beam. This end result is shown in the right bottom echogram. A dB setting of 58 was needed to accomplish this.

various parts of the surface. For instance, the maximum scleral signal obtained at 5:00 o'clock is weaker than the maximum signal obtained at 6:00. In this case the 6:00 maximum signal is the stronger one and is to be chosen as standard. The minimum system sensitivity required to display the maximum spike of the respective surface in the height defined by the horizontal measuring line is the end point of each measurement. Figure 7 illustrates the technique of achieving this end point in determining the maximum signal of a fibrovascular membrane, using the Kretz technik 7200 MA. These end points are digitally indicated in tenths of a decibel, when using the Mini A-scan.

The minimum system sensitivity needed to display the maximum membrane echo signal in the defined height is then compared with the minimal system sensitivity to achieve the same end point for the strongest maximum ocular wall spike. Since the sclera is a stronger reflector than a detached retina, and the detached retina a stronger reflector than a fibrovascular vitreous membrane, the required minimal system sensitivities are highest for the membrane, and lowest for the sclera. A **difference** between the system sensitivity setting needed (a) to bring the maximum echo signal from the examined large surface to the height of the measuring line and (b) to obtain the corresponding setting for the ocular wall spike of **15 dB or less** proves that the membraneous structure is **detached retina**. On the other hand, the membraneous structure is recognized as being a vitreous membrane when the difference in dB settings is greater than 20. The same technique is applied, in addition, to the pre-scleral layer (defined as the first independent echo spike of the ocular wall complex). If the retina is attached, this pre-scleral signal is produced by the retinal surface; its typical difference to the ocular wall standard is 10–12 dB. If, however, the retina is detached, then the pre-scleral signal is produced by the pigment epithelium which reflects weaker than an attached retina. The resulting difference to the standard signal is 14 dB or greater. A difference of 13 dB is borderline.

Quantitative Echography II is a way to accurately measure the reflectivity of a large surface within the living eye. It is usually applied in the differentiation between detached retina and dense fibrovascular membranes [44, 48], when its result is called the A_4 sign (see below). Both produce 100% high spikes at Tissue Sensitivity. This becomes evident during a Quantiative Echography I evaluation: the maximum spike obtained at Tissue Sensitivity using a Standardized A-scan instrument will be 100% high whether the surface stems from a detached retina or a very dense fibrovascular membrane. However, the left ascending limb clarifies the underlying structure: it is smooth, sharply rising and contains very few if any high-frequency nodules in the case of retinal detachment. The left limb appears rugged or at least does not rise sharply and contains numerous high-frequency nodules when obtained from a fibrovascular membrane. Ossoinig has termed this differential diagnostic sign the A_1 sign [48]. It is the easiest, most available and most sensitive of the four A-scan and four B-scan differential criteria which he found useful for the differentiation of retinal detachments from dense fibrovascular membranes in eyes with dense vitreous hemorrhage and severe proliferative changes as frequently encountered in severe diabetic retinopathy and severe ocular trauma. Quantitative Echography II provides another A-scan differential criterium, the A_4 sign [48]. It is more time-consuming than the other differential criteria but has the highest specificity and therefore is used as judge in borderline cases when the other differential criteria are weak or contradictory.

References

[1] K.C. Ossoinig. Acoustic diagnosis of intraocular and orbital tumors – experimental and

clinical examinations with the A-scan technique (Ger) In W Buschmann and I Hildebrandt (eds) Diagnostica Ultrasonica in Ophthalmologia (Proc of SIDUO I, Berlin, 1964) Wiss Z Humboldt-Univ Berlin, Math -Nat R 1965,14 185-191

[2] K C Ossoinig Discussion to Buschmann "Echography of intraocular tumors" (Ger) In W Buschmann and I Hildebrandt (eds) Diagnostica Ultrasonica in Ophthalmologia (Proc of SIDUO I, Berlin, 1964) Wiss Z Humboldt-Univ Berlin, Math -Nat R 1965,14 167-169

[3] K C Ossoinig Echography of tumors of the eye – clinical and experimental studies with the A-scan method (Ger) Klin Monatsbl Augenheilk 1965,146 321-337

[4] K C Ossoinig and H Steiner Standardization in echography – a model for the diagnosis of intraocular tumors (Ger) In W Buschmann and I Hildebrandt (eds) Diagnostica Ultrasonica in Ophthalmologia (Proc of SIDUO I, Berlin, 1964) Wis Z Humboldt-Univ Berlin, Math -Nat R 1965,14 129-133

[5] K C Ossoinig and K Seher Echographic studies of microscopic structures – clarification of the echo origin in tumors (Ger) I Theoretical considerations Graefes Arch Ophthalmol 1966,171 17-24

[6] K C Ossoinig and H Steiner Standardization in echography of the eye (Ger) Graefes Arch Ophthalmol 1966,169 241-249

[7] K C Ossoinig Ultrasonic diagnosis of the eye – an aid for the clinic (review) In H Gernet (ed) Ultrasonics in Ophthalmology (Proceedings of the Munster Symposium, 1966) Karger Basel/New York, 1967, pp 116-133

[8] K C Ossoinig Further experiences with models as aids for the ultrasonic diagnosis of intraocular tumors (Ger) Graefes Arch Ophthalmol 1967,174 1-8

[9] K C Ossoinig A new ultrasound instrument for ophthalmology (Ger) Graefes Arch Ophthalmol 1967,171 312-317

[10] K C Ossoinig and K Seher Studies on the histopathological basis of echograms (Ger) In A Oksala and H Gernet (eds) Ultrasonics in Ophthalmology (Proc of the Munster Symposium, 1966) S Karger, Basel/New York, 1967, pp 103-109

[11] K C Ossoinig, K Seher and F Kaufmann Echographic studies of microscopic structures II Phenomenon observed in echographic examinations of citrated blood (Ger) Graefes Arch Ophthalmol 1967,173 327-338

[12] K C Ossoinig Additional experiences with phantoms as aids in the ultrasonic diagnosis of intraocular tumors Graefes Arch Ophthalmol 1968,174 1-8

[13] K C Ossoinig Tomographic B-scan echography of the orbit (Ger) In J Vanysek (ed) Proc of SIDUO II, Brno 1967 Acta Fac Med Univ Brunensis 1968 35 117-123

[14] K C Ossoinig Basics, methods and results of ultrasonography used in the diagnosis of intraorbital tumors In K A Gitter et al (eds) Ophthalmic Ultrasound (Proc of the 4th International Congress of Ultrasonography in Ophthalmology, Philadelphia) C V Mosby, St Louis, 1968, pp 282-293

[15] K C Ossoinig Method of B-Scan echography of the eye and orbit In J Vanysek (ed) Proc of SIDUO II, Brno 1967 Acta Fac Med Univ Brunensis 1968,35 125-132

[16] K C Ossoinig First experiences with the combined A-scan and B-scan echography of orbital tumors (Ger) Wien Klin Wschr 1968,80(4) 72-74

[17] P Till and K C Ossoinig Echography of retinoblastoma (Ger) In Ber Dtsch Ophthalmol Ges 1969,69 203-209

[18] J Boeck and K C Ossoinig Relationship between the histological structure and the echograms – basis for a non-traumatic tissue differentiation (Ger) Klin Monatsbl Augenheilk 1969,155 687-695

[19] K C Ossoinig Routine ultrasonography of the orbit In M A Wainstock (ed), Ultrasonography in Ophthalmology International Ophthalmol Clin Vol 9(3) Little, Brown & Co , Boston, 1969, pp 613-642

[20] K C Ossoinig Basics, methods and results of ultrasonography used in the diagnosis of intraorbital tumors In K A Gitter et al (eds), Ophthalmic ultrasound (Proc of the 4th International Congress of Ultrasonography in Ophthalmology Philadelphia, 1968) C V Mosby, St Louis, 1979, pp 294-393

[21] K C Ossoinig and P Till Methods and results of ultrasonography in diagnosing intraocular tumors In K A Gitter *et al* Ophthalmic Ultrasound (Proc of the 4th International Congress of Ultrasonography in Ophthalmology, Philadelphia, 1968) C V Mosby, St Louis, 1969, pp 294–300

[22] K C Ossoinig and P Till Echo-ophthalmography (description of an exhibit, Ger) In Ber Dtsch Ophthalmol Ges 1970,70 605–613

[23] J Boeck and K C Ossoinig Fundamentals of non-traumatic tissue differentiation by ultrasound Part III Histological structures and ultrasonograms In J Boeck and K C Ossoinig (eds), Ultrasonographia Medica (Proceedings of the 1st World Congress on Ultrasonic Diagnostics in Medicine and SIDUO III, Vienna, 1969) Vol 1 Verlag Wiener Med Akademie, Vienna, 1971, pp 411–417

[24] R Gerstner and K C Ossoinig A new high-frequency echograph for the differential diagnosis of tissues (Ger) In J Boeck and K C Ossoinig (eds), Ultrasonographia Medica (Proceedings of the 1st World Congress on Ultrasonic Diagnostics in Medicine and SIDUO III, Vienna, 1969) Vol 1 Verlag Wiener Med Akademie, Vienna, 1971, pp 55–60

[25] K C Ossoinig Basics of echographic tissue differentiation I Experimental and clinical examinations of the influence of system parameters on the diagnostic value of echograms (Ger) In J Boeck and K C Ossoinig (eds) Ultrasonographia Medica (Proceedings of the 1st World Congress on Ultrasonic Diagnostics in Medicine and SIDUO III, Vienna, 1969) Vol 1 Verlag Wiener Med Akademie, Vienna, 1971, pp 155–168

[26] K C Ossoinig Basics of echographic tissue differentiation II Acoustic behavior of biological structures (Ger) In J Boeck and K C Ossoinig (eds) Ultrasonographia Medica (Proceedings of the 1st World Congress on Ultrasonic Diagnostics in Medicine and SIDUO III, Vienna, 1969) Vol 1 Verlag Wiener Med Akademie, Vienna, 1971, pp 419–439

[27] K C Ossoinig Basics of clinical echo-opthalmography IV Clinical standardization of equipment and techniques (Ger) In J Boeck and K C Ossoinig (eds) Ultrasonographia Medica (Proceedings of the 1st World Congress on Ultrasonic Diagnostics in Medicine and SIDUO III, Vienna, 1969) Vol 2 Verlag Wiener Med Akademie, Vienna, 1971, pp 83–118

[28] K C Ossoinig Basics of clinical echo-ophthalmology (text book, Ger) Verlag Wiener Med Akademie, Wien

[29] K C Ossoinig Clinical echo-ophthalmography In F C Blody (ed) Current concepts of ophthalmology Vol 3 C V Mosby Company, St Louis, 1972, pp 101–130

[30] K C Ossoinig and P Till Clinical standardization in ophthalmology I In L Filipczinski (ed) Ultrasonics in Biology and Medicine (Proc of the Conference on Ultrasonics in Biology and Medicine, Warsaw) PWN Polish Scientific Publishers, Warsaw, 1972, pp 173–182

[31] P Till and K C Ossoinig Clinical standardization in ophthalmology II In L Filipczinski (ed) Ultrasonics in Biology and Medicine (Proc of the Conference on Ultrasonics in Biology and Medicine, Warsaw, 1970) PWN Polish Scientific Publishers, Warsaw, 1972, pp 233–238

[32] K C Ossoinig A new standardized instrument for echo-ophthalmography Proposals for the standardisation of important instrument parameters (Ger) In M Massin and J Poujol (eds), Diagnostica Ultrasonica in Ophthalmologia (Proc of SIDUO IV, Paris, 1971) Centre National d'Ophtalmologie des Quinze-Vingts, Paris, 1973, pp 131–137

[33] K C Ossoinig Preoperative differential diagnosis of tumors with echography I Physical principles and morphological background of tissue echograms In F C Blodi (ed) Current Concepts in Ophthalmology Vol 4 C V Mosby, St Louis, 1974, pp 264–280

[34] K C Ossoinig Preoperative differential diagnosis of tumors with echography II Instrumentation and examination techniques In F C Blodi (ed) Current Concepts in Ophthalmology Vol 4 C V Mosby, St Louis, 1974, pp 280–296

[35] K C Ossoinig Preoperative differential diagnosis of tumors with echography III Diagnosis of intraocular tumors In F C Blodi (ed) Current Concepts in Ophthalmology Vol 4 C V Mosby, St Louis, 1974, pp 296–314

[36] K C Ossoinig and F C Blodi Preoperative differential diagnosis of tumors with echography IV Diagnosis of orbital tumors In F C Blodi (ed) Current Concepts in Ophthalmology Vol 4 C V Mosby, St Louis, 1974, pp 313–341

[37] K C Ossoinig Quantitative echography – an important aid for the acoustic differentiation of tissues In M de Vlieger et al (eds) Ultrasonics in Medicine (Proc of the 2nd World Congress on Ultrasonics in Medicine, Rotterdam, 1973) Excerpta Medica, Amsterdam, 1974, pp 49–54

[38] K C Ossoinig Quantitative echography – the basis for tissue differentiation J Clinical Ultrasound 1974,2(1) 33–46

[39] P Till Solid tissue model for the standardization of the echo-ophthalmograph 7200 MA (Kretztechnik) Docum Ophthalmol 1976,41 205

[40] K C Ossoinig and J H Patel A-Scan instrumentation for acoustic tissue d fferentiation II Clinical significance of various technical parameters of the 7200 MA unit of Kretztechnik In D White and R E Brown (eds) Ultrasound in medicine Vol 3B Plenum Press, New York, 1977, 1949–1954

[41] K C Ossoinig and J H Patel A-scan instrumentation for acoustic tissue differentiation III Testing and calibration of the 7200 MA unit of Kretztechnik In D White and R E Brown (eds) Ultrasound in Medicine Vol 3B Plenum Press, New York, 1977, pp 1955–1964

[42] J H Patel and K C Ossoinig A-scan instrumentation for acoustic tissue differentiation I Signal processing in the 7200 MA unit of Kretztechnik In D White and R E Brown (eds) Ultrasound in Medicine Vol 3B Plenum Press, New York, 1977, pp 1939–1947

[43] P Till and K C Ossoinig First experiences with a solid tissue model for the standardization of A- and B-scan instruments in tissue diagnosis In C D White and R E Brown (eds) Ultrasound in Medicine) Engineering Aspects Vol 3B Plenum Press, New York, 1977, pp 2167–2174

[44] K C Ossoinig Standardized echography basic principles, clinical applications and results In R L Dallow (ed) Ophthalmic Ultrasonography Comparative Techniques Int Ophthal Clin Vol 19(4) Little, Brown & Co , Boston, 1979, pp 127–210

[45] P Till Testing of ultrasonic probes and their suitability for tissue differentiation with the help of the solid tissue model (Ger) Klin Mbl Augenheilk Vol 176 F Enkeverlag, Stuttgart, 1980, pp 337–340

[46] K C Ossoinig The significance of the S-shaped amplifier characteristics in echographic tissue diagnosis In J M Thijssen and A M Verbeek (eds) Ultrasonography in Ophthalmology [Proceedings of the 8th SIDUO Congress] Docum Ophthal Proc Series Vol 29 Dr W Junk Publishers, The Hague, 1981, pp 441–443

[47] P Till and V Scheiber Reliability and accuracy of the TM (tissue model) for the calibration of standardized A-scan instrumentation In J M Thijssen and A M Verbeek (eds) Docum Ophthal Proc Series Vol 29 Dr W Junk Publishers, The Hague

[48] K C Ossoinig, G Islas, G E Tamayo and C Tamburelli Detached retina versus dense fibrovascular membrane Standardized A-scan and B-scan criteria In K C Ossoinig (ed) Ophthalmic Echography [Proceedings of the 10th SIDUO Congress] Docum Ophthal Proc Series Vol 48 Martinus Nijhoff/Dr W Junk Publishers Dordrecht/Boston/Lancaster, 1987, pp 275–284

[49] K C Ossoinig Standardized echography of the optic nerve (1st SIDUO Jules Francois Memorial Lecture), in P Till (ed) Ophthalmic Echography 13 (Proc SIDUO XIII), Docum Ophthal Proc Series Vol 55 Kluwer Academic Publishers, Dordrecht/Boston/Lancaster 1993, pp 3–99

[50] K C Ossoinig Standardized ophthalmic echography of the eye, orbit and periorbital region A comprehensive slide set and study guide, 1985

The Diagnosis and Differential Diagnosis of Neoplastic Lesions of the Extraocular Muscles with Standardized Echography*
Invited Lecture

KARL C. OSSOINIG

(Iowa City, USA)

1. Introduction

The evaluation of extraocular muscles has become one of the most important applications of Standardized Echography: according to latest statistics, about 50% of all cases seen in an Echography Clinic are likely to be (peri)orbital in nature, when the full capacity of Standardized Echography is realized, i.e., when (immersion) axial eye length measurements as well as diagnostic evaluations of the posterior and anterior eye segments, and of the orbital and periorbital regions are included. Disorders of the extraocular muscles (with or without associated optic nerve problems) make up more than 75% of these orbital patients. Thus the echographic identification of extraocular muscle patterns and the recognition of lesions affecting the muscles has become the single most frequent task of Standardized Echography, provided that the echographic practice is not limited to a narrower field, for instance to the diagnosis of vitreoretinal diseases only.

Among the diseases that affect extraocular muscles Graves' orbitopathy ranks clearly first: Graves' orbitopathy was shown to be the primary cause of the muscle thickening in about 70% of all patients who were evaluated in recent years in the Echography Service of the Department of Ophthalmology at the University of Iowa for exophthalmus and who were found to have thickened extraocular muscles as the primary or only cause of their exophthalmus. In addition to diagnosing this disease process reliably, Standardized Echography is very helpful in grading it objectively, in recognizing optic nerve compression early and promptly, and in providing unique quantitative data for an optimal management of Graves' orbitopathy. Idiopathic (acute) orbital myositis ranks second with almost 18%, and tumors, which are the underlying cause of muscle thickening in about 5%, rank third.

Orbital tumors, which are confined to the space within muscle sheaths and which affect primarily or solely extraocular muscles, are rare. Neverthe-

*This study was supported in part by an unrestricted grant from Research to Prevent Blindness, Inc

J M Thijssen, H C Fledelius and S Tane (eds), Ultrasonography in Ophthalmology 14, xxxiii–lvii
© 1995 *Kluwer Academic Publishers, Dordrecht*

less, their echographic diagnosis can have important consequences for the management of such a patient: the tumor in the orbit may be the first and only manifestation of cancer existing elsewhere in the body; the correct diagnosis of the orbital metastasis may be crucial to quickly detect and treat the primary tumor with a minimum of diagnostic effort and expense; the echographic diagnosis may save a patient unnecessary surgery and initiate timely and optimal treatment without a biopsy, e.g., in the case of a known primary carcinoma that has become metastatic to an extraocular muscle; on the other hand, Standardized Echography may act as a reliable and accurate guide in determining the optimal (easiest and quickest) approach for a needed biopsy (e.g., when a lymphatic tumor is diagnosed); finally, Standardized Echography is an ideal tool for follow-up evaluations and for checking on treatment results.

In order to successfully apply Standardized Echography to the diagnosis and management of diseases of the straight and oblique extraocular muscles, a clear understanding of their anatomy and topography, and a complete knowledge of their acoustic properties are indispensable prerequisites. Likewise, echographers must learn to master the basic scanning techniques and must have the special examination techniques for the display of the various measuring points and zones at their command to be able to quickly and precisely measure extraocular muscles and to reliably differentiate the pathologies underlying a muscle thickening or thinning. Echographers must also have a thorough knowledge of the artefacts and pitfalls involved in the echographic display, measurement and differentiation process. Any effort to document the echographic findings in a meaningful, understandable, comparable, and repeatable way must follow a standard approach.

The detection of disorders affecting solely or mostly extraocular muscles is primarily based on an evaluation of muscle thickness. Both the A-scan and B-scan techniques are employed to screen the straight and oblique extraocular muscles for abnormal thickness in what is called the basic scanning of extraocular muscles. Marked thickening of a muscle is easily detected with either A-scan or B-scan, especially when comparing the corresponding muscles in both orbits of a patient. If the thickening (or thinning) of an extraocular muscle is minor, however, the A-scan method is required since it provides precise measurements of maximum muscle thicknesses at defined measuring points.

The differential diagnosis of muscle disorders is accomplished with the Standardized A-scan method applying primarily techniques of Quantitative Echography I which furnish crucial information on internal structure, reflectivity and sound attenuation of the diseased muscle(s). Through its measurements A-scan also provides the diagnostically important information of where a muscle is thickened primarily. In addition, Kinetic A-scan Echography indicates whether a thickened muscle is vascularized and to what degree. Topographic B-scan Echography contributes to the differential diagnosis by clarifying the exact location, outline and shape of a diseased muscle. In large neoplastic lesions of extraocular muscles, topographic B-scan information may be crucial to even recognize that the tumor is confined within the sheaths of a muscle. The finding that a tumor is muscle-related also has a bearing on the differential diagnostic process.

The A-scan patterns and techniques of measuring and evaluating extraocular muscles with Standardized Echography were introduced and expanded in the 1970's [1–3, 5, 10, 11]. Since then numerous contributions have been published on this subject [6–9, 12–14, 16–30]. This paper takes measurement and evaluation of diseased extraocular muscles one step further introducing objective, reliable, reproducible and comparable measuring points and zones for all straight and oblique extraocular muscles and defining useful criteria for the diagnosis, differential diagnosis and management of disorders affecting extraocular muscles with special reference to neoplastic lesions.

2. Detection of Muscle Disorders

Muscle disorders may be detected with basic scanning techniques using both A-scan and B-scan displays and are confirmed by precise measuring procedures with the Standardized A-scan method. Apart from neurogenic muscle pareses and cases of primary strabism which are not dealt with in this paper, an extraocular muscle is recognized as being abnormal when it is thicker by more than 0.1 to 0.2 mm at the muscle insertion, or more than 0.3 to 0.4 mm at the muscle belly, respectively, than the synonymous muscle in the fellow orbit of the patient. Instruments which utilize extremely small electronic measuring units (e.g., 0.03 mm in the Mini A-scan) and conditions which provide a sharp outline for the affected muscle such as acute (idiopathic) myositis allow the most precise measurements.

In more severe conditions such as severe cases of Graves' orbitopathy or orbital myositis, as well as in most neoplastic lesions of the extraocular muscles, abnormal muscles are recognized easily from their marked thickening already during the basic scanning with either A-scan or B-scan. Even in these cases precise measurements are, however, obtained for documentation, for grading of the severity, and for more reliable comparison during follow-up examinations. In cases of lesser severity such as mild Graves' orbitopathy or myositis, or in early stages of neoplasms, precise measurements of all straight and oblique extraocular muscles at defined measuring points are needed to detect a muscle disorder. Measurements of extraocular muscles require the A-scan method, to be reliable, accurate and clinically meaningful. B-scan is not suited for measurements because of the blooming phenomenon [31].

In Standardized A-scan displays the peaks of the echo spikes from the outer surfaces of the muscle sheaths (surface spikes) are used for thickness measurements of the extraocular muscles. In A-scans obtained with Standardized instruments at Tissue Sensitivity the position of these peaks is independent of the echo intensities (reflectivity of the echo-producing in-

xxxvi

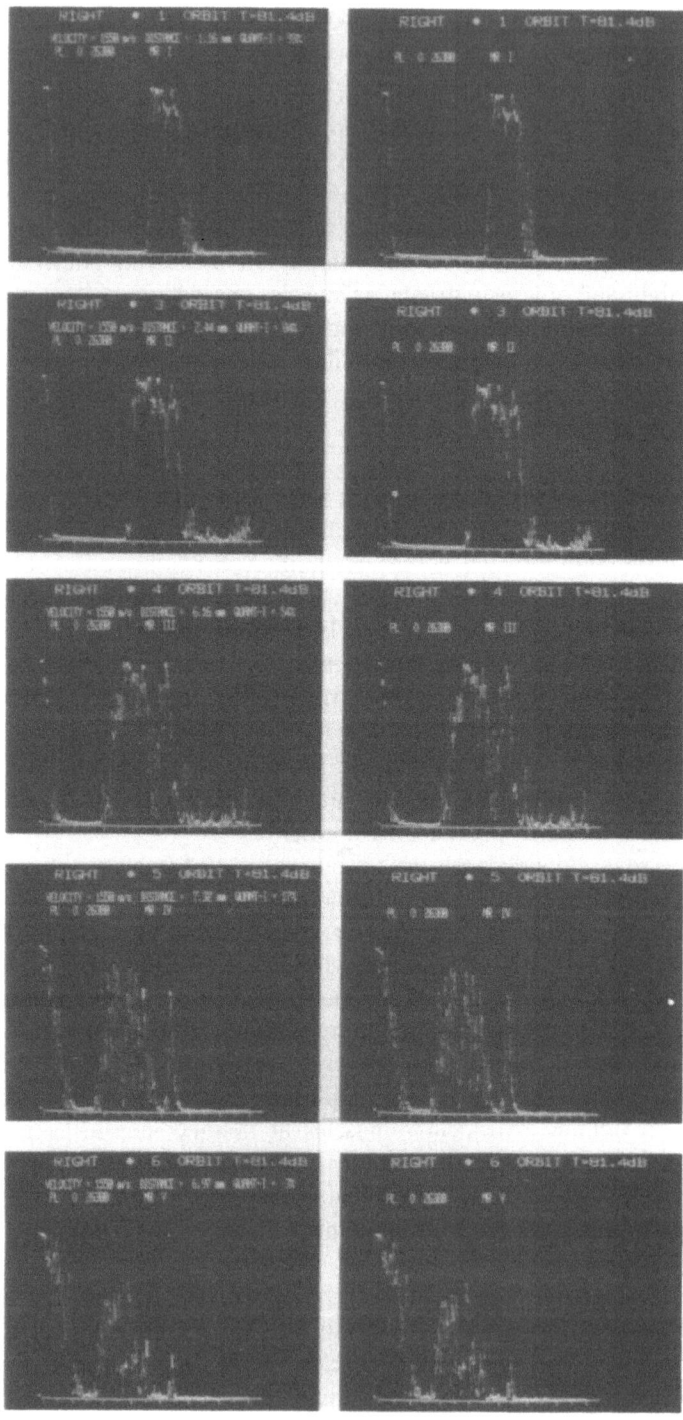

terfaces) and is clear-cut as long as the spikes are not 'overloaded'. Electronic gates are placed over the peaks so that the peaks come to lie at the extreme left end of each gate. Short (point-like) gates are ideal for this purpose (Fig. 1). In muscle echograms overloading rarely occurs at the Tissue Sensitivity setting of the Standardized A-scan instrument so that the muscle thickness can be measured with ease and great accuracy. Since Tissue Sensitivity is required to identify the muscle cross-sections in maximal width, this fact is very helpful and eliminates the need to identify maximal muscle width at one system sensitivity (i.e., high Tissue Sensitivity) and measure it at another (i.e., low measuring sensitivity), which may be necessary when other tissue structures, e.g., small intraocular tumors are to be measured reliably and accurately. Measurements of extraocular muscles are therefore quick and easy. They are reliable and accurate, and the measuring results are not dependent upon the depth location of the muscle cross-section measured, as long as maximal height of both surface spikes is displayed.

2.1. *Measuring Points and Zones*

The thickness of normal as well as abnormal extraocular muscles changes continuously throughout their course between insertions. For example, the thickness of a normal medial rectus muscle increases continuously from the most anterior segment of its inserting tendon toward its belly; it then decreases again continuously from its belly toward the annulus zinni (Fig. 2). Therefore measurements of various muscle segments other than the muscle's absolutely maximum thickness (normally at the muscle's belly), require the use of defined, comparable and repeatable measuring points and zones within which the (relatively) maximum muscle thickness is displayed and measured in order to make muscle measurements meaningful, comparable and repeatable.

Measuring points are defined as muscle segments of minimal extent such as the inserting portion of a tendon. **Measuring zones** are larger segments of a muscle, i.e., the muscle bellies, within which the maximum width needs to be searched for before a measurement is performed. At these measuring points and zones the relatively maximum muscle thicknesses can be displayed reliably, measured precisely, and compared in a meaningful way between the two orbits of a patient, between follow-up examinations of the same

---

Figure 1. Series of Standardized A-scan patterns (*Biovision S*) of a medial rectus muscle displayed in maximum width for measurement at the measuring points I, II and III, in the measuring zone IV, and at the measuring point V (from top to bottom; cf. Fig. 2). Both the lateral (left surface spike) and medial (right surface spike) surfaces of the muscle sheaths are displayed in maximal height indicating perpendicular sound beam incidence. On the left side the electronic gates are shown to be placed over the peaks of both surface spikes for measurement. On the right the same muscle patterns were displayed without the electronic gates for better visibility of the peaks of the surface spikes.

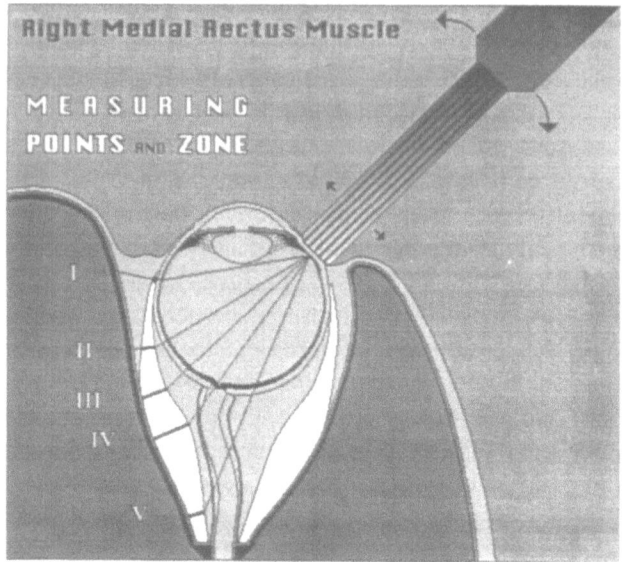

Figure 2. Schematic drawing illustrates the position of the probe, the direction of the beams and the measuring points I, II, III and V as well as the measuring zone IV used for thickness measurements of a medial rectus muscle.

patient, or between different patients. Figure 2 illustrates the measuring points and zone of the medial rectus muscle and the technique of measuring maximum muscle thicknesses at these defined segments.

One needs to realize that – similar to the situation of optic nerve measurements [31] – the ultrasonic beam is refracted toward the muscle body at the outer layers of the muscle sheaths reached first in an oblique direction. Because of this refraction it is possible even in the most posterior orbit to aim the sound beam in a perpendicular direction at the muscle surface and thus obtain truly crossectional muscle measurements.

Tables 1–4 list the measuring points and zones used for each of the 6 extraocular muscles highlighting those used to complement the basic scanning (Table 1), those used primarily in Graves' orbitopathy (Table 2) or in orbital myositis (Table 3), and the ones important for the diagnosis of neoplastic lesions of the extraocular muscles (Table 4). There are, however, situations when all available measuring points and zones (or other than those specified in the tables for the mentioned conditions) become useful or even important during the evaluation of a patient.

Medial, Lateral, and Superior Rectus Muscles. The medial, lateral and superior rectus muscles each offer 4 measuring points and 1 measuring zone (Tables 1–4). Figures 1 and 2 illustrate these defined measuring marks and

Table 1 Measuring points and zones for extraocular muscles

	Basic scanning				
	Point # I	Point # II	Point # III	Zone # IV	Point # V
Medial rectus	+	+	+	√	+
Lateral rectus	+	+	+	√	+
Superior rectus	+	−	+	√	+
Inferior rectus	+	+	±	√	+
Superior oblique	+	−	+	√	+
Inferior oblique	+	−	−	√	−

+, available, −, unavailable, points and zones
Check marks indicate those used to complement *basic scanning*

Table 2 Measuring points and zones for extraocular muscles

	Graves' orbitopathy				
	Point # I	Point # II	Point # III	Zone # IV	Point # V
Medial rectus	+	+	+	+	√
Lateral rectus	+	+	+	+	√
Superior rectus	+	+	+	+	√
Inferior rectus	+	+	±	+	√
Superior oblique	+	−	+	+	√
Inferior oblique	+	−	−	√	−

+, available, −, unavailable, points and zones
Check marks indicate those used to complement *Graves' orbitopathy*

Table 3 Measuring points and zones for extraocular muscles

	Orbital myositis				
	Point # I	Point # II	Point # III	Zone # IV	Point # V
Medial rectus	√	√	√	+	+
Lateral rectus	√	√	√	+	+
Superior rectus	√	√	√	+	+
Inferior rectus	√	√	√	+	+
Superior oblique	√	−	√	+	+
Inferior oblique	√	−	−.	√	−

+, available, −, unavailable, points and zones
Check marks indicate those used to complement *orbital myositis*

the beam paths leading to these measurements using a medial rectus muscle as an example.

Measuring point # 1 is the most anterior end of the inserting tendon. When the ultrasound beam is shifted posteriorly along the muscle (from its insertion into the globe toward the muscle belly), the muscle pattern not only widens but also shifts away from the ocular wall signals toward the

Table 4 Measuring points and zones for extraocular muscles

	Neoplastic lesions				
	Point # I	Point # II	Point # III	Zone # IV	Point # V
Medial rectus	+	+	+	√	+
Lateral rectus	+	+	+	√	+
Superior rectus	+	+	+	√	+
Inferior rectus	+	+	+	√	+
Superior oblique	+	−	+	√	+
Inferior oblique	+	−	−	√	−

+, available, −, unavailable, points and zones
Check marks indicate those used to complement *neoplastic lesions*

orbital bone spike(s). One has to find the beam direction that displays the muscle pattern halfway between the ocular and bony wall signals and then maximize its width through minimal angling of the beam across the muscle in order to display the **measuring point # II**. This measuring point 2 loses its identity, however, when a muscle gets so thick that it fills the space between the ocular wall and the bony orbital wall entirely. This is often the case in large neoplastic lesions of the muscles (Fig. 6A). When the beam is angled slightly more posteriorly the muscle pattern shifts further toward the right and becomes situated adjacent to (preceding) the bony wall spike. This right surface spike initially has full height (100% of the display height). As the beam is shifted further posteriorly, the bony wall spike decreases in height even though it may still be maximized. The most posterior beam direction that still allows the right surface spike to be 100% high specifies the **measuring point # III**. In other words, the measuring point III is the most posterior muscle portion that is displayed in front of a right surface spike of 100% height at Tissue Sensitivity of the Standardized A-scan instrument. Even minimal further posterior angling of the sound beam will result in a drop of the height of the maximized right muscle surface spike (or bone spike) from the required 100% of the display height. The muscle belly provides a measuring zone rather than a point: **measuring zone # IV**. To find the maximal width of the muscle within this zone for a reliable and precise measurement requires angling of the beam not only across, but also along, the muscle. The most posterior portion of the muscle within the orbital apex is measured again as a point: this **measuring point # V** is displayed by first angling the beam posteriorly into the apex, while following the muscle pattern, as far as this is possible without loosing its surface spikes from the display. Once this is achieved, the beam is angled minimally across the muscle to display its maximum thickness together with maximal (though low) height of the two surface spikes.

Inferior Rectus Muscle. The inferior rectus muscle differs from the other straight muscles in several important ways:

(a) Unless marked proptosis is present, the inserting tendon cannot be displayed reliably in straight gaze direction since the probe cannot be placed sufficiently behind the upper limbus as the superior orbital rim gets in its way. Since, however, a tendon does not increase in thickness during a contraction of the muscle, this difficulty can be avoided by letting the patient look slightly downward when displaying the measuring point I of the inferior rectus muscle. It frequently suffices to have the patients lift their chin.

(b) Unlike the other straight muscles, the inferior rectus muscle often remains separated from the slanted orbital floor by fat tissues in the anterior and mid-orbits and may fully approach the bony orbital wall only in the most posterior orbit. Therefore the measuring point III may lose its identity when measuring inferior rectus muscles. This is particularly true of relatively thin inferior rectus muscles. The thicker an inferior rectus muscle gets, the more likely it comes into contact with the periorbita more anteriorly and the more useful its measuring point III becomes.

(c) An important pitfall in measuring the inferior rectus muscle is the fact that this muscle passes near the inferior orbital fissure and may even cross over the most posterior part of the fissure. The pattern obtained from the inferior fissure, however, may resemble that of the muscle belly and thus be confused with it. The best way to avoid the mistakes of measuring fissure depth instead of muscle thickness or of measuring both together is to observe the displayed pattern during a dynamic forward/backward scanning with the beam. If, indeed, the pattern corresponds to the inferior rectus muscle, it will show the typical shift toward/from the ocular wall signals. If, on the other hand, the pattern is obtained from the inferior fissure, it will promptly disappear during the dynamic scanning in both (anterior as well as posterior) directions. This shifting pattern should always be tested before proceeding with the measurement of an inferior rectus muscle.

Superior Oblique Muscle. The superior oblique muscle offers 3 measuring points and 1 measuring zone (Tables 1–4): the measuring point I is provided by the inserting tendon which is located way behind the superior rectus muscle insertion near 12 o'clock. This is a most useful measuring point in the diagnosis of orbital myositis which frequently involves the superior oblique muscle. It is found by placing the probe on the bulbar conjunctiva at 6:00 o'clock behind the limbus and by searching for a tiny, but clear-cut reflectivity defect in the episcleral zone around the 12:00 o'clock meridian at or behind the equator. Once this pattern is found, minimal angling and shifting of the beam in all directions is performed in order to maximize the width of the pattern and to display the two surface spikes of the tendon in maximal height. The *measuring point II* is too difficult to find for the superior oblique muscle since the tendon approaches the bony orbital wall at the trochlea in a direction which is almost opposite to the main course of the muscle body.

The next useful measuring point is III. It is found by placing the probe on the bulbar conjunctiva opposite the trochlea, i.e., between limbus and equator of the globe at the 7:30 o'clock meridian OD, and at the 4:30 o'clock meridian OS. The beam is than shifted posteriorly and anteriorly always angling it also across the meridian where the trochlea is expected to be located in an effort to find the pattern of the most anterior portion of the superior oblique muscle. Once a muscle pattern is found, the beam is angled anteriorly in an attempt to keep the pattern displayed. When doing so the pattern of the superior oblique muscle stays next to the bone signal until it suddenly disappears when the beam passes beyond the trochlea. The measuring point III is then identified, when the most anterior portion of the superior oblique muscle is found and maximized in width with maximally high left and right surface signals. Unlike the straight extraocular muscles, the superior oblique muscle has its most anterior end still in touch with the bone, and this is the measuring point III.

The measuring zone IV of the superior oblique muscle (i.e., at its belly), and its measuring point V (i.e., its most posterior portion near its insertion into the annulus zinni) are displayed with a different approach: the medial rectus muscle serves as guiding structure. The sound beam is shifted posteriorly along the medial rectus muscle into the orbital apex. There the beam is angled slightly superiorly in order to display another muscle pattern which is the most posterior portion of the superior oblique muscle. The measuring point V is then specified by displaying the widest portion with maximized (though low) surface spikes on each side. As is true of all straight extraocular muscles the measuring point V of the superior oblique muscle too is its most frequently measured muscle segment since it is the significant one in diagnosing and grading Graves' orbitopathy (Table 2). The measuring zone of the muscle belly on the other hand is of greatest importance in other conditions of the muscles such as hyperemia and tumors (Table 4). The measuring zone IV of the superior oblique muscle is usually found by angling the beam forward after locating its measuring point V. Another although more difficult way to find this measuring zone is to shift the beam posteriorly from the measuring point III of the superior oblique muscle.

Inferior Oblique Muscle. The inferior oblique muscle is measured at one point, i.e., at its insertion into the globe (measuring point I) and in one zone, i.e., at its belly around the 6:00 o'clock meridian (measuring zone IV). The measuring point I is best found by placing the probe behind the limbus opposite the insertion of this muscle, i.e., at 2:00 o'clock in OD and at 10:00 o'clock in OS. The beam is first aimed at the inserting tendon of the lateral rectus muscle which serves as a guiding structure. Once this is identified dynamically by shifting the beam back and forth in order to confirm the shifting character of the muscle pattern, the beam is angled slightly more inferiorly and posteriorly in an attempt to display another (muscle) insertion pattern which stems from the scleral insertion of the inferior oblique muscle. The belly of the inferior oblique muscle is its measuring zone IV. This zone is utilized much more frequently than the measuring point I, not only in the

Table 5. Normal range for extraocular muscle thickness.

	Measuring point # I	Measuring zone # IV
Medial rectus	<1.2 mm	<6.4 mm
Lateral rectus	<1.1 mm	<5.8 mm
Superior rectus	<0.8 mm	<6.8 mm
Inferior rectus	<0.8 mm	<4.5 mm
Superior oblique	<0.8 mm	<4.0 mm
Inferior oblique	<1.0 mm	<4.3 mm

completion of the basic A-scanning, but in diagnosing or following up almost any type of lesion including neoplasms of this muscle (Tables 1–4). For the measurement, the probe is placed on the skin of the lower lid at 6:00 o'clock using plentiful 2% methylcellulose as coupling agent. The beam is first aimed into the globe displaying a typical globe pattern. Probe and beam are then angled inferiorly until the globe pattern disappears as the beam leaves the globe. While the beam is angled more inferiorly yet, the probe is pressed slightly against the globe so as not to by-pass the inferior oblique muscle belly, which hugs the globe, with the beam. Slight back and forth angling of the beam serves to display both surface signals of the muscle, i.e., the signals from its anterior (left surface spike) and posterior sheath surfaces (right surface spike) in maximal height.

When measuring the thickness of extraocular muscles, the following considerations are important:

(a) The comparison between right and left orbits is much more meaningful and clinically significant than the actual numbers as measured in mm are (Table 5), because the normal range of muscle thicknesses is quite wide and overlaps greatly the abnormal range. In contrast, the comparison between the corresponding muscles in the two orbits of a patient is a highly sensitive indicator of whether a muscle is normal or abnormal.

(b) When the measurements differ only slightly between the two orbits, repeat measurements of the thinner muscle (with the aim of getting a wider measurement of this muscle and thus disproving thickening of the corresponding muscle in the fellow orbit that was measured wider previously) is an effective technique for optimizing measuring accuracy and for avoiding mistakes.

(c) One should always measure extraocular muscles with the patient's eyes in **primary gaze** direction. If this is not possible the two orbits, nevertheless, need to be compared in strictly symmetric gaze directions.

2.2. *Documentation of Echographic Measurements*
There is enormous need for quantitative documentation of in vivo measurements of extraocular muscles and other orbital structures in order to have baseline data to be able to compare during follow-up examinations, to learn more about the natural course of disorders, to gauge the effectiveness of

treatment, etc. Orbital imaging with CT and MRI has been attempted to satisfy these needs but in addition to their prohibitive cost both fail to provide measurements of the orbital structures that are accurate, comparable and repeatable to any useful degree. Standardized Echography is an ideal tool to achieve just that: its well defined and standardized dynamic measuring procedures allow the reliable and accurate measurement of a great many orbital structures including several segments of all 6 extraocular muscles, of the optic nerve structures, the periorbita, the lacrimal gland etc., all with a high degree of precision that remains unmatched by any other diagnostic method.

Orbital and Muscle Profiles. The maximum (posterior) thicknesses of all extraocular muscles in an orbit together with the thickness of optic nerve sheaths, periorbita, and lacrimal gland may be documented as *orbital profile.* Such a profile may be documented either by arranging and mounting the individual echogram photos or prints from each orbit in the topographic order in which the corresponding structures appear to the examiner facing the patient [31; Figs. 3 and 4A,B] or by having the instrument print out the entire profile or at least the relevant measuring data involved.

Orbital profiles of this kind serve the documentation of measuring data in various conditions. Such documentation is particularly useful in the diagnosis and management of patients with Graves' orbitopathy when the measuring points V are used [31] and with neoplasms of the extraocular muscles when the measuring zones IV are used, for the following purposes: (a) to establish the primary diagnosis; (b) to document the echographic measurements providing the muscle index (see below) for the purpose of grading the severity of the disease; (c) to determine the natural course or the effectiveness of therapy of the disease through follow-up evaluations; and (d) to document the echographic measurements on which the superonasal index is based. This index alerts the examiner to the possibility of existence or imminence of optic nerve compression (see below). Muscle profiles may also be used for the diagnosis and management (e.g., follow-up of effectiveness of radiation therapy) of neoplasms affecting the extraocular muscles (Figs. 3A,B and 4A,B).

Muscle Index (MI). The muscle index of an orbit is calculated by dividing the sum total of the maximal thicknesses of all 6 extra-ocular muscles in an orbit by 6. For the grading of Graves' orbitopathy the MI is calculated from the maximum thicknesses of the muscles as measured at their measuring point # V (straight and superior oblique muscles) and measuring zone # IV (inferior oblique muscle), respectively (Table 2). Table 6 lists the ranges of posterior MI's for the normal population and for different degrees of severity in Graves' orbitopathy (grades I–III).

In other conditions than Graves' orbitopathy, other measuring points or zones may be preferable. The measuring of zone IV is the preferred muscle

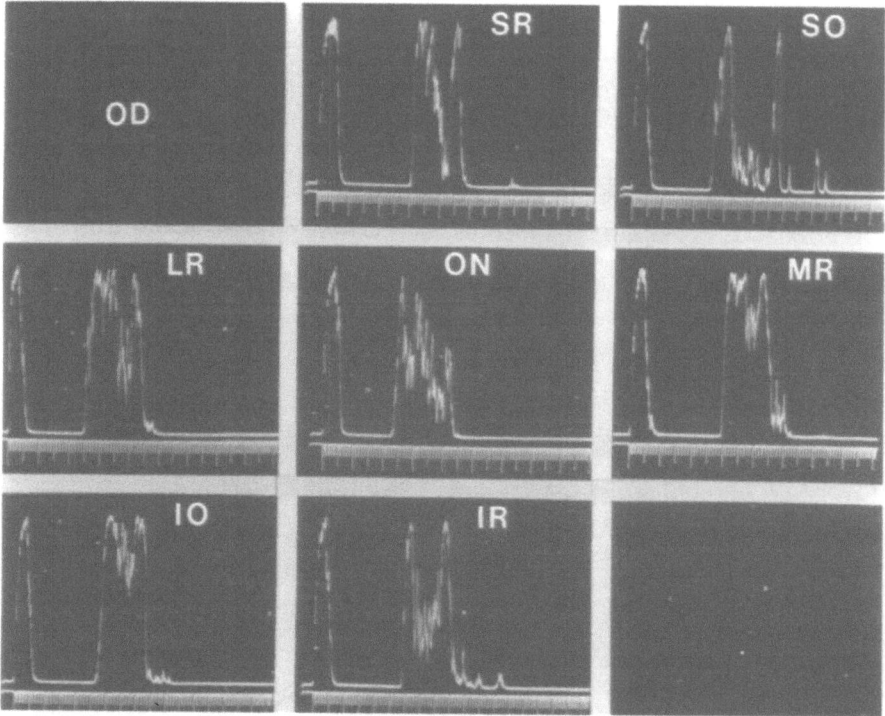

Figure 3A. Orbital (muscle) profile showing maximum muscle thicknesses (measured within their measuring zone IV) of the right orbit of patient with metastatic carcinoma involving mostly the superior oblique (SO), superior rectus (SR), and inferior rectus (IR) muscles. Both the lateral rectus (LR) and inferior oblique (IO) muscles are minimally thickened whereas the medial rectus muscle (MR) appears normal. ON is cross-section of right optic nerve (*Kretz 7200 MA*).

segment for calculating a muscle index in neoplasms of the extraocular muscles. The measuring points I–III are usually chosen to calculate a muscle index in a patient with orbital myositis.

Superonasal Index (SNI). The superonasal index of an orbit is calculated by dividing the sum total of the maximum thicknesses of the medial and superior rectus, and the superior oblique muscles by 3.

This quantitative data is very helpful in detecting patients with severe (sometimes clinically not so severe in appearance) Graves' orbitopathy who are in the danger of developing, or already have, compression of an optic nerve (CON). SNI's below 6.5 have never been found in association with active CON in patients with Graves' orbitopathy. SNI's near or above 7.0 (Graves' orbitopathy grade IV), however, have frequently been associated with CON. Thus a SNI of ≥7.0 places patients at risk of developing compressive optic neuropathy if they do not already have morphological (echographic)

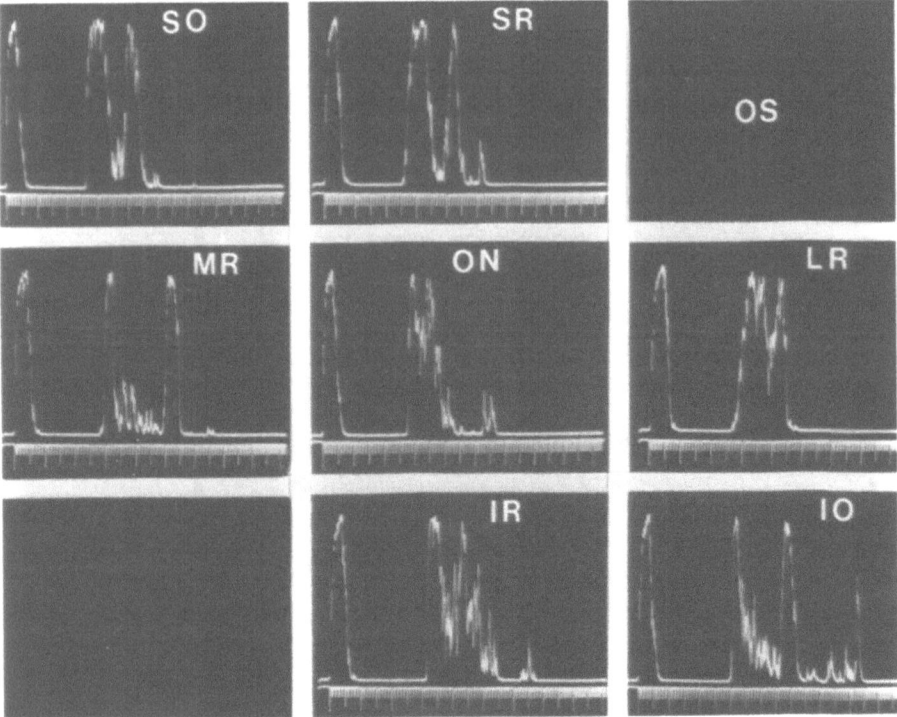

Figure 3B. Orbital (muscle) profile of left orbit of patient with metastatic carcinoma (same patient as in Fig. 3A) involving mostly the medial rectus (MR), inferior oblique (IO), superior oblique (SO), and superior rectus (SR) muscles. The inferior rectus muscle (IR) is mildly thickened, whereas the lateral rectus muscle (LR) appears of normal thickness. ON is optic nerve cross-section (Kretz 7200 MA).

signs of CON [31] (Graves' orbitopathy grade V). If the morphological signs of CON are aggravated by loss of optic nerve function (i.e., at least two of the following tests are abnormal: visual acuity, visual field, computed flicker fusion, color vision, relative afferent pupillary defect), the patient's Graves' orbitopathy is graded as VI.

In neoplasms of the extraocular muscles optic nerve compression may be caused by excessive thickening of a single muscle in an orbit. While in these cases the SNI is irrelevant, the exercise of the optic nerve and the decrease or disappearance of the subarachnoidal fluid surrounding the retrobulbar optic nerve after such an exercise (as is part of the routine evaluation of patients with Graves' orbitopathy with a SNI of $\geqslant 7$ [31]) is proof of optic nerve compression by the tumor.

3. Differential Diagnosis of Muscle Disorders

For the differentiation of lesions affecting predominantly or solely extraocular muscles both the B-scan and A-scan methods are used.

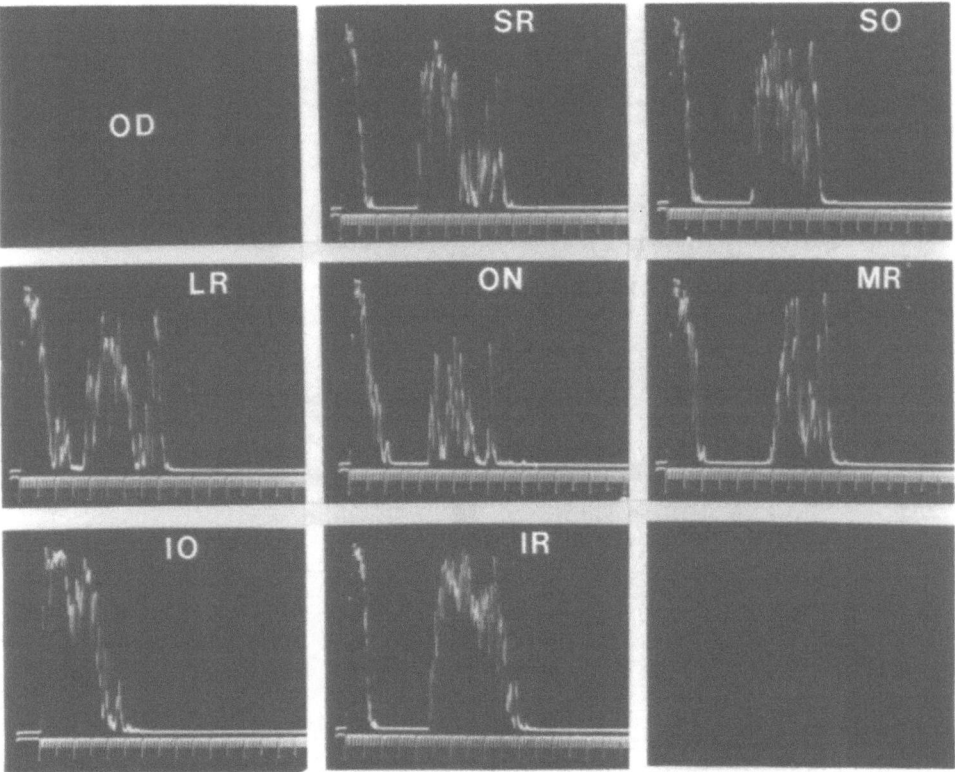

Figure 4A. Orbital (muscle) profile of right orbit of same patient shown in Fig. 3A obtained 6 months later (after radiation therapy). Note that the superior oblique and inferior rectus muscles are much less thickened and higher reflective than before. Other muscles (e.g., the medial rectus and superior rectus muscles) have become thicker as the patient's coexisting Graves' orbitopathy got worse (Kretz 7200 MA).

B-scan displays, especially acoustic long-sections, of extraocular muscles reveal marked swelling of a muscle. Such swelling becomes obvious in particular when the corresponding muscles of both orbits of a patient are compared. In cases of marked muscle thickening B-scans also readily demonstrate which muscle portions are predominantly affected. Anterior muscle segments are thickened predominantly in cases of myositis, whereas the posterior segments. are primarily thickened in Graves' orbitopathy. Hyperemia of muscles (e.g., in orbital congestion due to A–V fistulas) and, especially, large neoplasms located within the muscle sheaths often affect the entire muscle body. In addition, this *Topographic Echography* reveals the shape of neoplasms in extraocular muscles which then often have pear-like or nodular appearance or show a bumpy contour of the affected muscle (Figure 5).

A-scan displays not only are much more sensitive in revealing minor

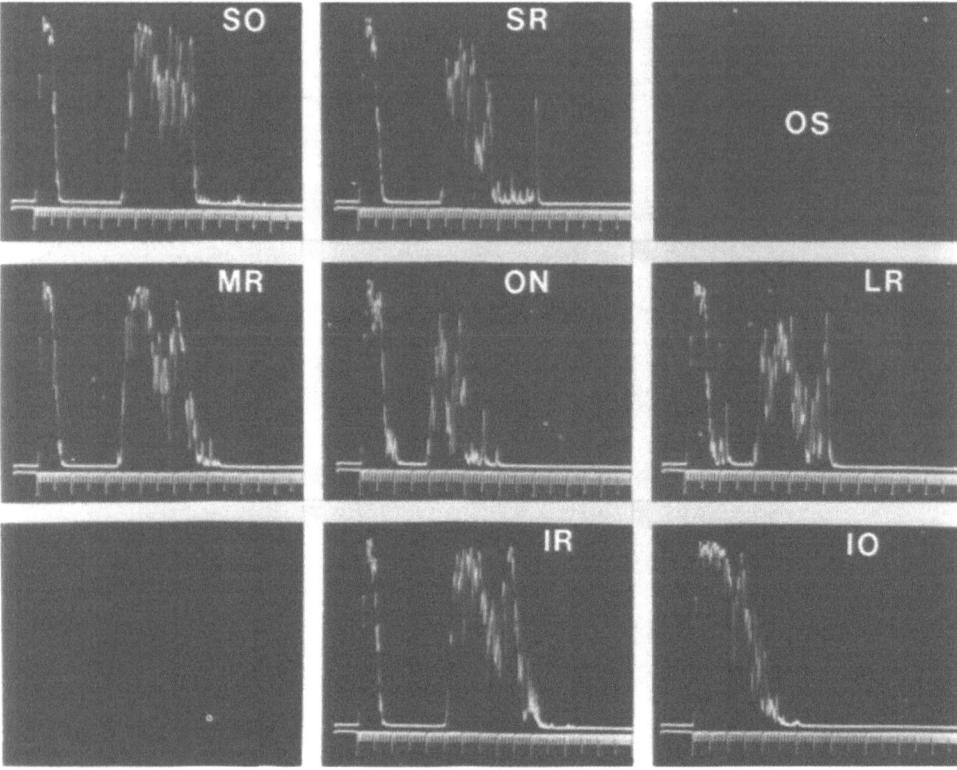

Figure 4B. Orbital (muscle) profile of left orbit of same patient shown in Fig. 3B obtained 6 months later (after radiation therapy). Note that the initially thickest muscles, i.e., the medial rectus, inferior oblique and superior oblique muscles are much less thickened and higher reflective. Other muscles, especially the superior rectus muscle now are thicker than before due to the patients coexisting Graves' orbitopathy. The superior rectus muscle also became higher reflective (not as recognizable from the pattern in this figure, which has been obtained in most posterior orbit at measuring point V (Kretz 7200 MA).

Table 6. Muscle index (MI) for diagnosis and grading of Graves' orbitopathy.

Normal range:	3.5–5.0
Mild Graves' orbitopathy (grade I):	4.5–5.4
Moderate Graves' orbitopathy (grade II):	5.5–6.4
Severe Graves' orbitopathy (grade III):	≥6.5

thickening of extraocular muscles and thus are the primary method of detecting most cases of orbital myositis and of Graves' orbitopathy, they also contribute essentially to the differentiation of lesions of the extraocular muscles. This is achieved, first of all, through precise measurements of different muscle segments (see above). In orbital myositis the inserting ten-

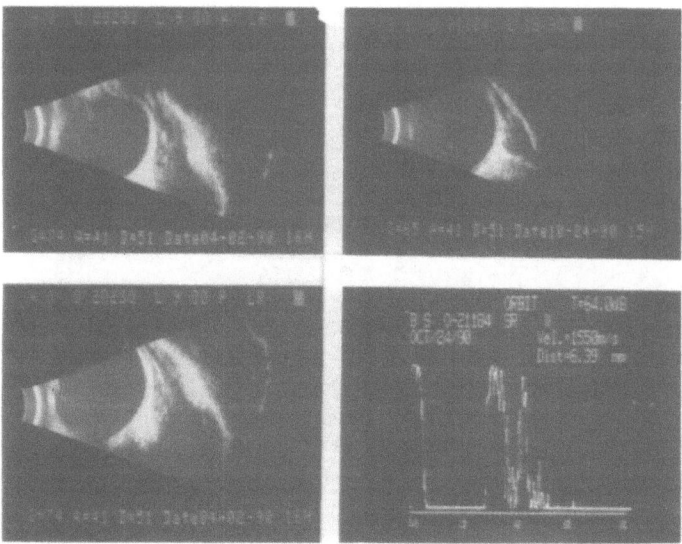

Figure 5. Longitudinal B-scan (Ophthascan S) patterns from right lateral rectus muscle (insertion shown superiorly in top left echogram, posterior belly next to optic nerve shown in left bottom echogram) thickened in a pear-like shape because of carcinoma metastatic from prostate cancer. The right top echogram shows anterior longitudinal section of right superior rectus muscle in a different patient with carcinoma thickening this muscle in a nodular fashion with bumpy contour; this carcinoma was metastatic from a breast tumor. The A-scan echogram (Mini A-scan) at the right bottom shows the low reflectivity of this moderately thickened superior rectus muscle.

don and most anterior portion of a muscle are mostly affected and thus the measuring points I, II and III are most relevant. In addition, the internal reflectivity is markedly decreased and the reflectivity of the large surfaces of the muscle sheaths is enhanced. In Graves' orbitopathy, the posterior segments of muscles (all straight and the superior oblique muscles) are most thickened and the measuring points V (measuring zone IV of the inferior oblique muscle) are the segments measured. In hyperemia of extraocular muscles as well as in tumors which are confined to the space within the muscle sheaths, e.g., metastatic carcinomas, lymphomas, sarcoidosis, leucemia or inflammatory pseudotumors, often the entire muscle bodies are affected and usually the measuring zone IV is the most useful one for documenting and following their size.

In addition to these measurements, *Quantitative Echography I* – by indicating the internal structure and sound attenuation, but especially by revealing the internal reflectivity – contributes greatly to the differentiation of disease processes which cause muscle thickening (Table 7; Figs. 3–7). *Kinetic A-scan echography* too is of help by clarifying and quantitating internal lesion vascularity (Fig. 7A).

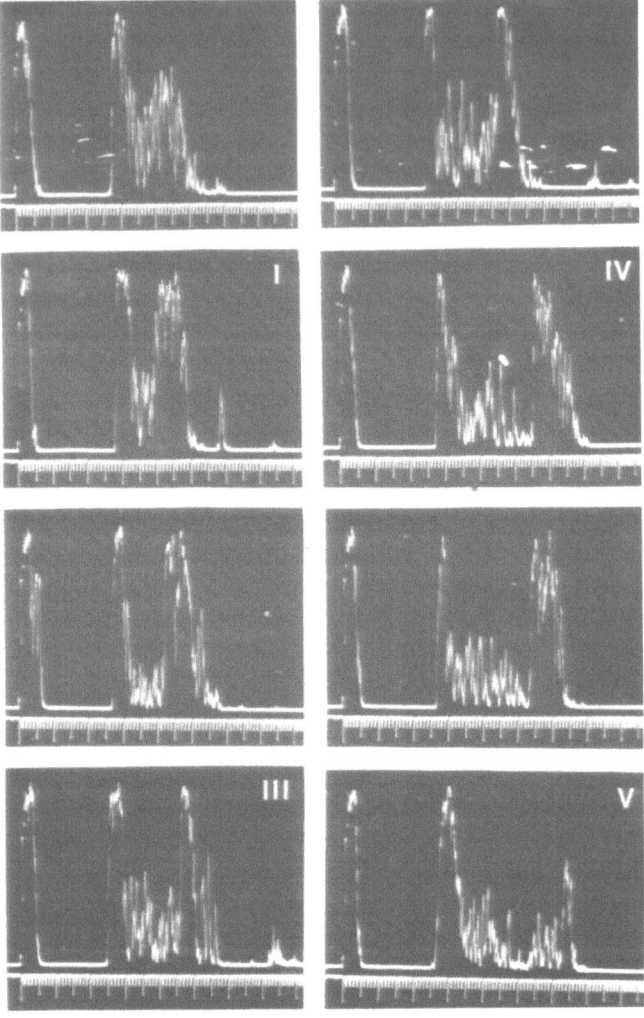

Figure 6A. Series of Standardized A-scan echograms (*Kretz 7200 MA*) showing maximal cross-sections of left medial rectus muscle (anterior portion left: inserting tendon to anterior belly – from top to bottom; posterior portion right: belly to apex – from top to bottom) thickened by carcinoma metastatic from prostate tumor. The marked echograms correspond to the measuring points I, III and V, and to the measuring zone IV. Because of the excessive thickening of the muscle its measuring point II is not applicable.

Acoustic Key Differential Criteria. With Standardized Echography, particularly with the help of quantitative A-scan techniques, a specific diagnosis of the underlying pathology of a muscle thickening (or thinning) is often possible aiding greatly in the management of these patients. For the differentiation of pathologies underlying thickening of the extraocular muscles,

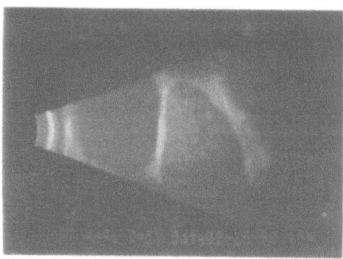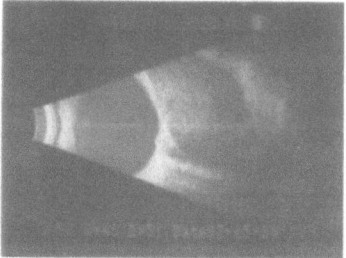

Figure 6B. Longitudinal B-scan sections (Ophthascan S) from left medial rectus muscle excessively thickened by metastatic carcinoma (same case as in Fig. 6A). The left echogram shows anterior portion of muscle (insertion seen superiorly); the right echogram shows posterior belly impinging on optic nerve (optic nerve seen inferiorly).

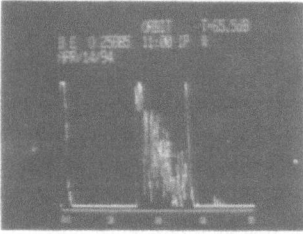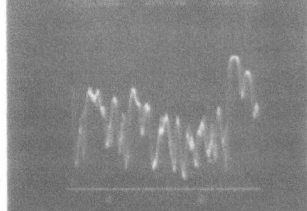

Figure 7A. Standardized A-scan echograms (Mini A-scan) from left superior rectus muscle (at measuring point III) in a patient with metastatic carcinoid. The left echogram was obtained prior to biopsy, center echogram was obtained almost $3\frac{1}{2}$ years later. Note the minor increase in internal reflectivity presumably due to the radiation treatment. The right echogram was obtained at initial visit with maximum zoom applied in order to maximize the picture repetition frequency on the screen and so optimize real-time display of vascular motion of tumor spikes (blurred appearance in photograph). Also note the large angle kappa.

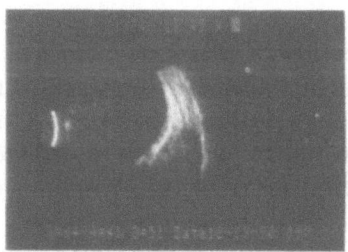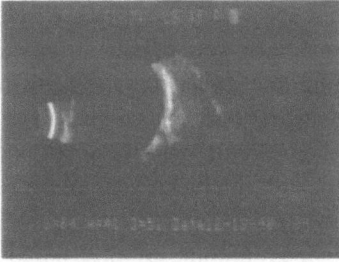

Figure 7B. Longitudinal B-scan echograms (Ophthascan S) from thickened right lateral rectus muscle of same patient shown in Fig. 7A. The left echogram shows normally thin inserting tendon and most anterior portion of lateral rectus muscle superiorly and the markedly thickened muscle belly inferiorly. The right echogram shows the muscle belly with its most posterior nodular portion coming close to optic nerve (inferiorly in echogram).

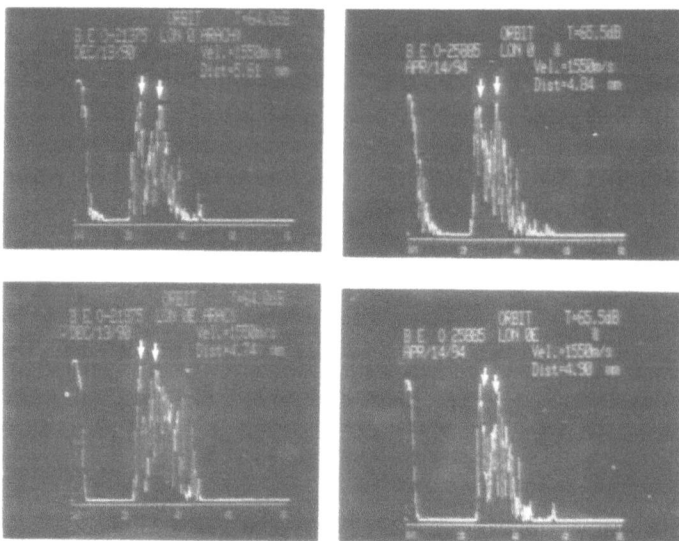

Figure 7C. Standardized A-scan echograms (Mini A-scan) showing maximized retrobulbar arachnoidal optic nerve diameters of the left orbit. Arrows point at peaks representing the lateral (left) and medial (right) arachnoidal surfaces. The left top echogram was obtained at initial visit prior to optic nerve "exercise" (arachnoidal diameter = 5.61 mm). The left bottom echogram was obtained during the initial visit following optic nerve exercise (arachnoidal diameter has decreased to 4.74 mm indicating mild optic nerve compression by the tumor). The right top echogram (obtained $3\frac{1}{2}$ years later) shows the pre-exercise arachnoidal diameter of the same (left) optic nerve to be 4.84 mm. The right bottom echogram was obtained at this later visit following optic nerve exercise (arachnoidal diameter has increased minimally to 4.90 mm indicating absence of optic nerve compression).

the **internal reflectivity** plays the key role (Table 7). In general it holds true that lesions confined within the sheaths of extraocular muscles display an internal reflectivity which is a level lower than that of their counterparts in the orbital tissues outside the muscle sheaths. For instance, carcinoma metastatic to the orbital fat tissues is high-reflective (producing high V-patterns in the A-scan echograms at Tissue Sensitivity of the Standardized A-scan instrument [4, 7]), whereas the same tumor is low-reflective when metastatic to the muscle tissues and limited to the space within the muscle sheaths (Fig. 6A). This situation is similar to the two different reflectivities of the same cell densities in vitreous (higher reflectivity) and subvitreal (lower reflectivity) hemorrhages.

When evaluating the internal structure, reflectivity and sound absorption of lesions of the extraocular muscles (Quantitative Echography I), the following specifics must be observed:

(a) The surface signals from the muscle sheaths must be maximized through perpendicular sound beam exposure just as is necessary for the thickness measurements of the muscles. These maximal surface spikes are

Table 7. Quantitative echography I of extraocular muscle disorders (spectrum of internal muscle reflectivities).

← l o w	REFLECTIVITIES	high →
← MYOSITIS		GRAVES' ORBITOPATHY →
	HYPEREMIA / CONGESTION	
LYMPHOMATOUS TUMORS		
LEUKEMIC INFILTRATE		
	METASTATIC CARCINOMA	
	CARCINOID	
SARCOID		
	HEMATOMA	
	← NORMAL MUSCLES →	

excluded from the evaluation of internal structure, reflectivity and absorption.

(b) The internal structure (distribution of spike heights) should be evaluated in the anterior half of all straight and the superior oblique muscles. When displaying the posterior half of these muscles, the sound beam traverses the posterior ocular wall so obliquely that because of total reflection of part of the beam at the ocular wall (acoustic shadowing) too much ultrasonic energy is lost as to reliably indicate the internal muscle structures.

(c) This phenomenon of ocular wall shadowing is even more critical when the internal reflectivity of muscles is to be evaluated. For this quantitative evaluation only the anterior third of these muscles should be examined. For the display of their anterior third the ultrasonic beam can be aimed fairly perpendicularly at the ocular wall. In such sound beam directions the ocular wall does not attenuate either the proceeding beam or the returning echoes to any measurable degree.

(d) For the evaluation of sound absorption within a muscle, the system sensitivity may have to be altered (usually raised) away from Tissue Sensitivity in order to display medium high internal muscle signals for an adequate quantitative evaluation of the angle kappa. This is not necessary when the tumor pattern displays about medium spike height at Tissue Sensitivity as is the case in carcinoid (Fig. 7A).

Figs. 3, 4, 5 and 6 illustrate the typical A-scan and B-scan patterns obtained from the most frequently encountered neoplasm in extraocular muscles, i.e. **metastatic carcinoma**: while the B-scans show the typical tumor patterns (pear-shape, nodular shape or at least bumpy muscle contour), the A-scans reveal a heterogenous internal structure caused by the low signals from the carcinoma cells and interspersed higher (but no more than medium high) connective tissue septa signals. Metastatic carcinomas cause little if any sound attenuation. Lymphomatous tumors (malignant lymphoma and inflammatory pseudotumors alike) tend to have an even lower internal reflectivity than metastatic carcinomas. In contrast to carcinomas, they also are clearly (though mildly) vascular.

Figures 7A and B illustrate the typical A-scan and B-scan patterns of a carcinoid metastatic to extraocular muscles of both orbits in a patient. While this tumor is extremely rare, this case example illustrates the tremendous potential of Standardized Echography in differentiating orbital tissues including disease processes of extraocular muscles.

The patient whose echograms are illustrated in Figs. 7A, B and C had initially been diagnosed as suffering from euthyroid Graves' orbitopathy on the basis of his bilateral painless exophthalmus and the CT findings of several thickened extraocular muscles, two years prior to the first echographic examination. The diagnosis of carcinoid metastic to the lateral rectus muscle OD and the superior rectus muscle OS was made with Standardized Echography on the basis of medium to high internal reflectivity, large angle kappa and marked internal vascularity. These acoustic properties of carcinoid had previously been established in a case of orbital metastasis [15]. Although the internal reflectivity in the published case had been clearly higher, it was concluded from our experience with metastatic carcinoma, that within the muscle boundaries a metastatic carcinoid would have lower reflectivity than elsewhere in the orbit (see discussion above). The echographic diagnosis of carcinoid was confirmed thereafter by an orbital biopsy and histopathological examination. During the preoperative echographic examination, the left optic nerve was found to be compressed by the large tumor in the superior rectus muscle (Fig. 7C, left). Following a debulking of the left orbital mass during the biopsy the echographic signs of compressive optic neuropathy [31] disappeared and have not yet recurred (Fig. 7C, right). The orbital tumors were treated palliatively with radiation. While at first no primary tumor could be detected in spite of extensive radiological testing, the primary tumor was located in the ileum later and was surgically removed. Echographic follow-up examinations were done on a yearly basis since the first visit and showed in 4 years (a) only minimal growth of the orbital tumors and (b) slightly increased internal reflectivity of the radiated tumors.

The diagnosis (and differential diagnosis) of disorders of the extraocular muscles is geared primarily toward the **comparison of corresponding muscles** in the two orbits of a patient whether plain A-scanning and B-scanning or precise measurements are used. This certainly is the method of choice to obtain reliable, accurate, comparable and repeatable results. In addition, quantitative, topographic and kinetic acoustic differential criteria, especially the **inner** reflectivity of the muscles are used to obtain a differential diagnosis of the muscle disorder detected.

References

[1] K.C. Ossoinig and F.C. Blodi. Preoperative differential diagnosis of tumors with echogra-

phy IV Diagnosis of orbital tumors In F C Blodi (ed) Current Concepts in Ophthalmology Vol 4 C V Mosby, St Louis, 1974, pp 313-341

[2] L McNutt Ultrasound of Graves' orbitopathy (seminar) Department of Ophthalmology
Univ of Iowa Hospitals, Iowa City, USA, 1975

[3] K C Ossoinig A-scan echography and orbital disease In Proc of 2nd International
Symposium on Orbital Disorders Mod Probl Ophthalmol 1975,14 203-235

[4] K C Ossoinig and P Till Ten-year study on clinical echography in orbital disease In J
Francois and F Goes (eds), Ultrasonography in Ophthalmology Bibl Ophthal , No 83
Karger, Basel, 1975, pp 200-216

[5] L C McNutt, S L Kaefring and K C Ossoinig Echographic measurement of extraocular
muscles In D White and R E Brown (eds) Ultrasound in Medicine Vol 3A Plenum
Press, New York, 1977, pp 927-932

[6] K C Ossoinig The role of clinical echography in modern diagnosis of periorbital and
orbital lesions In G Bleeker (ed) Proc of 3rd Int Symp on Orbital Disorders, Amsterdam 1977 Dr W Junk Publishers, Amsterdam, 1977, pp 496-540

[7] K C Ossoinig Echography of the eye, orbit and periorbital region In P H Arger (ed)
Orbit Roentgenology J Wiley & Son, New York, 1977, pp 224-269

[8] B L Hodes, L Frazee and S Szmyd Thyroid orbitopathy an update Ophthalmic Surgery
1979,10(11) 25-33

[9] B L Hodes and D E Shoch Thyroid ocular myopathy Transactions of the American
Ophthalmological Society 1979,77 80-103

[10] K C Ossoinig Standardized echography basic principles, clinical applications and results
In R L Dallow (ed) Ophthalmic Ultrasonography Comparative Techniques Int
Ophthal Clin Vol 19(4) Little, Brown & Co , Boston, 1979, pp 127-210

[11] K C Ossoinig The technique of measuring extraocular muscles In H Gernet (ed)
Diagnostica Ultrasonica in Ophthalmologia (Proc of SIDUO VII, Muenster 1978) R A
Remy Verlag, Muenster , 1979, pp 166-172

[12] H J Shammas, D S Minckler and C Ogden Ultrasound in early thyroid ophthalmopathy
Arch Ophthalmol 1980,98 277-279

[13] H W Skalka The use of ultrasonography in the diagnosis of endocrine orbitopathy Neuro-
Ophthalmol 1980,1 109-116

[14] H Shibata, Y Masuyama, Y Nishimoto and A Sawada Echography in orbital myositis
Docum Ophthal Proc Series, Vol 29 Dr Junk Publishers, The Hague, 1981, pp 343-
352

[15] R Divine, R Anderson and K C Ossoinig Metastatic carcinoid unresponsive to radiation
therapy presenting as a lacrimal fossa mass In Ophthalmology 1982,89(5) 516-520

[16] K C Ossoinig A new echographic sign for the reliable diagnosis of Graves' disease (Ger)
In Klin Monatsbl Augenheilk 1982,180 189-197

[17] S R Byrne and J S Glaser Orbital tissue differentiation with standardized echography
Ophthalmology 1983,90(9) 1071-90

[18] K C Ossoinig Advances in diagnostic ultrasound In Henkind et al (eds) Acta XXIV
(Internat Congress of Ophthal , San Francisco 1982) J B Lippincott Co , Philadelphia,
1983, pp 89-114

[19] K C Ossoinig and G Hasenfratz The role of standardized echography in the diagnosis
and treatment of orbital myositis [German] Fortschritte der Ophthalmologie
1983,80(6) 475-81

[20] K C Ossoinig and V Hermsen Myositis of extraocular muscles diagnosed with standardized echography In J S Hillman and M M LeMay (eds) Ophthalmic Ultrasonography
Dr W Junk Publishers, The Hague, 1983, pp 381-392

[21] S Tane and A Komatsu Echographic measurements of extraocular muscles in normal
persons and in patients with thyroid orbitopathy In Henkind et al (eds) Acta XXIV
(Internat Congress of Ophthal , San Francisco 1982) J B Lippincott Co , Philadelphia,
1983, pp 128-131

[22] K C Ossoinig Ultrasonic diagnosis of Graves' ophthalmopathy In C A Gorman et al

(eds) The Eye and Orbit in Thyroid Disease Raven Press, New York, 1984, pp 185–211

[23] H J Shammas Atlas of ophthalmic ultrasonography and biometry (textbook), 1984, pp 230–233

[24] L Tychsen, D Tse, K C Ossoinig and R Anderson Trochleitis with superior oblique myositis 1984 In Ophthalmology 1984,91(9) 1075–1079

[25] R Rochels Ultrasound diagnosis in ophthalmology (textbook, Ger), 1986, pp 92–96

[26] G Hasenfratz Standardized echography in Graves' disease In K C Ossoinig (ed) Ophthalmic Echography (Proc SIDUO X) Documenta Ophthalmol Proc Series 1987,48 557–564

[27] W L Wan, M R Cano and R L Green Orbital myositis involving the oblique muscles – an echographic study Ophthalmology 1988,95(11) 1522–1528

[28] K C Ossoinig The role of standardized ophthalmic echography in the management of Graves' ophthalmopathy In C R Pickardt and K P Boergen (eds) Graves Opthalmopathy – Developments in Diagnostic Methods and Therapeutical Procedures Vol 20 Devel Ophthalm Basel, Karger, 1989, pp 28–37

[29] S F Byrne and R L Green Ultrasound of the eye and orbit (textbook) 1992,10 353–392

[30] A D Dick, V Nangia and H Atta Standardized echography in the differential diagnosis of extraocular muscle enlargement Eye 1992,6 610–17

[31] K C Ossoinig Standardized echography of the optic nerve (1st SIDUO Jules Francois Memorial Lecture) In P Till (ed) Ophthalmic Echography 13 (Proc SIDUO XIII) Doc Ophth Proc Series 1993,55 3–99

1.1. Processing and Analysis of Echograms: A Review

J.M. THIJSSEN and J.T.M. VERHOEVEN

(Nijmegen, the Netherlands)

Abstract. The conditions for quantitative echography are outlined. First the calibration, data-acquisition and pre-processing are discussed. The preprocessing is necessary to remove the influences of beam-diffraction and focussing, of the instrument setttings, as well as of the attenuation, from the radiofrequency (rf-) signals. The first part of the analysis of echographic data concerns the acoustospectrography, quantifying the frequency dependence of the attenuation and of the backscattering by tissues. The second part of the analysis comprises the assessment of the texture of echographic images (first and second order grey level statistics). The echographic images are processed for improving the detection and subsequent differentiation of pathology (primarily of tumours). Two main categories of processing are distinguished: speckle reduction methods and parametric imaging methods. The quality of these algorithms is assessed by the calculation of the "Lesion Signal-to-Noise-Ratio" (SNR_L), which describes the detectability of a lesion by an ideal observer. Parametric imaging comprises the two-dimensional presentation of locally derived acoustic- or image-texture parameters.

Key words: Ultrasonic tissue characterization, image processing, acoustospectrography, filtering, texture analysis, parametric imaging.

1. Introduction

The application of computerized methods to echographic signals and images is called ultrasonic tissue characterization. This work started in the seventies (Lizzi *et al.* 1976, Kuc *et al.* 1976) and it was concerned with the analysis of the radio-frequency echograms, i.e. the signals derived from the transducer after a linear amplification step. The data are generally analysed in the frequency domain, hence, the term acoustospectrography adequately describes the processssing methods. Both the frequency dependence of the attenuation coefficient (Kuc and Schwartz 1979) and of the backscattering

J.M. Thijssen, H.C. Fledelius and S. Tane (eds.), Ultrasonography in Ophthalmology 14, 1–8.
© *1995 Kluwer Academic Publishers, Dordrecht.*

spectrum (Lizzi *et al.* 1983, Coleman *et al.* 1985, Feleppa *et al.* 1986) are quantified in this approach.

A second approach concerns the analysis and processing of the echo-graphic images. These video signals are the demodulated (rectified and low-pass filtered) rf-signals. The analysis results were limited by the dependence of the image texture on the performance characteristics of the employed echographic equipment and on the control settings used during the examination. The first problem was investigated by experiments and simulations (Oosterveld *et al.* 1985). Clinical applications of video signal analysis, either separately (Trier and Reuter 1973, Decker *et al.* 1973, Thijssen and Verbeek 1981, Thijssen *et al.* 1981), or combined with acoustospectrography (Romijn *et al.* 1991, Thijssen *et al.* 1991) are promising.

The processing of echographic images is performed to reach one of the two alternative goals: either to suppress the speckle noise in the images for improving the detection of lesions (Trahey *et al.* 1986, Bamber and Daft 1986), or to enhance the lesion contrast by parametric imaging (see also: Loupas *et al.* 1989, Kotropoulos *et al.* 1993, Verhoeven and Thijssen 1993). The parametric imaging may be based either on a parameter derived from the image texture (Verhoeven *et al.* 1991), or alternatively from a local acoustospectrographic analysis (Lizzi *et al.* 1981, Insana *et al.* 1990, Romijn *et al.* 1991). In these latter cases the displayed information is not available to the observer in conventional (B-mode) echograms and a significant gain in diagnostic efficacy can be anticipated.

2. Acquisition and Processing

2.1. *Calibration*
This is a preliminary action that has to be performed for each transducer or scanning probe to be used in the acquisition phase. The calibration is needed to be able to correct the echographic data for the transducer performance characteristics and the control functions of the scanner (Romijn *et al.* 1991).

2.2. *Data Acquisition*
The acquisition software consists of four parts: the acquisition of rf-data, the storage, the coordinate transformation and the ROI selection. The acquired data can be continuously seen on the screen of the workstation in a rectilinear image display (Euclidian coordinates), after simple rectification. After acceptance, the data are stored on disk and processed. When a sector scanner is used it is necessary to convert the real-time image to polar coordinates.

2.3. *Pre-Processing*
The assumptions made when analyzing echographic signals are: linear amplification, plane wave propagation of the ultrasound (far field approximation, no depth dependence), homogeneous and isotropically scattering medium, fixed and known ultrasound propagation speed. The next step concerns the

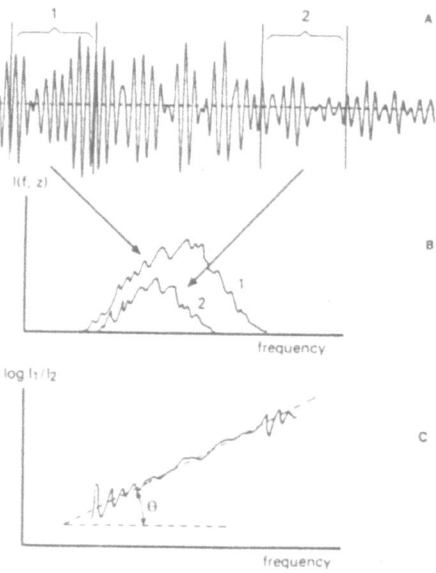

Figure 1. A. Radiofrequency echogram, depth windows 1 and 2. B. Amplitude spectra corresponding to windows 1 and 2. C. Attenuation coefficient vs. frequency.

corrections of the data for the TGC using the look-up table, the calculation of spectra by a Fourier Transform from 50% overlapping segments along each scan line, which are obtained by a Hanning window function. Subsequently, a correction of the thus obtained spectrogram is performed to remove the depth dependence (beam diffraction), by using the stored correction spectra. After AM-demodulation the final B-mode image is obtained.

3. Analysis/Processing

3.1. *Acoustospectrography*
Two acoustic characteristics of the tissues are extracted from the rf-signals by processing in the frequency domain: the already mentioned attenuation coefficient and the backscattering characteristics. The estimation of the attenuation coefficient is discussed first. The back-scattered spectrogram is estimated from every rf-echoline within a region-of-interest (ROI). The spectrogram consists of an ensemble of spectra obtained from a time window that is shifted over the rf-scanlines (Fig. 1A). When two spectra obtained at different depths, e.g. 1 and 2 in Fig. 1B, are compared the effects of attenuation become evident: the total energy decreases with increasing depth and in addition the higher frequencies are stronger attenuated. By taking the logarithm of the ratio of the spectra a straight line is approximately obtained which indicates that the attenuation coefficient is proportional to the frequency (Romijn *et al.* 1991).

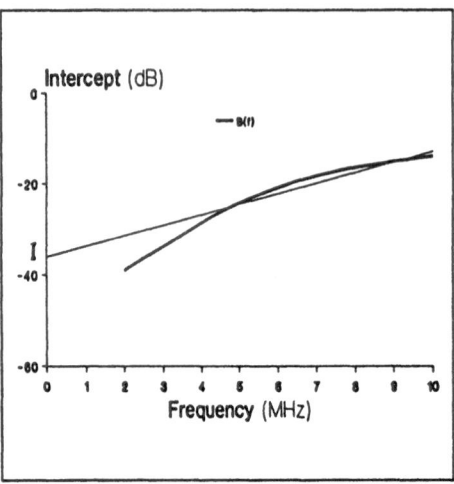

Figure 2. Backscattering spectrum vs. frequency; straight line fit in transmitted frequency range (2–10 MHz), characterized by slope S and intercept I.

The next phase in the analysis of the spectral information is performed after correction of the spectrogram for the frequency dependent attenuation, which in this respect is to be considered as the final preprocessing step. The spectra forming the spectrogram, which is already laterally averaged over the scanlines within the ROI, can now be averaged also over the depth range. So, for each ROI one spectrum results which summarizes the backscattering properties of the tissue. As is shown in Fig. 2 a straight line can be fitted to this spectrum over the range of frequencies available by using a particular transducer. In the example of Fig. 2 this range covers the frequency band 2–10 MHz. The linear fit is characterized by a slope S and an intercept I.

The 2-dimensional images obtained after preprocessing and demodulation of the rf-echolines can be characterized as "noisy". The reception by the transducer of acoustic waves scattered by homogeneous media containing randomly distributed scattering sites, yields a summation of randomly phased echo-wavelets. Due to the quasi-monochromatisme an interference pattern is formed.

The scattering from the previously defined medium can be characterized as diffuse scattering (i.e. non-coherent), and the texture is identical to a speckle pattern, as is produced by laser light. Therefore, image characteristics can statistically be described by the properties of both the gray-level histogram and the spatial autocovariance function (ACVF). Because the diffraction correction can be performed in the depth direction only, the latter analysis has to be restricted to the depth range.

The gray-level histogram is quantified by its mean μ and the signal-to-noise ratio (SNR), the latter is defined as the ratio of the mean over the standard deviation (μ/σ). The ACVF can be quantified by its full-width-at-

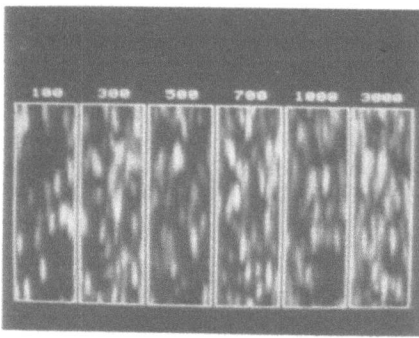

Figure 3. Simulated B-mode scans (normalized) for randomly scattering medium; number density of scattering structures are indicated (Oosterveld *et al.* 1985).

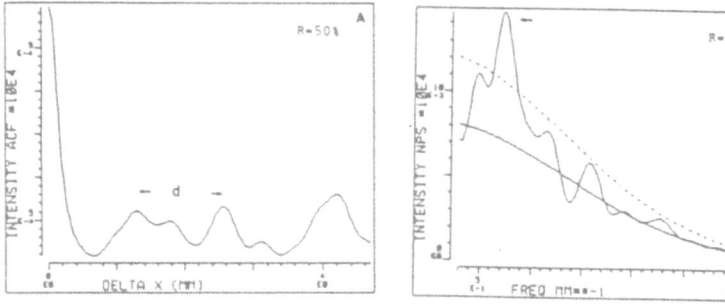

Figure 4. A. Axial autocovariance function of speckle for mixed random/structural scattering medium. B. Corresponding power spectrum. Structural dimension: d.

half-maximum (FWHM) value and it may be considered as an estimate of the average size of the speckle in the depth direction (Wagner *et al.* 1983). A theoretical analysis of these first and second order statistics can be found in literature (Wagner *et al.* 1983, Smith *et al.* 1983). Results of realistic simulations and experiments on the applicability to tissue typing were presented by Oosterveld *et al.* (1985). Figure 3 shows the effects of increasing the number density of the scatterers on the image texture.

Further sophistication of the texture analysis was introduced by Wagner and colleagues by separately quantifying the structural and diffuse scattering components underlying the texture (Wagner *et al.* 1988, Insana *et al.* 1986). This latter analysis is based on a composite model, in which any regularity of the structure of a tissue is represented by a structural scattering (coherent scattering), superimposed on the diffuse scattering assumed so far. In addition to the intensity components of the structural- and diffuse scattering, also the dimension of the structural component (matrix size) can be estimated (c.f. Fig. 4) by analyzing the Fourier transformed ACVF.

6

Table I.

Speckle reduction	Parametric imaging	Segmentation	Detection
Linear filter	Data analysis	Histogram analys.	Location
Non-linear filter	(acoustic, texture)	Gradient analysis	Size
Adaptive	Parameter encoding	Thresholding	Differentiation
Non-adaptive	Display	Morphologic filter	

4. Image Processing

The scheme of the approach for image processing is shown in Table I. The "speckle reduction" and parametric imaging phases are useful to enhance the contrast between the pathologic region, i.e. the lesion, and the surrounding tissue. The speckle reduction algorithms are aiming at an improvement of the intensity contrast of the lesion and/or at a reduction of the spatial noise caused by the speckle. The parametric imaging methods either make the results of the acoustospectrography available in a pictorial fashion, or produce an image of texture parameters. Therefore, the parametric imaging adds essentially new information to the conventional echographic B-mode images.

4.1. *Image Processing (Speckle Reduction)*
Speckle reduction is applied to echographic images to reduce the noisy appearance and to enhance the lesion detectability. If the reduction is achieved by a linear filter (e.g. a mean filter) it might be expected that both the terms A_c and A_L will be affected and the contrast and the pixel signal-to-noise ratio will change in an inverse fashion (Smith *et al.* 1983). This would imply that the lesion detectability (Thijssen *et al.* 1988) remains practically constant after filtering. Therefore, it is necessary to investigate nonlinear filters for processing of echographic images (c.f. Pitas and Venetsanopoulos 1990).

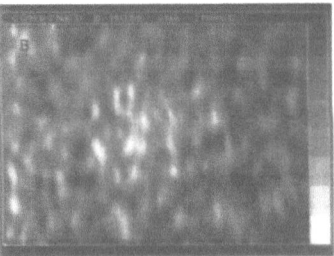

Figure 5. A. Simulated echogram containing isoechoic central lesion (number density $500\,cm^{-3}$, as compared to surrounding medium n.d. = $5000\,cm^{-3}$). B. Composite B-mode/SNR-image of A, central lesion becomes available.

4.2. *Parametric Imaging*

By definition this method implies the imaging of a parameter obtained by using a sliding window technique. A non-adaptive mean, or a median, filter would therefore belong to this category. However, also other statistical texture parameters can be used. Verhoeven *et al.* (1991) investigated the signal-to-noise ratio (SNR) of the B-mode echogram as an imaging parameter and they were able to show its potential to reveal iso-contrast lesions (Fig. 5).

Also acoustospectrographic parameters can be used to generate new images. The analysis of the local backscattering spectrum yields an estimate of the effective size of the scattering structures, which method has been termed acoustic staining of tissues (Lizzi *et al.* 1985, Insana *et al.* 1990a,b, Romijn *et al.* 1991). Also the attenuation coefficient was used as an imaging parameter (Lizzi *et al.* 1981, 1985, Romijn *et al.* 1991).

5. Conclusion

It may be concluded, that sufficient evidence can be found in the literature for the statement: echographic imaging can be significantly expanded and, when performed in real-time, image processing based on the analysis of rf- and B-mode signals will greatly improve the diagnostic potentials of echography.

6. References

Bamber, J C and Daft, C Adaptive filtering for reduction of speckle in ultrasonic pulse-echo images Ultrasonics 1986,24 41–44

Coleman, D J , Lizzi, F L , Silverman, R H , Helson, L and Tarpey J H , *et al* A model for acoustic characterization of intraocular tumors Invest Ophthal Vis Sci 1985,26 545–550

Decker, D , Epple, E , Leiss, W and Nagel, M Digital computer analysis of time-amplitude ultrasonograms from the human eye II – Data processing J Clin Ultrasound 1973,1 156–159

Feleppa, E J , Lizzi, F L , Coleman, D J and Yaremko, M M Diagnostic spectrum analysis in ophthalmology a physical perspective Ultrasound Med Biol 1986,12 623–631

Insana, M F , Wagner, R F , Garra, B S and Brown, D G Analysis of ultrasound image texture via generalized Rician statistics Opt Eng 1986,25 743–748

Insana, M F and Hall, T J Characterization of microstructure of random media using ultrasound Phys Med Biol 1990a,36 1373–1386

Insana, M F and Hall, T J Parametric ultrasound imaging from backscatter coefficient measurements image formation and interpretation Ultrasonic Imag 1990b,12 245–267

Kotropoulos, C and Pitas, I Nonlinear filtering of speckle noise in ultrasound B-scan images Ultrasonic Imag 15

Kuc, R , Schwartz, M and Von Micsky, L Parametric estimation of the acoustic attenuation coefficient slope for soft tissue IEEE Ultrasonics Symposium Proc, IEEE Cat No 76 CH 1120-SSU, 1976,44–47

Kuc, R and Schwartz, M Estimating the acoustic attenuation slope for liver from reflected ultrasound signals IEEE Trans Sonics Ultrasonics 1979,SU-26 353–362

Lizzi, F L , St Louis, L and Coleman, D J Applications of spectral analysis in medical ultrasonography Ultrasonics 1976,14 77–80

8

Lizzi, F L , Coleman, D J , Feleppa, E J , Herbst, J and Jaremko, M M Digital processing and imaging modes for clinical ultrasound In J M Thijssen and A M Verbeek (eds), Ultrasonography in Ophthalmology, Vol 8, Junk, The Hague, 1981,405–410

Lizzi, F L , Greenebaum, M and Feleppa, E J , *et al* Theoretical framework for spectrum analysis in ultrasonic tissue characterization J Acoust Soc Am 1983,73 1366–1373

Lizzi, F L , Coleman, D J and Driller, J Ultrasonic therapy and imaging in ophthalmology In A J Berkhout, L F van der Wal and J Ridder (eds), Acoustical Imaging, Vol 14, Plenum, New York, 1985,635–641

Loupas, McDicken, W N and Allan, P L An adaptive weighted median filter for speckle suppression in medical ultrasonic images IEEE Trans Circ Syst 1989,CAS-36 129–135

Oosterveld, B J , Thijssen, J M and Verhoef, W A Texture of B-mode echograms 3-D simulations and experiments of the effects of diffraction and scatterer density Ultrasonic Imag 1985,7 142–160

Pitas, I and Venetsanopoulos, A N Non-linear digital filters, Kluwer Academic Publ , Hingham, 1990

Romijn, R L , Thijssen, J M , Oosterveld, B J and Verbeek, A M Ultrasonic differentiation of intraocular melanomas parameters and estimation methods Ultrasonic Imag 1991,13 27–55

Thijssen, J M , Verbeek, A M , Romijn, R L , de Wolff-Rouendaal, D and Oosterhuis, J A Echographic differentiation of histological types of intraocular melanoma Ultrasound Med Biol 1991,17 127–138

Trahey, G E , Allison, J W , Smith, S W and Von Ramm, O T A quantitative approach to speckle reduction via frequency compounding Ultrasonic Imag 1986,8 151–164

Trier, H G and Reuter, R Digital computer analysis of time-amplitude ultrasonograms from the human eye I Signal acquisition J Clin Ultrasound 1973,1 150–154

Verhoeven, J T M , Thijssen, J M and Theeuwes, A G M Improvement of lesion detection by echographic image processing signal-to-noise ratio imaging Ultrasonic Imag 1991,13 238–251

Verhoeven, J T M and Thijssen, J M Improvement of lesion detectability by speckle reduction filtering a quantitative study Ultrasonic Imag 1993,15

Wagner, R F , Smith, S W , Sandrik, J M and Lopez, H Statistics of speckle in ultrasound B-scans IEEE Trans Sonics Ultrasonics 1983,SU-30 156–163

Wagner, R F , Insana, M F and Smith, S W Fundamental correlation lengths of coherent speckle in medical ultrasonic images IEEE Trans Ultrason Ferroel Freq Contr 1988,UFFC-35 34–44

Biophysics Laboratory
Department of Ophthalmology
University Hospital
P O Box 9101, 6500 HB Nijmegen The Netherlands

1.2. Acoustic Tissue Typing (ATT) by Sonocare (Sonovision, Computerized B-scan, STT 100). Our Experience and Results

LEONARDO FALCO, SABRINA UTARI, STEFANO ESENTE,
and NICOLA PASSARELLI

(Florence, Italy)

Abstract. Acoustic Tissue Typing (ATT) provides the possibility of distinguishing different types of tumors on the basis of spectral reflectance. Application of spectral analysis to ultrasound images has been fully investigated by Coleman who has also proven its validity. This method of "objective diagnosis" is no longer confined to the Cornell University laboratories since it has been incorporated to an ultrasound system which is now available on the market. The software program compares the frequency spectrum derived from the tumor being investigated with spectra of a data base related to the different types of tumors. This comparison leads to the estimation of a probability index for the specific lesion: spindle cell melanoma, epitheloid/-mixed melanoma, hemangioma, or metastatic carcinoma. The authors present their experiences with this new method in the diagnosis of intraocular tumors.

Key words: spectral analysis, ultrasound examination, intraocular tumor.

Introduction

Classical A/B-scan ultrasound examinations have made a marked contribution to the diagnosis of intraocular tumors. However, the electronic signal processing in echographic equipment leads to a loss of information regarding the structure under analysis (Coleman *et al.* 1991). This limitation even applies to the 'standardized' A-scan ultrasonograms.

The possibilities of effecting more accurate diagnoses of intraocular tumors are fully described in the literature. However, in many cases doubt may remain as to the nature of the lesion and it may be difficult for different examiners to obtain the same results.

Current ultrasound tumor diagnostic criteria involve the use of a terminology which introduces concepts of pathognomicity, compatibility and non-compatibility for certain types of tumors.

Compared with current diagnostic methods and the respective reporting

J.M. Thijssen, H.C. Fledelius and S. Tane (eds.), Ultrasonography in Ophthalmology 14, 9–14.
© 1995 *Kluwer Academic Publishers, Dordrecht.*

systems based on empirical observation and clinical experience, a new method (Acoustic Tissue Typing, ATT) classifies tumors objectively on the basis of spectral reflectance criteria using multivariate statistics to distinguish different types and subtypes of intraocular tumors (Coleman *et al.* 1987–90–91). Spectral analysis defines some frequency characteristics related to tumor tissue cytoarchitecture. Vascularization, scatter size, fibrosis, necrosis and melanin content are considered important tissue features and are indirectly incorporated in the ATT system to determine probability indices (Lizzi *et al.* 1983, Coleman and Lizzi 1983, Feleppa *et al.* 1986).

The aim of our study was to evaluate the diagnostic and clinical potential of ATT in intraocular tumors. The preliminary results were presented and discussed at the WFUMB (Congress of World Federation for Ultrasound in Medicine & Biology, Copenhagen, September 1991) (Falco *et al.* 1992), this paper presents a broader survey and some considerations on the results obtained to date.

Materials and Methods

The Acoustic tissue typing (ATT) uses radio frequency echo signals before the signals are processed. The signals are analyzed mathematically in the frequency domain using the Fourier transform after having been compared with a spectral calibration model. This method of correcting equipment factors makes it possible to reproduce the results.

We used the Sonovision Computerized B-Scan STT-100 (Sonocare, Inc.) which recently appeared on the market; the technical data are readily available.

A 10 MHz focused probe with a bandwidth from 5 to 15 MHz was used to analyze frequency spectra with the ATT system. A window, available in various sizes, is placed over the area of the tumor to be studied. The window must be as large as possible and positioned over the most homogeneous part of the tumor tissue.

The spectral analysis is performed by taking the mean of the spectra in each line in the window, referred to the system's calibration spectrum.

The spectral analysis system is based on the Fourier Transformation which separates each signal into its sinusoidal components. Spectral analysis is represented in a diagram as amplitude, expressed in decibels, as a function of the frequency. The diagram shows the amplitude on the abscissa and the frequency on the ordinate.

The ATT uses three parameters to classify different types of intraocular tumors: spectral slope, spectral intercept and the statistical variability in estimating the point of intercept (residual). These parameters vary from tumor to tumor. They are statistically analyzed simultaneously to define the distinguishing feature which highlights the difference between the most common types of tumors.

The different types of tumors are represented graphically and three dimensionally (Feleppa *et al.* 1986). The boundary area common to various types of tumors represents uncertain diagnoses. Approximately 10% of the tumors fall within this area of overlapping.

Tumors which can be recognized by the spectral analysis system on the basis of their cytoarchitecture are divided into the groups according to Callender's classification: type B = spindle cell malignant melanoma; type E = mixed epitheloid cell malignant melanoma; met = metastatic carcinoma; and hemang = choroidal hemangioma.

The spectral analysis of each window under study is compared with those typical of various known tumors represented in the frequency spectrum.

In cases where there is no match in the memory, the system defines the lesion as out-of-range and therefore does not define the tissue characteristics.

According to Coleman *et al.* (1987–90–91) the acoustical features of different types of melanomas associated with their dimensions are very useful for prognostics. For instance, those classified as type B (spindle cell melanoma) are known for greater post-treatment regression as opposed to type E (epitheloid and mixed melanoma).

The patients who came under our observation were examined with different ultrasound instruments: Sonomed B3000, Sonovision STT-100 (Sonocare, Inc.) that use the ATT method. Our first step was a classic ultrasound diagnosis (Sonomed B3000, Sonovision STT-100) and then we re-examined all the patients using the ATT (Sonovision STT-100) method.

Our study covered 26 patients; in 13 cases the clinical diagnosis was MM and in 13 there was no definite diagnosis. The lesions ranged from a minimum of 1.3 mm to a maximum of 15.6 mm (mean 5.15 mm) in size.

Results

We examined 26 patients using traditional ultrasound and ATT system tests (Table 1). In 13 cases we arrived at clinical diagnoses of malignant melanoma (m.m.) of the choroid which were all substantiated by traditional ultrasonograms.

In 13 cases the clinical diagnoses were uncertain and remained so even after traditional ultrasonography. The results obtained with the ATT system tests are shown in Table 1.

Of the 13 cases that were clinically and ultrasonographically uncertain, the ATT showed 3 to be hemangiomas, 8 to be m.m. and 3 metastatic carcinomas. In the 21 cases of m.m., ATT showed 15 to be type e and 6 to be type b.

Discussion

The reliability of the ATT method has been fully described by Coleman (1983–87–90–91).

In our study we obtained a clinical and/or histological (2 cases) confirma-

Table 1. Lesions indicated with E were clinically and by classical ultrasound positive for melanoma. For the melanoma type (second and third rows) the left number is the maximum index, the second number is the minimum index and the third number is the sum of maximum and minimum index.

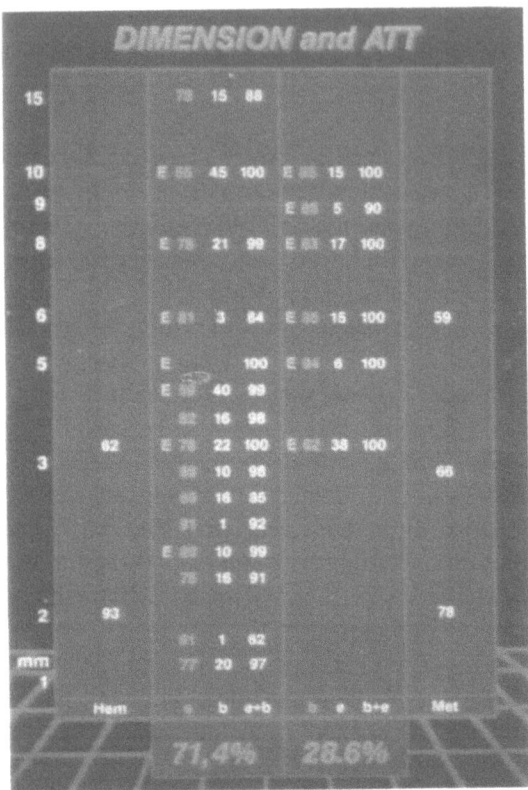

tion of 50% of the cases subjected to ATT. The follow-up on the other cases did not make it possible to confirm the ATT diagnosis.

We did not, in any of the cases, see any correlation between the size of the lesions and the ATT diagnosis. In the very small lesions, for example, the probability index was sometimes very high for a cellular type, and in larger lesions at times the probability index was not a determining factor in indicating a certain type of tumor.

For the melanomas we added the two indices of probability (Type e + type b or vice versa) since neither clinical examinations nor classic ultrasonograms permit this type of distinction to be made. This type of evaluation that may be somewhat controversial and which would seem to diminish the diagnostic potential of ATT, actually allows us to compare the ATT and 'classic' ultrasonogram findings for a further confirmation of the diagnosis. In fact, the

Table II. Sum of the two melanoma types. (Second, third rows) The first number in these rows is the maximum probability index for a certain type of melanoma. The second is the sum of this with the second (minimum probability index).

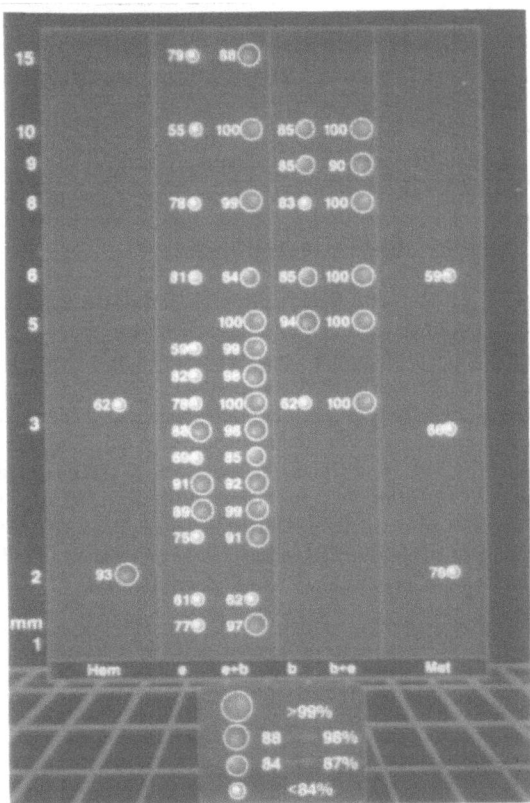

sum of the two cell types yielded a generic index of probability for melanoma in 57.15% of the cases (Type e + type b or vice versa) that ranged 100 to 99%; from 98 to 88% in 28.57%; from 87 to 84% in 9.52%; and less than 8% in 4.76% (Table 2).

Follow-up examinations and the acquisition of new cases will certainly provide the best responses to our observations.

Comments

We feel obliged to make a statement in order not to create confusion about ATT.

The method of summing the two indices of probability (type e + type b or vice versa) is our own method. Neither the manufacturer nor Coleman

14

provide any indications about it. The significance of these sums is limited to the manner in which it is presented in the text.

References

Coleman, D.J. and Lizzi, F.L. Computerized ultrasonic tissue characterization of ocular tumors. Am. J. Opthalmol. 1983;96:165–175.

Coleman, D.J., Rondeau, M., Silverman, R.H. and Lizzi, F.L. Computerized ultrasonic biometry and imaging of intraocular tumors for the monitoring of therapy. Tr. Am. Ophth. Soc. vol. LXXXV, 1987;49–81.

Coleman, D.J., Silverman, R.H., Rondeau, M.J., Lizzi, F.L., McLean, I.W. and Jakobiec, F.A. Correlations of acoustic tissue typing of malignant melanoma and histopathologic features as predictor of death. Am. J. Ophthalmol. 1990;110:308–398.

Coleman, D.J., Silverman, R.H., Lizzi, F.L. and Rondeau, M.J. The relationship of ultrasound tissue characterization parameters and clinical indicators for uveal malignant melanoma. Proceedings of International Symposium on Intraocular Tumors, Falco L., Esente S. (ed.) Medical Books, Palermo, 1991;159–163.

Falco, L., Esente, S., Passarelli, N. and Utari, S. Our experience in the diagnosis of intraocular tumors by a B-Scan computerized system and angiodynography (Doppler). Preliminary results. Proceedings 6 WFUMB. Acta Ophthalmologica Vol. 70, Supplement 1992;204:76–80.

Feleppa, E.J., Lizzi, F.L., Coleman, D.J. and Yaremko, M.M. Diagnostic spectrum analysis in ophthalmology: a physical perspective. Ultrasound Med. Biol. 1986;12:623–631.

Lizzi, F.L., Greenebaum, M., Feleppa, E.J., Marek, E. and Coleman, D.J. Theoretical framework for spectrum analysis in ultrasonic tissue characterization. J. Acoustic. Soc. Am. 1983;73:1366–1373.

Centro Oculistico, Corso Italia n. 2
Florence, Italy

1.3. Processings for Echographic Three-Dimensional Display in Ophthalmology: A Survey

MASAYASU ITO

(Tokyo, Japan)

Abstract. Three-dimensional (3D) display attracts many people engaged in medical imaging, since it is useful for comprehension and measurement of the structure, and the functions of tissue through its image. 3D display is a broad interdisciplinary issue, but much attention is focused on ultrasound 3D echography, specially in ophthalmology in this paper. Several related 3D technologies are reviewed and current state of the arts and problems including image processings will be discussed. Finally future trends in 3D images will be described.

Key words: Echography, three-dimensional imaging

1. Introduction

The main purpose of 3D display is to make it possible to comprehend and measure the structure and functions of the body through the image (Hermann 1990). The fundamental but important geometrical characteristics are volume, area, length, location and relative distance.

In addition, we need more information about complex structures, such as morphology, shape factor, topological property, anatomical and pathological relations, and spatial relation among lesions. On the other hand, space-time relation is an important function. This may lead to a real-time 3D display in the future [1].

At present we can consider four different 3D imaging techniques; perspective view, stereoscopic view using parallax, hologram and special optical machines. 3D structure can be easily projected on 3D display, and is mostly used, since the other three are not practical in diagnosis from the view points of system size, cost, handling and other factors.

In order to implement 3D display, we collect 3D data or 3D array of values. The values may be physical values or characteristics, whatever they are. In ultrasound application, structure and function may be better represented as qualitative and quantitative information. The former includes physi-

J.M. Thijssen, H.C. Fledelius and S. Tane (eds.), Ultrasonography in Ophthalmology 14, 15–18.

cal context, tissue type, shape and others. The latter includes organ dimensions, tissue properties such as attenuation, speed, refraction, and others.

In the following sections, present ultrasound three dimensional display techniques are reviewed.

2. Construction of 3D Image

3D constructions are sorted into three categories, surface rendering, volume rendering, and simultaneous display of two characteristics in 3D fashion.

In surface rendering, the shape of an object is represented as a wire frame or the surface can be represented approximately as the overlay of cross sections (called boarder sweeping method) or the patches of surface elements with ray tracing. At first, the surface of an object should be detected from 3D data. If the boarder is not well-defined, wire frame image does not work well. This surface rendering is applied to a object, having a well-defined surface such as a smooth organ. Surface can be usually detected by thresholding an intensity. However, an automatic decision of the boarder or the surface is difficult and it is often defined manually. In the future, it will be better to introduce a multidimensional feature-space partition method, considering such features as texture and acoustic characteristics.

In volume rendering [2], 3D array elements are each able to be assigned colors and opacity with luminance and chromaticity and thus will become a general purpose 3D display method. The surface of a diffuse tumor is not well-defined and the shape of a region is uncertain a priori. Therefore, volume rendering will be best in its display functions. but it needs a large capacity of memories and a complex hardware system to speed up the process.
1. shape and structure,
2. morphology and function, say shape and tissue parameters,
3. multimodality images, say X-ray and Ultrasound image.

3. Ophthalmic Ultrasound 3D Imaging

3.1. *Principle*
Recent techniques and researches in ophthalmic ultrasound 3D imaging will be explained next.

Volumetric data are collected by a linear array probe for fast scan or by a single probe for high resolution scan. The B-mode image plane may be spiral or parallel, as long as it can collect enough data for reconstruction [3, 4, 5]. Before constructing 3D image, we have to consider the following limitations and necessary processings; resolution, artifacts, noise, tissue movement and boundary detection method. Needless to say, resolution cannot be better than that of the 3D array.

One of the the most fundamental but important processes is a smoothing of the collected 3D data before detecting a boundary or a surface [6]. When we construct a 3D image from the boundaries of two dimensional smoothed images, sharp objects located perpendicular to the two dimensional surfaces are not displayed clearly and displayed sometimes in discontinuous shape. If a 3D smoothing like a median-median filter [7] is applied, such a sharp object can be obtained even among noises. In this process, we take median value for each of 13 directions, and take again the median value of the 13 directions. Blood vessels of the liver were also clearly displayed by this smoothing.

3.2. 3D Information

Tissue has 3D information such as shape and structure. Structure can be represented noninvasively by tissue characterizing parameters. When we are interested in only a shape, it can be displayed by a boarder sweeping and depth coding method, which can be also rotated and/or tilted.

Structure may be displayed together with its shape. Then we find the relation between the shape and its structure. We can, of course, construct a B-mode image to view more than one scan plane.

Various parameters such as acoustic parameters can be displayed. Furthermore, superimposed 3D imaging can be useful in therapy. For example, 3D shape and temperature distribution in ultrasonic hyperthermia treatment is reported in [8]. A simultaneous display of a reconstructed B-mode image of pseudo color and the shape is reported [9], where B-mode image of an oblique plane different from the scanning ones is reconstructed from 3D data. If the oblique plane is close to perpendicular to the viewing angle, we can see the cross section more easily.

Among applications, geometric measurement and visualization of tissue structure are main subjects. Besides tissue characterization, treatment planning and monitoring are also important applications.

4. Further Remarks

Future trends in 3D medical imaging are summarized well in the reference [10]. It says that mapping of morphological information and functions gives very useful diagnostic information.

In order to accelerate 3D medical imaging, accurate and reproducible methods for any diagnostic information should be developed. They must be robust, independent of a patient, position and image registration. How can we identify a reference marker for this purpose in ophthalmic region? It may be an actually existing marker (showing an absolute position or a well-known object) or some intrinsic key feature. This is the key to success in every image diagnosis. Other relations such as stationary and moving, local and global are also interesting subjects to be investigated [10].

Finally, virtual reality will be introduced in 3D world with a multidisciplinary research on medical computer graphics and tissue characterization.

18

References

[1] Gabor T Herman A Survey of 3D Medical Imaging Technologies, IEEE Engineering in Medicine and Biology, 190,9 15-17

[2] Arie Kaufman, Reuven Bakalash, Daniel Cohen and Roni Yagel A Survey of Architectures, for Volume Rendering, IEEE Engineering in Medicine and Biology, 1990,9 18-23

[3] Y Yamamoto, Y Sugata, M Tomita and M Ito, Three dimensional scan using a single transducer and image construction, Ultrasonography in Ophthalmology 12, Kluwer Academic Publishers, 455-460, 1990

[4] Y Sugata, Y Yamamoto and M Ito Three dimensional display of ocular region using an array transducer, Ultrasonography in Ophthalmology 12, KIuwer Academic Publishers, 461-466, 1990

[5] M M Yaremko, A E Dumke, R Silverman, F Lizzi and D J Coleman Three-Dimensional Ultrasonic Tissue Characterization and Imaging, Fourteenth International Symposium on Ultrasonic Imaging and Tissue Characterization, June 1989

[6] M Ito, T Shiina, Y Sugata and Y Yamamoto Two and three dimensional image processings applied to ophthalmic region, Ultrasonography in Ophthalmology 12, Kluwer Academic Publishers, 449-453, 1990

[7] Takashi Mochizuki, Masayasu Ito and Kenkich Tachikawa Ultrasonic Image Processing Using a Three-Dimensional Median Filter, Japanese Journal of Applied Physics, 1991,30 228-230

[8] A E Dumkek, F Lizzi, D J Coleman, A L Rosado and R Silverman, Three-Dimensional Imaging of Tissue Structure for Treatment Planning and Monitoring, Fourteenth International Symposium on Ultrasonic Imaging and Tissue Characterization, June 1989

[9] M Ito and Y Yamamoto, Construction of Ultrasonograms by Spiral Scan and Three-Dimensional Display of a Tissue, Japanese J of Medical Electronics and Biological Engineering, 1986,24,7 43-48

[10] Jean Louis Coatrieux, Christine Toumoulin, Christian Hamon, Limin Luo, Future Trends in 3D medical Imaging, IEEE Engineering in Medicine and Biology, 1990,9 33-39

Tokyo University of Agriculture and Technology
Department of Electronics and Information Engineering
2-8-1 Harumi-cho, Fuchu-shi
Tokyo 183, Japan

1.4. Three Dimensional Reconstruction of Video-Recorded Ultrasound Images: Up-dates

LEONARDO FALCO, GIANLUCA PALADINI,* STEFANO ESENTE, NICOLA PASSARELLI, SABRINA UTARI.

(Florence, Italy)

Abstract. We present a new technique for the three-dimensional reconstruction of ultrasound images, describing the image acquisition process and the software used. We discuss the useful applications of such technique for discriminating between normal and pathological anatomical structures, as well as for an accurate volumetric measurement of intra-ocular lesions.

Key words: Echography, Three dimensional, Ultrasound, Volume.

Introduction

The modern diagnostic needs create a constant incentive towards research in ultrasound imaging [1]. The 'new generation' ultrasound equipment has given us, thanks to the processing of US images, new diagnostic capabilities [2, 3, 4]. In the past, a few commercial products allowed a so called 'Isometric' or 'Pseudo Three Dimensional' image representation [5]. Later on, such type of representation has been abandoned; however, a further examination of recent literature [6, 1, 7, 8, 9] shows that many authors have been interested in the 3D (three-dimensional) reconstruction of ultrasound images. Until now there were no commercial products available for such 3D reconstruction; in the future Sonocare expects to provide a software for its Sonovision STT-100 Computerized B-Scan, for volumetric reconstruction based on studies made by Coleman [10]. In this paper we present our personal experience in 3D reconstructions using a software package, called VXL3D, which uses a new technique for volumetric acquisition and 3D visualization of US images [12–14].

Materials and Methods

All the echographic examinations have been performed using a Sonomed B-3000 and a Sonocare Sonovision STT-100 Computerized B-Scan and recorded on videotape (VHS). The 3D reconstruction has been achieved using VXL3D

J.M. Thijssen, H.C. Fledelius and S. Tane (eds.), Ultrasonography in Ophthalmology 14, 19–24.
© *1995 Kluwer Academic Publishers, Dordrecht.*

(© Nuova Paladini s.r.l. 1991), a software package with the following features:
- Real time digital image acquisition and Cine-Vision playback from a video source
- Interactive masking of the region of interest
- Adaptive speckle filtering
- Tissue classification based on gray level histogram thresholding
- Interactive 3D reconstruction
- Optical disk database storage

The video output of the ultrasound equipment is connected to a simple personal computer, IBM compatibile, which utilizes a video frame-grabbing board to accept both NTSC and PAL video standards. Such a board can digitize and store images of resolution up to 720×512 pixels, and store them on optical disk at the mean rate of 5 frames per second. Live digitized video is overlayed on the computer screen, so that there is no need for a second monitor. The board is also capable to display up to 16.7 million colors, necessary for three-dimensional color shaded graphics. For convenience, the video signal can be video recorded on tape: the computer can then be connected to the VCR during playback. The software runs under the Microsoft Windows environment, and provides a user-friendly interface based on simple mouse-driven commands [13, 14].

Image Acquisition

During the image acquisition process, the echographer scans the eye of a patient free-hand, with a linear and constant motion for about 10 seconds, while recording the resulting images onto a VHS videotape recorder (NTSC or PAL). Later on, the video tapes of interesting cases can be used for 3D reconstruction: the videotape recorder is connected to a PC, and the scanning sequence of frames is digitized. A 10 s scan yields about 50 sections, which are enough for an accurate 3D reconstruction; however, the software is able to record up to 256 sections. During the masking process, an outline can be drawn around the region of interest and can be applied automatically to the entire sequence of frames, in order to eliminate elements which might obstruct the view in three-dimension. The speckle filtering and removal option has been implemented not only to obtain better quality, noise-free images, but also to allow a more accurate region classification for three-dimensional reconstruction during the tissue classification step.

Tissue Classification

We have implemented a tissue classification method based on the observation of the gray level histogram [11]: since the gray levels in a US image have a Rayleigh distribution, each peak in the histogram implies a different tissue. These peaks are usually overlapping, however, the speckle filter improves

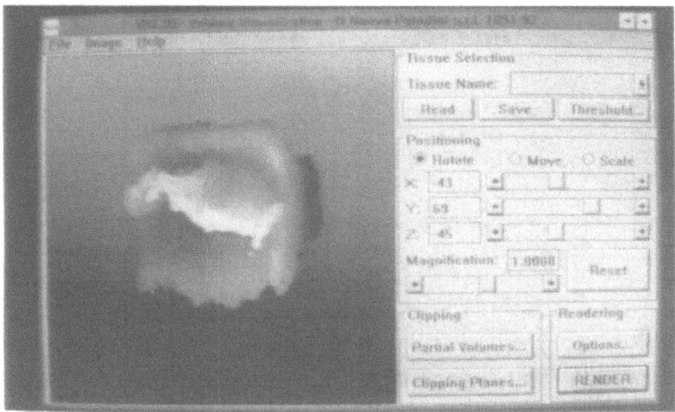

Figure 1. 3-D view of the posterior segment, containing a retinal detachment.

the discrimination of such peaks by reducing their width. It is therefore possible to separate the image into a few distinct areas and extract these automatically from the background, specifying some ranges of gray level values belonging to each tissue, and assign to each thresholded region a specific color and transparency value.

Volume Visualization

After the data has been filtered and classified, it is ready for a three-dimensional reconstruction. The user can rotate, magnify, move, scale each axis of the 3D volume using mouse-driven controls. Each shaded 3D image requires from 20 seconds to 1 minute to be computed, depending on the number of slices and their resolution, using a back-to-front projection algorithm with depth and transparent gradient shading. The maximum volume resolution is a cube of $256 \times 256 \times 256$ voxels, while the 3D rendered image is 512×512 pixels with 16.7 million colors. Other options include arbitrary cutting planes, volume sub-sectioning, and interactive modification of the region classification parameters. The software stores on optical disk all the images of each US exam which include image stills, motion images, and 3D reconstructions.

We rendered several 3D ultrasound images obtained from different ocular pathologies. In Fig. 1 we present an example of a 3D image showing a retinal detachment, while Fig. 2 shows the same case, rotated around the vertical axis. Figure 3 shows one of the 60 sections used for the 3D reconstruction; one can see the mask used (250×168) to clip out uninteresting parts, which then do not appear in the 3D reconstruction. Figure 4 shows a photograph of a melanoma of the iris. Figure 5 shows the same tumor in three-dimensions as seen from posterior.

22

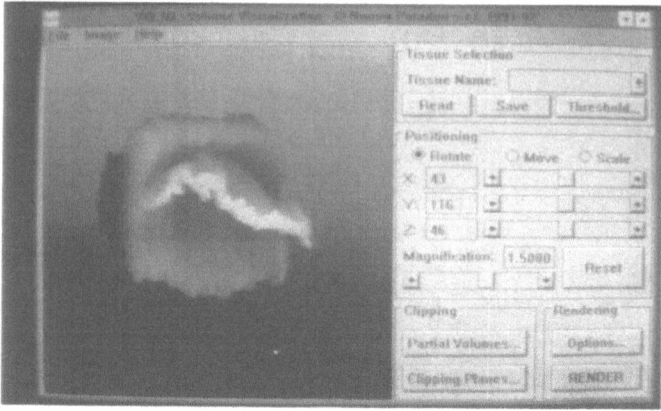

Figure 2. Same case as Fig. 1, after rotation of the volume.

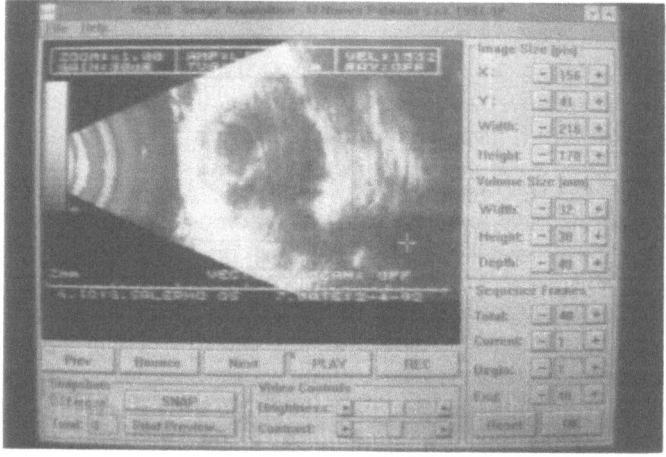

Figure 3. One out of 60 sequential scans used for the 3-D display of Figs 1 and 2. The segmentation "box" is circumventing the area of interest.

Summary

Using the VXL3D package, a sequence of analog ultrasound images, recorded on videotape, can be converted into digital form and processed in order to remove speckle artifacts. A mask which defines the region of interest can be applied to the entire sequence of frames. Subsequently, each different tissue can be classified interactively by selecting a range of thresholding values in the gray level histogram. A fast three-dimensional reconstruction allows to visualize the volume of data in any orientation and with arbitrary slicing planes. The software can be used with any equipment having a video

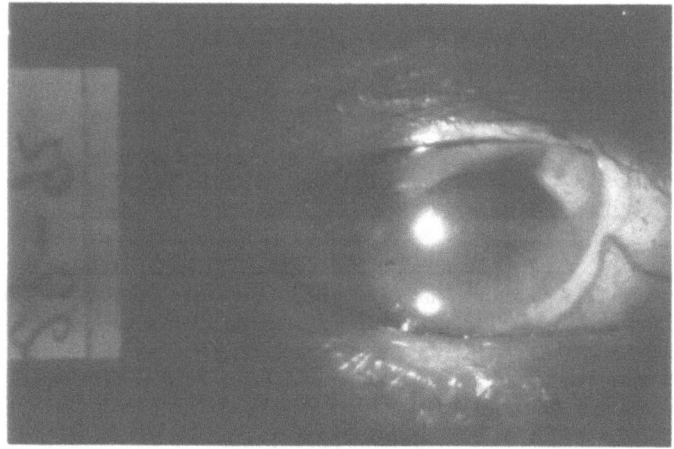

Figure 4. Eye with iris tumor.

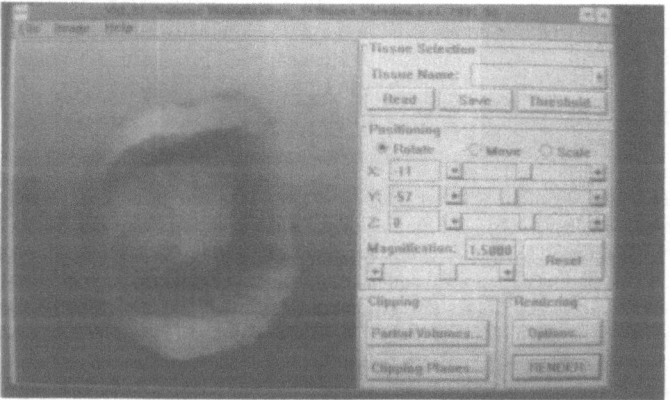

Figure 5. 3-D display of iris tumor, as seen from posterior.

output. Possible future applications of this system could be in the diagnostic discrimination of vitreous-retinal membrane structures, and in a better understanding of the morpho-pathological relations between different structures. Furthermore, the volume computation of neoplastic structures could increase the precision of evaluation for conservative treatment.

References

[1] E. Motolese, G. Addabbo, B. Daniello, N. Panterra, and M. Di Luzio. Ricostrizione tridimensionale in ecoftalmologia. Boll. Ocul. 1991, 70, N. 5, 1023–1032.
[2] L. Falco, C. Mazzini, and F. Passani. The Ophthascan B (Biophysic Medical) a new A⁻ and B⁻ scan unit. Docum. Ophthal. Proc. Series 51. Ultrasonography in Ophthalmology,

11 (J.M. Thijssen, J.S. Hillman and P.E. Gallenga, Eds.) Kluwer Academic Publishers, Dordrecht 1988, 25–30.

[3] L. Falco, S. Esente, N. Passarelli, and A. La Torre. RGB output: our experience. Docum. Ophthal. Proc. Series 53. Ultrasonography in Ophthalmology, 12 (R. Sampaolesi, Ed.) 1990, 487–489.

[4] L. Falco, S. Esente, N. Passarelli, S. Utari, and V. Mazzeo. Differential diagnosis of vitreoretinal membrane and in vivo thickness of detached retina using ultrasonic processing. 3rd International Congress on vitreo-retinal surgery. Rome, 1991, Proceedings in press.

[5] D.J. Coleman, F.L. Lizzi, and R.L. Jack. Ultrasonography of the eye and orbit. Lea and Febiger, 1977, Philadelphia, 78–79.

[6] R. Guthoff, D. Von Domarus, J. Draeger, and A. Bien. Tumor volume calculation by ultrasonographical data in the evaluation of regression patterns in ruthenium-treated melanomas. Doc. Ophthalmol. Proceeding series 53. (R. Sampaolesi, Ed.), Ultrasonography in Ophthalmology. Kluwer Academic Publishers, Dordrecht, 1990, 3–14.

[7] Y. Yamamoto, Y. Sugata, M. Tomita, and M. Ito. Three dimensional display of the ocular region. Improvement of the scanning method. Doc. Ophthalmol. Proceedings Series 48. (K. C. Ossoinig Ed.), Ophthalmic Echography. Martinus Nijhoff/Dr W. Junk Publishers, Dordrecht, 1987, 207–214.

[8] Y. Yamamoto, M. Kubota, Y. Sugata, S. Matsui, and M. Ito. Three dimensional ultrasonography of ocular region. Doc. Ophthalmol. Proceedings Series 51. (J. M. Thijssen, S. Hillman, P.E. Gallenga, Ed.) Kluwer Academic Publishers, Dordrecht 1988, 11–18.

[9] Y. Sugata, Y. Yamamoto, and M. Ito. Three dimensional display of ocular region using an array transducer. Doc. Ophthalmol. Proceedings Series 53. (R. Sampaolesi, Ed.) Ultrasonography in Ophthalmology. KIuwer Ac. Publishers, Dordrect, pp. 461–466, 1990.

[10] D.J. Coleman, R.H. Silverman, M.J. Rondeau, and F.L. Lizzi. 3D Volume Rendering of Ocular Tumors. 6th World Congress in Ultrasound. Copenhagen, Sept. 1991. Proceedings in press.

[11] D. Freedman and P. Diaconics. On the histogram as a density estimator: L2 Theory. Z. Wahrscheinlichkeitstheorie verw. Gebiete, Vol. 57, pp. 453–476, 1981.

[12] L. Falco, G. Paladini, S. Utari, S. Esente, and N. Passarelli. Ricostruzione tridimensionale computerizzata (VXL3D) di immagini ecografiche registrate su cassetta (VHS). Proceedings VI S.I.E.O. Congress, Clin. Ocul. n.4, 216–219, 1992.

[13] S. Esente, L. Falco, and G. Paladini. Le reconstruction en trois dimensions par ordinateur des images echographiques enregistrees sur cassette VHS. LXXXXVIII Congress Societé Francais D'Ophtalmologie. Paris 1992. (Proceeding in press).

[14] L. Falco, G. Paladini, S. Esente, and S. Utari. 3D reconstruction of intraocular tumors ultrasound images recorded on cassette: our experience. International Symposium on Ocular Tumors. New York 1992. (Oral presentation).

Centro Ocnlistico, s.r.l.
Florence, Italy
*Nuova Paladini s.r.l.
Florence, Italy.

1.5. Comparison of Ultrasonography, Computed Tomography and Magnetic Resonance Imaging in the Diagnosis of Orbital Tumors

GUO-XIANG SONG

(*Tianjin, China*)

Abstract. The merits of ultrasonography, computed X-ray tomography (CT) and magnetic resonance imaging (MRI) for the detection and characterization of orbital tumors was investigated. This study is based on sixty orbital tumors which were verified by histopathology. CT and MRI were superior in detecting tumors (100 percent), as compared to ultrasonography (91.7 percent). Internal structure of tumors is more optimally presented by ultrasonography.

Key words: Tumor, orbit, ultrasonography, computed tomography, magnetic resonance imaging

Introduction

Orbital tumors mostly are found in the retrobulbar space, with proptosis as the only early clinical sign. This sign, however, may be caused by many orbital diseases; it was difficult to differentiate the early conditions in the past. Since ultrasonography (US), computed tomography (CT) and magnetic resonance imaging (MRI) are used in this area, despite the opacity of the eye-ball wall and other orbital structures, the tumors can be shown early. This has been a great breakthrough in the diagnosis of orbital lesions. This paper describes 60 orbital tumors which underwent comparative examinations of these three techniques, in an attempt to find the advantages of each method, in order to obtain the best combination of imaging techniques.

Materials and Methods

This study group comprises 60 selected cases of orbital tumors, which were confirmed by pathologic examination in all cases. The group consisted of 10 hemangiomas, 9 meningiomas, 9 pseudotumors, 4 peripheral nerve tumors, 3 optic nerve gliomas, 3 dermoid cysts, 3 malignant tumors of lacrimal gland, 2 fibrohistiocytomas, 2 hematomas, 2 mucoceles, 2 xanthomatosises, 2

J.M. Thijssen, H.C. Fledelius and S. Tane (eds.), Ultrasonography in Ophthalmology 14, 25–27.

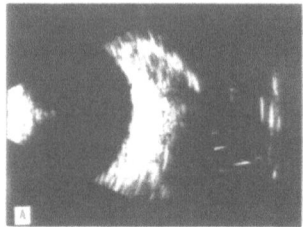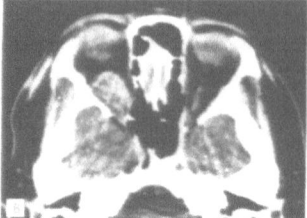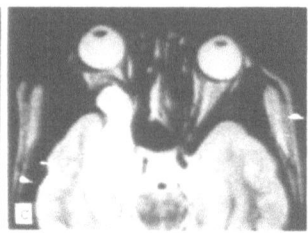

Figure 1 A 27-year-old woman with an neurolemmoma in her right orbit A, US shows a retrobulbar poor echo tumor B, CT scan detects a intraconal mass of the right orbit C, MR image on T2WI shows the tumor entering the middle cranial cavity

paranasal sinus carcinomas, 2 metastatic carcinomas and each one of chemo-dectoma, liposarcoma, rhabdomyosarcoma, malignant lymphoma, alveolar soft part sarcoma, cystcercosis, and fibrous dysplasia. Each case was examined by US, CT and MRI. US was performed by using Ultrascan digital B IV with 10 MHz probe, CT scans were obtained with Somatom DR3 System and MRI was performed using Magnetom, a 1.0 T superconducting magnet unit, TR/TE = 500/15–20 ms on T1WI and 2000–2500/90 ms on T2WI.

Results and Discussion

I. *Discovery rate of tumors.* US, CT and MRI all have a high rate of discovery in regard to orbital tumors, but they differ in different location. Of 60 tumors, 55 tumors (91.7%) were detected by US and due to the limited transmission of high frequency ultrasound, the remaining 5 tumors, which were located in the orbital apex, were not demonstrated by US. CT and MRI revealed all the tumors, a discovery rate of 100%. These two imaging modalities were extremely helpful in the assessment of the orbital apex tumors.

II. *Posterior extent of tumors.* Orbital tumors, especially optic nerve tumors, may extend posteriorly into the optic canal and cranial cavity. Partial volume effect and beam hardening artifacts prevent delineation of intracanal-icular and neighbouring cranial base lesions with CT. In this respect, MRI is more advantageous to US and CT (Fig. 1).

III. *Internal structure of tumors.* US can show acoustic interfaces of lesions, which resemble histologic features to some degree, whereas CT and MRI mainly show the outline of a lesion. To reveal the internal structure of tumors, US is better than CT and MRI (Fig. 2).

IV. *Characterization and localization.* US represents histologic structure, as CT and MRI show the secondary changes of lesions, so these three techniques offer similar results in characteristic diagnosis, however in localiz-ation, CT and MRI are superior to US (Figs. 1, 2).

V. *Relationship between the tumors and optic nerve.* After a careful US scanning, the relationship between tumors and optic nerve was demonstrated

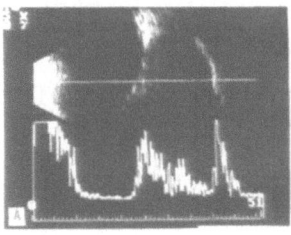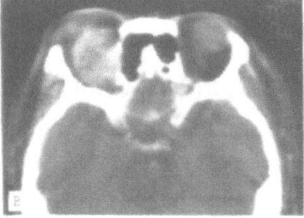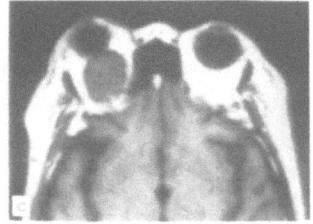

Figure 2. A 64-year-old man with a hemangioma in his right orbit. A, B-scan and A-scan US detect a retrobulbar tumor with its acoustic texture. B, C, CT and MR scan only show the outline of this tumor.

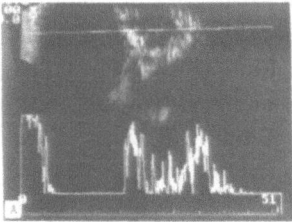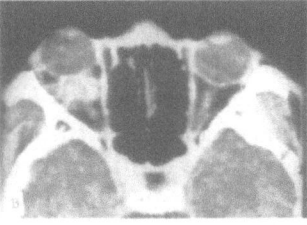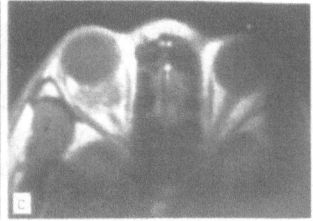

Figure 3. A 33-year-old man with a venous angioma in his right orbit. A, B-scan US discover a tumor upon the optic nerve. B, C, CT and T1-weighted image do not show the exact relationship between the optic nerve and tumor.

(Fig. 3) in all cases and for most tumors this relationship was confirmed by MRI, whereas in CT, only in one third of 60 cases tumors in relation to the optic nerve was shown.

In general, US and CT scanning are sufficient to evaluate orbital tumors. If diagnostic difficulty is encountered, MR imaging might be necessary.

Department of Ophthalmology
2nd Teaching Hospital
Tianjin Medical College
Tianjin, China 300211

1.6. Imaging of the Anterior Segment of the Eye by a High Frequency Ultrasonograph

YASUO SUGATA, MASAYASU ITO, YUKIO YAMAMOTO
and KEIJI KATO
(*Tokyo, Japan*)

Abstract. We tried to visualize the anterior segment of the eye with a newly developed high frequency ultrasonograph. This system consists of an imaging unit equipped with a personal computer and a scanner with a water chamber. The transducer of polyvinylidene fluoride (PVDF-2020, 30 MHz, 6 mmϕ, focussed to 25 mm) is manually driven linearly in the chamber through a release wire. The focus plane is set 1 mm below the aperture membrane. The scanner is held by hand on the ocular surface via methylcellulose as the coupling medium. A lateral range of 10 mm is scanned and the penetration depth is 4 mm, with a precision of 0.2 mm. Cornea, sclera, iris and ciliary body are distinguished. The configuration of the iridocorneal angle and peripheral anterior synechia are well visualized. This compact high frequency ultrasonograph is useful to observe the anterior segment of the eye especially in the out-patient glaucoma ward.

Key words: High frequency ultrasonography, glaucoma, anterior segment.

Introduction

A conventional ophthalmic B-mode ultrasonograph using 3–10 MHz is generally employed to investigate intraocular or retrobulbar lesions. However, it is difficult to visualize the anterior segment of the eye for its anatomical complexities, despite the efforts using an immersion technique [1]. Higher frequencies are required for these purposes. Sherar and Pavlin realized to visualize microscopic configuration of ocular tissues using a 50 to 80 MHz B-scan ultrasound backscatter microscope in their series of papers [2–7]. We proposed a compact B-mode ultrasonograph using 20–30 MHz by the direct application of an endovascular ultrasonograph to visualize the surface structure of the anterior segment of a living eye [8, 9].

J.M. Thijssen, H.C. Fledelius and S. Tane (eds.), Ultrasonography in Ophthalmology 14, 28–32.
© 1995 *Kluwer Academic Publishers, Dordrecht.*

Method

The system consists of an imaging unit with a personal computer and a scanner with a water chamber. The transducer of polyvinylidene fluoride (PVDF, 20–30 MHz, 6 mmϕ, focussed to 25 mm) placed in the chamber is driven linearly through a release wire by hand. The focus plane is set 1 mm below the aperture membrane. The hand held scanner is placed on the ocular surface, after installation of topical anesthesia, via methylcellulose as a coupling medium. The patient lies supine. The scanning range is 10 mm with a penetration depth of 4 mm, and a resolution of 0.2 mm.

Results

When the scanner is placed on the back of a hand, the echographic image of the surface vein and the tendon sheath underneath is visualized (Fig. 1). To investigate the discriminative power, the supporting loop of an intraocular lens (polypropylene, 0.15 mm ϕ) was depicted under the peripheral iris (the strong dual echoes in Fig. 2). The echoes from the central part of an intraocular lens (polymethylmetacrylate, center thickness 1.05 mm) was detected below the iris (Fig. 3). The penetration depth seems to be about 4 mm from the surface, with 0.2 mm axial resolution, though the sound velocity was not known in those cases. Of the structures of the anterior segment of the eye, corneal stroma showed the lower reflectivity, sclera showed homogeneous high reflectivity, and ciliary body, choroid and iris showed equally high reflectivity. The surface structure of the ciliary body could not be detected (Fig. 4), because of high absorption by intermittent tissues. A narrow but open angle was shown in a case of plateau iris (Fig. 5). The very narrow anterior chamber angle with a visible channel (Fig. 6) seems to support the maintaining of normal intraocular pressure in a case after glaucoma operation. The echogram after iridectomy was shown as the discontinued iris (Fig. 7). An anterior iridocorneal synechia was also drawn well (Fig. 8) in another case of glaucoma. The rubeotic iris showed a straight appearance (Fig. 9) in an advanced diabetic patient.

Discussion

This ultrasonographic system is the product of direct application of an endoscopic ultrasonograph developed for vessels or esophagus (Aloka). The scanner was adapted to imaging of surface structures by direct contact as for skin or eye. This compact B-mode echograph for the surface structures nicely images the configurations of the ocular chamber angle. But histological structures, as Schlemm's canal, the layer structure of cornea, or the epithelial layer of iris or ciliary body, could not be distinguished. Because of lower penetration power of this system, due to the higher attenuation by intervening tissues, the ciliary surface could not be depicted. The surface of crystalline

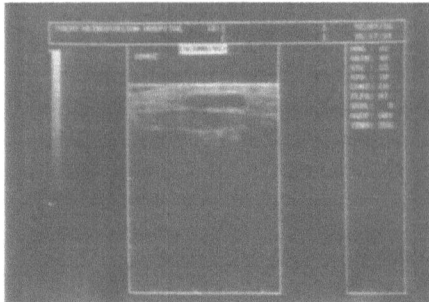

Figure 1. The echogram of the surface vein and the tendon sheath of the back of a hand.

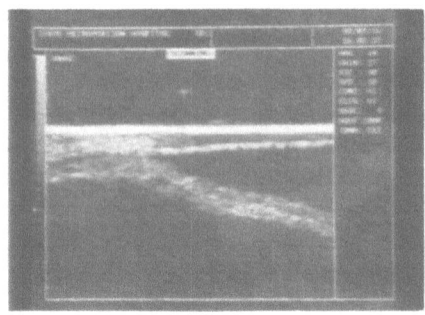

Figure 4. The structure of the anterior segment of the eye.

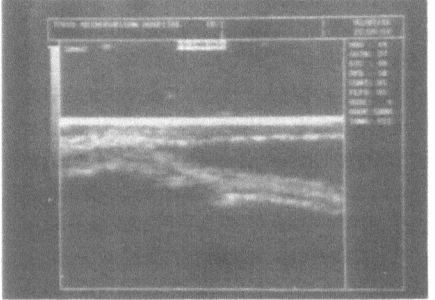

Figure 2. The echogram of a supporting loop of an intraocular lens.

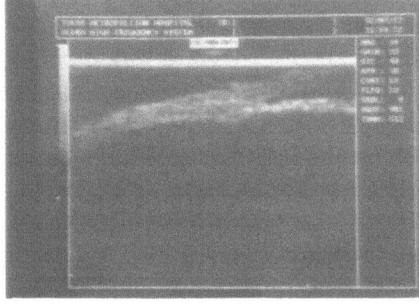

Figure 5. A narrow angle in the plateau iris syndrome.

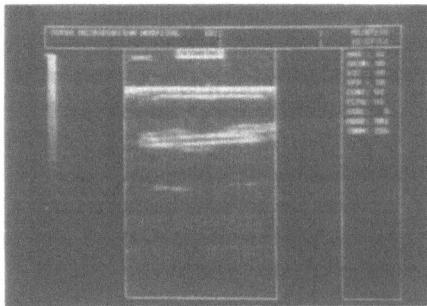

Figure 3. The echogram of an intraocular lens.

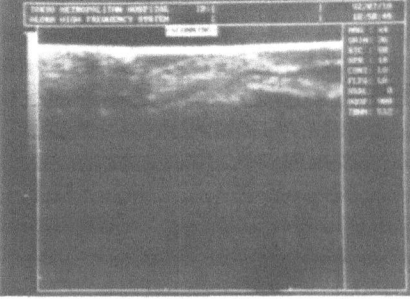

Figure 6. A narrow angle in a glaucomatous eye after operation.

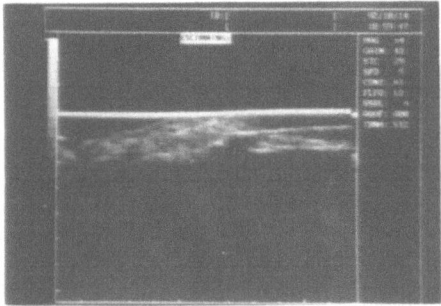

Figure 7. The area of peripheral iridectomy.

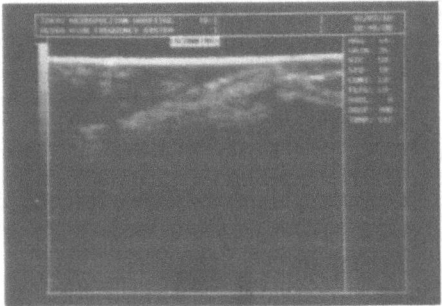

zure 8. The anterior synechia of a secondary glaucom

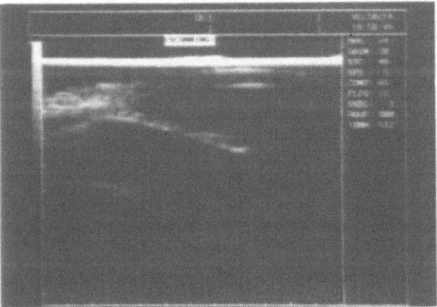

Figure 9. The echogram of a rubeotic iris in a diabetic patient.

lens was difficult to detect unless the surface was kept perpendicular to the sound beam. The hand-held scanner is rather heavy, so it is difficult to maintain a soft and stable contact to the ocular limbus without distorting the anatomy. Thus, it requires an assistant to handle the release wire to scan the transducer and the control panel of this equipment. This system is still useful in many respects for the glaucomatous eye in the daily clinic to get knowledge of angle structures, which can not be resolved by the conventional echographs. Further improvements are intended towards achieving higher power and automatically driven mechanical scanning.

References

[1] A.M. Verbeek. Diagnostic ultrasonography of the anterior segment of the eye. In P. Till (ed.), Ophthalmic Echography, Kluwer Academic Publ. Dordrecht, 1993, pp. 421–430.

[2] M.D. Sherar, M.B. Noss and F.S. Foster. Ultrasound backscatter microscopy images the internal structure of living tumor spheroids. Nature 1987;330:493–495.

[3] C.J. Pavlin, M.D. Sherar and F.S. Foster. Subsurface ultrasound microscopic imaging of the intact eye. Ophthalmology 1990;97(2):244–250.

[4] C.J. Pavlin, K. Harasiewicz, M.D. Sherar and F.S. Foster. Clinical use of ultrasound biomicroscopy. Ophthalmology 1991;98(3):287–295.

[5] C.J. Pavlin, K. Harasiewicz and F.S. Foster. Ultrasound biomicroscopy of anterior segment structures in normal and glaucomatous eye. Am. J. Ophthalmol. 1992;113:381–389.

[6] C.J. Pavlin, R. Ritch and F.S. Foster. Ultrasound biomicroscopy in plateau iris syndrome. Am. J. Ophthalmol. 1992;113:390–395.

[7] C.J. Pavlin, J.A. McWhae, H.D. McGawn and F.S. Foster. Ultrasound biomicroscopy of anterior segment tumors. Ophthalmology 1992;99(8):1220–1228.

[8] K. Kato, C. Kasai, T. Matsunaga, M. Ito, Y. Sugata, and Y. Yamamoto. High frequency ultrasound imaging system for ophthalmology. JSUM Proceedings 1992;60(31):117–118.

[9] Y. Sugata, M. Ito, Y. Yamamoto, C. Kasai and K. Kato. Development of high frequency ultrasound imaging system and imaging of the anterior segment of the eye. JSUM Proceedings 1992;60(150):357–358.

Dr. Yasuo Sugata
Department of Ophthalmology
Metropolitan Komagome Hospital
Honkomagome 3-18-22
Bunkyo-ku, Tokyo 113, Japan.

1.7. Annular Array Probe for Ocular Tissues Imaging

SADANAO TANE, MAKOTO TSUCHIYA, MARIKO
HASHIMOTO and YOTARO KIMURA
(*Kawasaki, Japan*)

Abstract. The ocular region was examined by echography using a high resolution annular array probe. The following results were obtained: (1) Homogeneous and clear images of the ocular region with excellent axial resolution and lateral resolution. (2) The occurrence of artifacts, which are specific to ultrasonograms, was relatively low, and images showing the precise shape of the eyeball without distortion were obtained. (3) Since the distance between the transducer and eye surface was relatively long, adequate images of the anterior ocular region were obtained, as with the sector scanning procedure by the immersion method. (4) As a result of long focal zone, each site of the eyeball could be distinctly and homogeneously visualized.

Key words: Annular array transducer, multifocus imaging, resolution

Introduction

We have recently used in a trial a hand-held, large diameter, annular array probe for the purpose of examining superficial tissues. This study was particularly aimed at the goal of improving image resolution. We applied this device to ophthalmologic diagnosis.

Equipment and Technique

The main specifications of this probe are as follows:
Shape of probe: Concave annular array.
Frequency: 7.5 MHz.
Diameter of transducer: 36 mm.
Number of transducer elements: 12.
Axial resolution: 0.25 mm (-12 dB).
Lateral resolution: 0.5 mm (-12 dB).

This probe, owing to electronic beam forming, provides an ideal pencil shape of the echo-beam and a long focal zone. It is also able to move by

J.M. Thijssen, H.C. Fledelius and S. Tane (eds.), Ultrasonography in Ophthalmology 14, 33–37.
© *1995 Kluwer Academic Publishers, Dordrecht.*

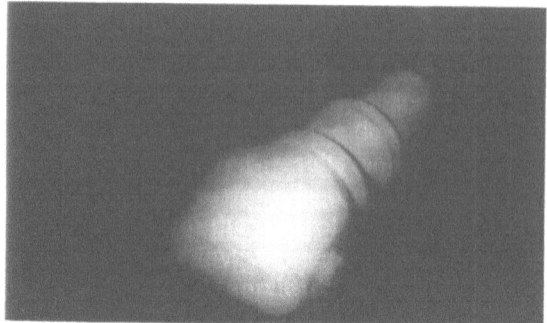

Figure 1. The annular array probe.

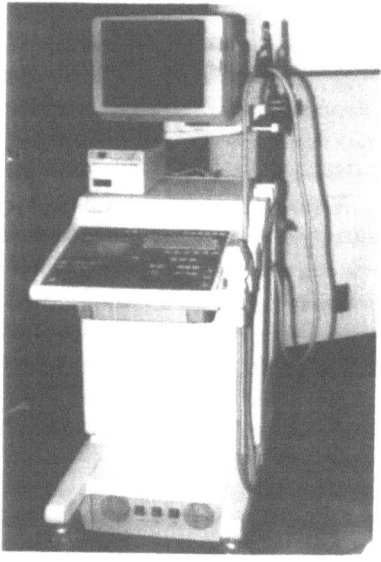

Figure 2 Sonolayer SSA-250 type equipment

software control the focus on 2 different sites, i.e. intrabulbar and intraorbital. In addition, two foci could be used simultaneously in one image, although at half the normal frame rate. This is a major characteristic of the probe.

The external appearance of the annular array probe and display apparatus are shown in Figs. 1 and 2, respectively. When it was used for examination, scopisol was applied to the palpebra. The tip of the probe slightly touched the closed palpebrae. While the palpebrae were still closed, the patient was instructed to move the eyes to the right and left. Kinetic diagnosis was performed by examination of the mobility of intraocular membranous lesions.

The image-receiving apparatus used was Sonolayer SSA-250 type equipment. The images were recorded on video tape, and frozen images were also photographed.

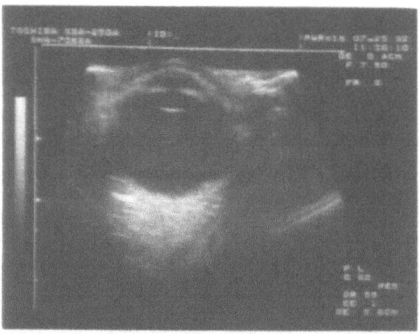

Figure 3. B-scan ultrasonogram of normal eye.

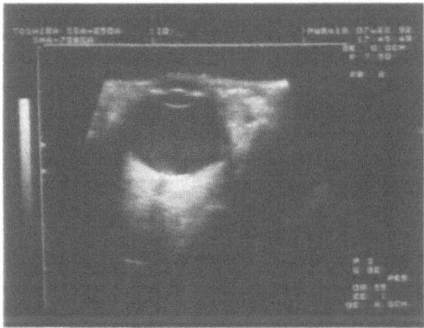

Figure 4. B-scan ultrasonogram of the eye with vitreous hemorrhage.

Results

The ocular region was examined by echography using this probe in 10 patients. Typical echograms are shown in following pictures.

Figure 3 is the B-scan ultrasonogram of a normal eye. Focus depths were 12 mm and 22 mm. The shapes of the whole eyeball, palpebra, cornea, iris, and facies anterior lentis and facies posterior lentis were distinctly visualized without deformation (52-year-old male patient).

The B-scan ultrasonograms of eye with vitreous hemorrhage is shown in Fig. 4. Focus depths were 16 and 22 mm. Hemorrhage from the vicinity of the optic disc spread into the vitreous, and vitreous membrane formation was partly observed. The echo of the retrobulbar optic nerve was also clear (68-year-old male patient).

Figure 5 shows the B-scan ultrasonographic findings of vitreous membrane formation in familial exudative vitreous retinopathy (Focus depths: 9 and 22 mm). A membranous echo was clear, and a somewhat oscillatory movement was observed on kinetic diagnosis (63-year-old male patient).

36

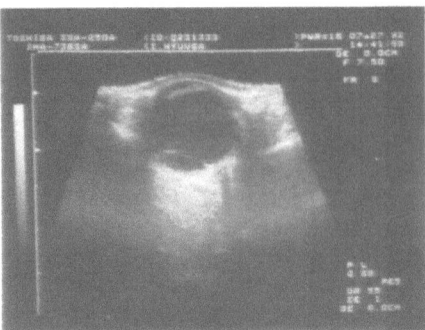

Figure 5. B-scan ultrasonogram of the eye with familial exudative vitreous retinopathy.

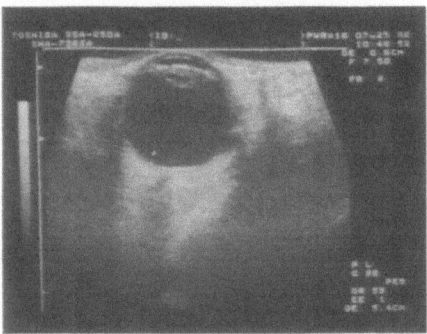

Figure 6. B-scan ultrasonogram of the eye with senile cataract.

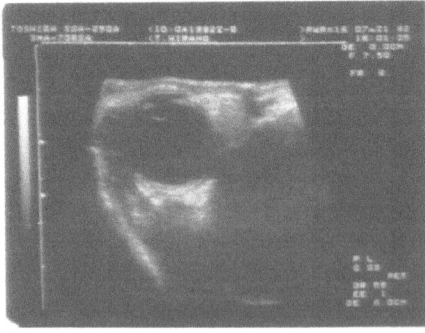

Figure 7. B-scan ultrasonogram of the eye with intraorbital arteriocavernous anastomosis malformation.

Figure 6 shows the B-scan findings of an eye with senile cataract with severe posterior capsule opacity (84-year-old female patient).

Figure 7 shows the B-scan ultrasonogram of intraorbital arteriocavernous anastomosis malformation. The condition of vessel malformation was clearer than that on the image taken with the Ophthasonic equipment (Focus depths: 28 and 40 mm).

Department of Ophthalmology, St. Marianna University, School of Medicine
2-16-1 Sugao
Miyamae-ku. Kawasaki-shi, Kanagawa-ken, 213
Japan.

2.1. Eye Size, Refraction, and Ocular Morbidity

An Ultrasound Oculometry Review

HANS C., FLEDELIUS*

(Hillerød, Denmark)

Given the opportunity of presenting a review on oculometry, my title for the Tokyo 1992 abstract book was as given above. Coming down to facts, however, it proved impossible within a single lecture to cover the full subject: The amount of ultrasound work in the field is far too voluminous and varied.

Instead, after a few general flashbacks, I will concentrate on more selected topics.

About Ultrasound Oculometry in General

Mundt and Hughes (1956) were the first to present the very foundation of ultrasound oculometry: an axial echogram showing the four main reflections, as ascribed to the front surface of the cornea, the two lens surfaces, and the vitreo-retinal interface. Establishing the ultrasound velocities in ocular tissues would allow translation of screen units, in time, into actual metric distances.

Determining the relevant velocities, Jansson presented the pioneering work (1961) and one of the first oculometry investigations (1963). Yamamoto, Gernet, Francois, Weekers, Grignolo and Rivara, and others, deserve much credit for their continuous mapping during the first decade of oculometric anatomy, with a view not only to the diseased eye but also to physiological states. Further, pioneers like Goes and Luyckx of Belgium appeared among the team of authors headed by Delmarcelle (1976) who presented an extensive and valuable review of the oculometric world literature, in its widest sense, until the early 70's.

My interest in ocular dimensional anatomy was founded in the late 60's during a large-scale investigation of low birth weight children around the age of 10 years (thesis published 1976). In the same period Larsen (1971) presented cross-sectional data analysing eye growth till the age of 13. Tane & Kohno had a similar scope in their study of Japanese children (SIDUO IX, 1982). Thirteen years of age has been the magical limit set by Sorsby and

*Now at University Eye Dept, Riqshospitalet, 2100 Copenhagen Ø, Denmark.

J.M. Thijssen, H.C. Fledelius and S. Tane (eds.), Ultrasonography in Ophthalmology 14, 39–46.
© 1995 *Kluwer Academic Publishers, Dordrecht.*

coworkers in their remarkable studies of refraction during childhood (1957–1970), which led to the assumption that axial growth generally stops at that age. Mainly their results were based on optical eye size calculations, not measurements, and mainly they were cross-sectional.

We still have only little evidence based on eyes followed longitudinally, to settle finally the question about when the eye stops growing.

Eye Size and Morbidity

In his 1864-textbook Donders described the anatomical knowledge of hypermetropic eyes as small, myopic eyes as long, and emmetropia in between. From a clinical point of view he added that a myopic eye is not a healthy eye. In his 1985-monograph 'The Myopias' Curtin agreed: "every bit of myopia carries with it a bit of risk of retinal detachment".

Accordingly, it is not only a matter of inconvenience regarding visual comfort and expenditure on optical correction when myopia increases in a population, both in frequency and in diopters. In Taiwan this has been observed to a degree so impressive that it is recognized as a significant health problem and dealt with not only by ophthalmologists, but also by the government (cf. Fledelius & Goldschmidt 1988). Education is considered the main raw material of Taiwan, and schooling is long and intense. In the wake has followed a very high frequency of myopia (80% in high school students, 96% among medical students) and with mean and median values so high as around 4 diopters (Lin and coworkers 1990). Likewise, the health authorities of Singapore recognize the high and increasing myopia frequency in its population, with its large share of Chinese, as a problem to be dealt with (Chew 1990). For long it has been known that myopia is also very frequent in Japan, and in particular among the higher educated.

Perkins (1979) emphasized an overrisk in myopic subjects of not only retinal disease, but also of cataract and (open angle) glaucoma. Another interesting question is whether corneal and ocular pathology eventually will show up in those who have refractive surgery performed (radial keratotomy, excimer laser ablation). So far we have only a short follow-up time.

Concerning the very short eye we face the problem of narrow angle glaucoma, a significant health problem in Mongoloid races in particular (Chinese, Eskimos, etc., e.g. Alsbirk 1974; Congdon et al. 1992). In general, short eyes have thicker lenses than long eyes and less volume to have them in. So, with age-related lens thickening the risk of angle closure, acute or creeping, increases. Possibly the risk is counteracted by age-related degenerations with collapse of the vitreous structure (Brown & Hungerford 1982) in association with cataract-related lens thinning. Otherwise unusual longevity would present with much more angle closure than actually encountered.

Short eyes are over-represented in squint series. Some authors maintain the importance of including eye size when planning the extent of surgery on the extraocular muscles. The smaller the eye, the greater the effect of a given resection/recession, and the higher the risk of overcorrection (Gillies et Hughes 1984).

Myopia Pathogenesis, Axial Elongation

For more than a century 'school myopia' has been used as a term for childhood and adolescent myopia (Goldschmidt 1968). The label is explained by (a) age of onset, mainly during school years, and (b) the remarkable accumulation of myopia in high school students and academics. Now it has new actuality concerning Taiwan and other parts of Asia, as referred to already. Goldschmidt (1988) introduced the term 'educational stress', but so far science has not been able to pinpoint a precise mode of action.

In a 1980 small-scale clinical study I described the distensability of the young eye, as evident by axial elongation after trauma or disease. Among Danes a 14-year limit was actually suggested, an age limit close to the abovementioned Sorsby-limit of eye growth. Until then there is still plasticity of eyewall collagen and other supporting tissue. After that age the eyewalls are considered firm and fixed and generally will not give way during eye disease, or to other stress.

Concerning myopia in general, and on Taiwan in particular, this view does not hold. Lin (1990) thus reported axial elongation the whole way through teenage years alongside with the progression of myopia. Obviously, this is a general event in adolescent Taiwan-Chinese, and not the exception to a norm as in the emmetropia-dominated European refractive distributions. A related item of interest is adult myopia, arising at the age of 20–40 years, an event probably far more common than classically believed (*cf.* Fledelius 1986–1988). Here one would expect that index factors be of main importance, as compared to axial elongation. Axial elongation was, however, suggested from a study by McBrien & Millodot (1987).

Discussing underlying mechanisms, probably they mainly relate to 'intrinsic' factors in the microstructure of ocular tissues. Where are the polypeptide factors released? On what biochemical/neuronal level? And why cannot the collagen of a given eye 'resist' myopia, giving way to a given intraocular pressure, for instance? Reference is made to Raviola & Wiesel (1988). Further, external factors are to be considered as triggers, the educational situation in all its complexity and diffuseness being the classical example.

Looking for myopia types with more direct evidence concerning outside influences, two examples are available: a) deprivation (lid suture) myopia and b) myopia of prematurity.

The former topic was dealt with at the 1990 SIDUO conference (Fledelius 1993). Human counterparts to the lid suture myopia of experimental animals are rare according to eye clinic experience. Concerning the prevailing type of myopia, that of juvenile onset, there is not much reason to consider visual form-deprivation a general mechanism.

In the following, present knowledge about refraction and eye size around

Table 1. Eye dimensions according to age. Only average values are given, all in mm. Corneal diameter, corneal curvature radius, axial eye length, anterior chamber depth, and lens thickness

	Average size at term	Final or turning point values, age (y.)	Subsequent change
Corn diam.	9.3	11.5/age 2	–
Corn curv r.	6.9	7.7/age 2	–
Ax. length	17.2	23.5/13–15 y.	No, except in adolescent axial myopia
ACDepth	2.5	3.8/13–15 y.	0.1 mm decrease/decade
Lens thickn	3.8	3.5/13–15 y.	0.2 mm increase/decade

term-time will be reviewed and discussed, with reference to myopia of prematurity in particular, but of relevance also for refractive development and adjustment in general.

Normal Correlation of Refractive Components

Through polygenic inheritance the term infant is coded to a certain eye growth and refractive development. The axial eye length and the corneal power are the two main refractive components. Both are easily and accurately measured, by ultrasound and keratometry.

Obviously the third main refractive determinant is the lens, as given by its thickness and form (curvatures), by the refractive indices of its various compartments (the 'lenses within the lens'), and by its location on the optical axis. Only the latter is readily measured, by ultrasound or optically.

More recently, it has been customary to exploit the cataract IOL calculation formulas for indirectly estimating the lens power in situ. However, this is under the assumption that a) the complex natural many-layer lens be replaced by a thin optically regular artificial lens, and b) the applicability of the given calculation formula in the given subject.

Presumably, the genetic coding is directing the adaptation during infancy and childhood by correlating the various components in a way (feed-back systems?) leading to a comfortable refraction in most subjects. In the Western world, at least, refraction mainly is grouped closely around emmetropia. Corneal size and shape are usually regarded permanent from the age of two years while axial length increases until (at least) teenage years (Table 1). Under eye growth, the lens is stretched to its thinnest state between age 10 and 20. From then it gets thicker with advancing age unless cataract interferes (with a thinner lens being more common than nuclear lens thickening, *cf.* Fledelius 1992).

With the early arrest of corneal power change, obviously the other factors have to 'subordinate', one way or the other, to achieve the adaptation guided by the regulators inherent in the genetical code.

Undoubtedly, this subtle interplay is currently influenced by external factors and responses may be normal or abnormal. A view in focus to-day is that the perfection of retinal image formation is one of the triggers for adjustment (*cf.* discussion of lid suture myopia above). Fifteen years earlier, intraocular pressure would have been highlighted; for want of concise mechanisms every decade has its pathogenetic trend.

Steiger (1913) was the first to describe fully the variation of all optical components. Were they combined haphazardly, or in a correlated fashion, as convincingly elaborated by Sorby and coworkers? (1961, 1970). When correlation – usually only in a minor part – does not suffice, significant ametropia will appear.

About myopia in general, is it due to inheritance or environment? If both parents are myopic, no wonder that their children acquire myopia at school age. But where former generations were emme- or hypermetropic, myopia in their offspring usually induces a search for outside factors. Inheritance *and* environment appears the answer to the question.

Myopia of Prematurity

Oculometric features of myopia of prematurity were first described by Fledelius (1976) and Tane (1980), the main feature being a shorter eye length than expected from the degree of myopia. Obviously, the other components had not adjusted as usually seen in full-terms, *cf.* above. The corneae were recorded more curved and the lenses slightly thicker. Apparently the untimely delivery had exerted its (arresting) influence during a stage of eye development characterized by a marked growth and final modelling of anterior eye segment structures. Possibly such events go along with what might appear in the posterior eye segment as retinopathy of prematurity (ROP).

Further, however, we are left with the question whether there is a general arresting effect of pre-term birth, on both eye segments, also where early ROP never appeared, or was mild only and regressed without visual reduction. The question arose from my already mentioned thesis investigation undertaken around 1970. The oculometric features in 10-year-old children were similar to those described above for myopia of prematurity: eyes were a little shorter, corneae more curved, and lenses slightly thicker, as apparent for instance from comparison of emmetropic eyes with normal vision in children aged 10 years, of low birth weight and of normal birth weight respectively. The oculometric differences according to the degree of maturity at delivery equalled those according to sex. Ex-prematures related to full-terms as girls to boys.

How many of these children had had ROP? With birth year about 1960 only guesses can be made. At that time mainly blindness due to retrolental fibroplasia caught attention, and not the mild cases with uneventful regression. Decades had to pass before routine observation for early ROP became standard. Restricted oxygen therapy to premature infants being the prevailing attitude, presumably ROP was not a common feature in Danish newborns then. Admittedly this statement is founded on more present epidemiological knowledge, and obviously with the clear reservation that deductions are hampered by the immense changes (improvements) regarding neonatal care over the subsequent span of years.

Assuming an influence on the growth curve of the eye, does it happen around the pre-term delivery, or is it timely delayed the same way as documented regarding ROP? An answer to the question presupposes measuring data from infants around term time, and a normal ocular growth curve to evaluate the data against.

An authorized growth curve is not available, but can be compiled from several sources: pathology institute material (abortions and stillbirths, Ehlers *et al.* 1974) together with pre- and post-term ultrasound recordings (e.g. Larsen 1971, Delmarcelle *et al.* 1976, and own data). Again reservations should be made, material and methods being quite different. For instance, part of the 'live' data is from infants of pre-term birth who – for that very reason – may have deviated from norm. Some rough data can however be given: axial growth from foetal week 16 to 28 is from about 7 to 14 mm (average increase 0.58 mm per week), and from week 28 to 40 (term-time) average weekly growth is 0.27 mm. At exactly week 40 the growth rate is estimated to 0.16 mm per week.

With measuring data available from prematurely born infants, for the first time we should be able to state how early the presumed (general) growth-arresting influence of pre-term birth can be demonstrated. Is it obvious already around expected term? From my 1992-material, at first glance the answer seems to be: no. Corrected week 40 axial lengths appeared similar in the pre-term and full-term group of that study. Those of lowest gestational age (30 weeks and less) at birth, however, including the main part of infants with regressed ROP of lower stages, had not quite attained an axial length term-value as that shown in the 33–34 weeks gestational age group. As a clearer oculometry result, in the group of pre-terms there was a relative maintenance of foetal anterior chamber dimensions: a thicker lens and a shallower anterior chamber than met in coeval full-term controls.

As a kind of conclusion concerning the influence of pre-term delivery Table 2 is given. Comparing my 1976-statement of a general growth depression even in ex-prematures with no obvious ocular sequelae to the early – likewise general – catch-up demonstrated in the cross-sectional study of Grignola and Rivara (1968), and to my own 1992 report, a further divison of the 'normal' group is suggested. Possibly two subpopulations are encountered: some with a quite unaffected eye development, and some who show the above prematurity features of retarded growth.

Concluding Remarks

Ultrasound oculometry is an established discipline in ophthalmology of today. It has rendered important information about morphological aspects

Table 2. The growth of the eye and the influence of pre-term delivery as suggested from the present review

Retinopathy of prematurity	Growth and development of the eye	Final visual acuity (corrected)
No ROP	(a) Unaffected eye growth	Normal
	(b) A slight general growth depression	Normal
Regressed ROP stage 1–3	(c) Refraction normal, like (b) i.e. smaller eye dimensions than expected	6/6–6/9
	(d) Myopia of Prematurity, arrested growth of both eye segments, more foetal proportions	6/9–6/18
ROP 4–5	(e) Small deep-set eyes, due to growth arrest and involution. Axial length often 14–15 mm	± light sense

of eye disease and about physiological states and eye growth from infancy to adult. Often, measuring results are of practical importance for therapeutic decision-making.

In addition, a renaissance of ultrasound oculometry has appeared in the wake of modern cataract microsurgery, intraocular lens calculation being of obvious importance for the visual comfort to be achieved.

Further, widespread computer facilities allow compilation of immense data sets, for cataract patients and for other age groups as well. Exploited in the right way, this should open up for new epidemiological horizons.

References

Alsbirk, P.H. Primary angle-closure glaucoma, oculometry, epidemiology, and genetics in a high risk population. Acta Ophthalmol (Copenh) 1976;54:Suppl. 127.

Brown, N. and Hungerford, J. The influence of the size of the lens in ocular disease. Brit. J. Ophthalmol. 1982;102:359–63.

Chew, S.J. A perspective on myopia research in Singapore. 4th Int. Conf. Myopia, Singapore (March) 1990.

Congdon, N, Wong, F. and Tielsch J.M. Issues in the epidemiology and population-based screening of primary angle-closure glaucoma. Survey Ophthalmol. 1992;36:411–423.

Curtin, B. The Myopias. Basic Science and clinical management 1985, Harper and Row, Philadelphia.

Delmarcelle, Y., Francois, J., Goes, F., Collignon-Brach, J., Luyckx-Bacus, J. and Verbraeken, H. Biométrie oculaire clinique (oculométrie) 1976. Masson, Paris.

Donders, F. C. Die Anomalien der Refraktion und Akkommodation des Auges. 1866. Braumüller, Wien 1866.

Ehlers, N., Matthiesen, M.E. and Andersen, H. The prenatal growth of the human eye. Acta Ophthalmol. (Copenh) 1968;46:329–49.

Fledelius, H.C.: Prematurity and the eye. Thesis. Acta Ophthalmol. (Copenh) 1976;54:Suppl 128.

Fledelius, H.C. The distensability of the young eye. Docum. Ophthal. Proc. Ser. 1981;28:117–20

Fledelius, H.C. Myopia and diabetes mellitus. With special reference to adult-onset myopia 1986.

Fledelius, M.C. and Miyamoto, K. Diabetic myopia. Is it lens-induced? Acta Ophthalmol. (Copenh) 1987;65:469–73.

Fledelius, H.C. Refration and eye size in the elderly. Acta Ophthalmol. (Copenh) 1988;66:241–49.

Fledelius, H.C. and Goldschmidt, E. Myopia Workshop, Fredensborg 1987, editors. Acta Ophthalmol. 1988;66:Suppl. 185.

Fledelius, H.C. and Goldschmidt, E. Ultrasound biometry and deprivation myopia. 1990. SIDUO XIII, Wien (to appear in Conference report 1993).

Fledelius, H.C. The thin and the thick lens. A mini-review 1992. SIDUO XIV Conference, Tokyo, October.

Fledelius, H.C. Pre-term delivery and the growth of the eye. An oculometry study of eye size around term-time. Acta Ophthalmol (Copenh) 1992;70:Suppl 204,10–15.

Gillins, W.E. and Hughes, A. Results in 50 cases of strabismus after graduated surgery designed by A-scan ultrasonography. Brit. J. Ophthalmol. 1984;68:790–95.

Goldschmidt, E. On the etiology of myopia. An epidemiological study. Thesis, Munksgaard, Copenhagen, 1968.

Goldschmidt, E. Acta Ophthalmol. 1988;66:Suppl. 185, editorial comment

Grignolo, A. and Rivara, A. Observations biométriques sur l'oeil des enfants nés a terme et des prématurés au cours de la premiere année. Ann Oculist 1968;261:817–26.

Jansson, F. Measurements of intraocular distances by ultrasound. A survey based on papers 1961–63. Acta Ophthalmol. (Copenh) 1963;41:Suppl 74.

Larsen, J. The sagittal growth of the eye I–IV. Acta Ophthalmol. (Copenh) 1971;49:239–62, 427–53, 873–86.

Lin, L., Jan, J.H., Shi, Y.F., Hung, P.T. and Hou, P.K. Longitudinal study on the ocular refraction with its optical components among children in primary schools. 4th Int Conf Myopia, Singapore, March 1990.

McBrien, M.A. and Millodot, M. A biometric investigation of late onset myopic eyes. Acta Ophthalmol. (Copenh) 1987;65:461–68.

Mundt, G.H. and Hughes, W.F. Ultrasonics in ultrasound diagnosis. Amer. J. Ophthalmol. 1956;41:488–98.

Perkins, E.S. Morbidity from myopia. Sight Sav. Rev. 1979;49:11–16.

Raviola, E. and Wiesel, T.N. The mechanism of lid-suture myopia. In: Fledelius, H.C. and Goldschmidt, E. Myopia Workshop, Fredensborg 1987. Acta Ophthalmol. 1988;66:Suppl 185, 91–93.

Sorsby, A., Benjamin, B., Davey, J.B. and Tanner, J.M. Emmetropia and its aberrations. Med. Res. Counc. Spec. Rep. Ser. 1957;293, London.

Sorsby, A., Benjamin, B. and Sheridan, M. Refraction and its components during the growth of the eye from the age of three. Med. Res. Counc. Spec. Rep. Ser. 1961;301, London.

Sorsby, A. and Leary, G.A. A longitudinal study of refraction and its components during growth. Med. Res. Counc. Spec. Rep. Ser. 1970;309, London

Steiger, A. Die Entstehung der sphärischen Refraktion des menschlichen Auges. Berlin, 1913.

Tane, S. and Kohno, J. Ultrasonic biometry of the sagittal growth of eyes in children. Docum. Ophthalmol. Proc. Ser. 1983;38:277–93.

Eye Department
Central Hospital
Hillerød, Denmark

2.2. Echobiometric and Refractive Evaluation in Pre-Term and Full-Term Newborns

A. POLIZZI, S.M. PANARELLO, L. PISSARELLO, A. DOLCI,
P. VITTONE and M. ZINGIRIAN

(Genoa, Italy)

Abstract. The authors have evaluated the axial length and the refraction in 24 eyes of pre-term and 24 eyes of full-term newborns, during the first 9 months of life. A statistical difference (Student's test) was found between the two groups at the first observation (40th gestational week), when axial length was 15.59 SD 0.39 mm in pre-terms and 16.72 SD 0.50 in full-terms. No statistical significant difference was found at 9 months (end of the follow-up) between the axial length of the eye in the pre-term (20.10 SD 0.54 mm) and the full-term newborns (20.33 SD 0.80 mm). Therefore a statistical significant difference ($p < 0.001$) of the growth of the eye has been demonstrated in the pre-term group, when compared to the full-term group. Elongation of the eye appears to be due mainly to an increase of the vitreous chamber. The refractive state at the first observation was slightly myopic in the pre-terms ($-0.71D$, SD 0.48) and hyperopic in the full-terms ($+1.02D$, SD 0.51). At the end of the follow-up, the refraction was slightly hyperopic in both groups.

Key words: Echobiometry, axial length, pre-term newborns, full-term newborns.

Introduction

The eye undergoes a more extensive growth during the first twelve months of life than in subsequent periods [1–4].

In a previous study [5] of 20 pre-term and 20 full-term newborns the authors found an evident correlation between axial length, gestational age and body weight at birth.

The aim of this study was the prospective evaluation of eye axial length growth in pre-term and full-term newborns during the first nine months of life.

J M Thijssen, H C Fledelius and S Tane (eds), Ultrasonography in Ophthalmology 14, 48–52
© 1995 *Kluwer Academic Publishers, Dordrecht*

Materials and Methods

Twenty-four eyes of 12 pre-term newborns (6 males and 6 females, with gestational age from 26 to 33 weeks and birth weight from 820 to 1300 g) and 24 eyes of 12 full term newborns (6 males and 6 females, with birth weight from 2400 g) were the object of the study.

Echobiometry was carried out with a Sonomed A 2500 (vel = 1550 m/s) under topical anaesthesia on the full-term newborns within three days after birth and on the pre-term newborns in the 40th week of gestational age and then at 3, 6 and 9 months of age. At the same time retinoscopy was performed after mydriacyl 0.5% given twice.

Ophthalmoscopy was performed on the pre-term newborns to exclude those with retinopathy of prematurity.

Student's test was utilised to investigate any statistically significant difference between groups.

Results

Our results showed there was a significant statistical difference ($p < 0.001$) of eye growth between pre-term and full-term newborns at the end of the follow-up (nine months of age) (Table 1). There was a significant statistical difference between the male components of the two groups during follow-up ($p < 0.005$) and an even greater difference between the female components ($p < 0.001$) (Tables 2 and 3). The refraction, the anterior chamber depth, the lens thickness and vitreous length are shown in Tables 4 and 5. Tables 6 and 7 show results from correlation analyses including the various parameters under study.

Discussion

The axial eye length value at first examination (40th week) was shorter in the pre-term newborns and this was significantly statistically different ($p < 0.001$). At the end of the follow-up the axial eye length value was still slightly shorter in the pre-term newborns but there was no significant statistical difference ($p > 0.5$).

Table 1. Mean axial length (AL in mm) and difference ($\Delta\%$) of eye growth between pre-terms and full-terms during the follow-up. Standard deviation in this and all following tables is given between brackets.

	AL 40th Wk	AL 6 months	Δ (%)	AL 9 months	Δ (%)
Pre-terms ($n = 24$ eyes)	15.59 (0.36)	19.40 (0.65)	24.51 (3.71) $p < 0.001$	20.10 (0.54)	28.93 (2.93) $p < 0.001$
Full-terms ($n = 24$ eyes)	16.72 (0.50)	19.51 (0.76)	16.71 (4.42)	20.33 (0.80)	21.62 (4.17)

Table 2. Mean axial length (AL in mm) and difference (Δ%) of eye growth between pre-term and full-term males during the follow-up.

	AL 40th Wk	AL 6 months	Δ (%)	AL 9 months	Δ (%)
Pre-terms	15.63 (0.42)	19.60 (0.77)	25.38 (3.20)	20.24 (0.72)	29.52 (2.88)
(n = 24 eyes)			p < 0.005		p < 0.005
Full-terms	16.92 (0.52)	20.01 (0.62)	18.70 (5.04)	20.90 (0.63)	23.63 (4.26)
(n = 12 eyes)					

Table 3. Mean axial length (AL in mm) and difference (Δ%) of eye growth between pre-term and full-term females during the follow-up.

	AL 40th Wk	AL 6 months	Δ (%)	AL 9 months	Δ (%)
Pre-terms	15.54 (0.28)	19.21 (0.40)	23.64 (4.03)	19.77 (0.18)	28.35 (2.88)
(n = 24 eyes)			p < 0.001		p < 0.001
Full-terms	16.53 (0.39)	18.15 (0.50)	15.03 (2.82)	19.95 (0.48)	19.61 (2.93)
(n = 12 eyes)					

Table 4. Mean values of refraction (D), anterior chamber depth (ACD), lens thickness (LT) and vitreous length (VL) in the pre-terms during the follow-up.

	40th Wk	3 months	6 months	9 months
Refraction (D)	−0.71 (0.48)	−0.02 (0.10)	+0.78 (0.38)	+1.44 (0.46)
ACD (mm)	1.89 (0.15)	2.28 (0.29)	2.64 (0.28)	3.01 (0.34)
LT (mm)	4.34 (0.22)	4.40 (0.29)	4.12 (0.38)	4.17 (0.29)
VL (mm)	9.63 (0.57)	11.15 (2.59)	12.71 (0.65)	12.81 (1.77)

Table 5. Mean values of refraction (D), anterior chamber depth (ACD), lens thickness (LT) and vitreous length (VL) in the full-terms during the follow-up.

	40th Wk	3 months	6 months	9 months
Refraction (D)	+1.02 (0.51)	+1.05 (0.42)	+1.20 (0.46)	+1.15 (0.39)
ACD (mm)	2.03 (0.30)	2.73 (0.28)	3.00 (0.28)	3.27 0.20)
LT (mm)	3.78 (0.28)	3.52 (0.33)	3.59 (0.27)	3.39 (0.29)
VL (mm)	10.90 (0.46)	12.16 (0.61)	12.96 (0.52)	13.62 (0.55)

The eye growth of the pre-term newborns was significantly greater than that of the full-term newborns ($p < 0.001$) during the follow-up. The increase in the depth of the anterior chamber and the decrease in the lens thickness were less in the pre-term newborns. At the first examination the anterior chamber was shallower in the pre-term (1.89 mm vs 2.03 mm) and the lens axially thicker (4.34 mm vs 3.78 mm); at the end of the follow-up (nine months of age) the anterior chamber was still shallower in the pre-terms

Table 6. Correlation coefficients between refraction (D), weight (g), and lens thickness with birth weight and some axial eye distances (ACD, LT, AL in mm) in the pre-terms at 9 months of age.

		All (n = 24)	Males (n = 12)	Females (n = 12)
Refraction (D)	and birth weight (g)	−0.46***	−0.46**	−0.47**
	and LT	−0.35**	−0.19	−0.36*
	and ACD	0.48**	0.11	0.50***
	and AL	0.12	−0.09	0.21
LT (mm)	and AL	−0.32*	−0.33**	−0.27
	and VL	−0.31**	−0.41**	−0.12
Weight (g)	and birth weight (g)	−0.31**	−0.34***	−0.29*
r ≠ zero	p < 0.05*	p < 0.01**	p < 0.001***	

Table 7. Correlation coefficients between refraction (D), weight (g), and lens thickness with birth weight and some axial eye distances (ACD, LT, AL in mm) in the full-terms at 9 months of age.

		All (n = 24)	Males (n = 12)	Females (n = 12)
Refraction (D)	and birth weight (g)	−0.57***	−0.65***	−0.50***
	and LT	−0.28*	−0.22**	−0.34*
	and ACD	−0.26*	−0.26*	−0.25*
	and AL	0.03	0.05	−0.02
LT (mm)	and AL	−0.27*	−0.34*	−0.20
	and VL	−0.38**	−0.40**	−0.36*
Weight (g)	and birth weight (g)	0.22	0.22	0.18
r ≠ zero	p < 0.05*	p < 0.01**	p < 0.001***	

(3.01 mm vs 3.27 mm) and the lens still axially thicker (4.17 mm vs 3.39 mm) with significant statistical difference ($p < 0.001$).

The vitreous length growth of the pre-term newborns was significantly greater than of the full-term newborns ($p < 0.001$).

The refraction defects in the pre-term newborns at the first examination were slightly myopic (-1 D), while at the end of the follow-up they were hyperopic.

The increase in the depth of the anterior chamber and the decrease in the lens thickness was correlated with the refraction defect and was greater in the full-term newborns. However, the vitreous and axial eye lengths did not correlate with the refraction defect in either group.

Conclusion

Our findings on oculometry of the pre-term newborns confirmed the results of other authors [1, 6, 7] in the features of the anterior chamber (shallower anterior chamber and thicker lens) at the 40th week of life.

Our results on the development of the eye during the first 9 months of age, confirmed that the pre-terms present a growth significantly statistically greater than the full-terms and at the end of the follow-up the axial length was only slightly shorter than in the full-terms.

The refraction changes into hyperopia are, as was presumed, statistically correlated with anterior chamber depth increase and lens thickness decrease.

This phenomenon can be considered a compensation of the elongation of the eye.

In agreement with Fong [8] we think that the achievement of emmetropia phase depends on the co-ordinated growth of each refractive component of the eye.

References

[1] A. Grignolo and A. Rivara. Observations biométriques sur l'oeil des infants nés à terme et des prématurés au cours de la première année. Ann. Oculist. 1968;201:817–826.

[2] Y. Delmarcelle, J. François and F. Goes et al. Biométrie oculaire clinique. Paris: Masson, 1976.

[3] J.S. Larsen. The sagittal growth of the eye. IV. Ultrasonic measurement of the axial length of the eye from the birth to puberty. Acta Ophthalmol. 1971;49:873–886.

[4] J. François and F. Goes. Ocular biometry. Introductory lecture. Doc. Ophthalmol. Proc. Series 1981;29:135–164.

[5] S.M. Panarello, E. Priolo and G. Polizzi et al. Valutazione ecobiometrica del bulbo oculare nei neonati a termine e pretermine: studio preliminare. Clin. Ocul. Patol. Ocul. 1991;12:177–178.

[6] H.C. Fledelius. Eye size of the premature infant around presumed term. Doc. Ophthalmol. Proc. Series 1990;53:165–172.

[7] H.C. Fledelius. Pre-term delivery and the growth of the eye. An oculometric study of the eye size around term-time. In H.C. Fledelius and P.K. Hansen (eds.), Ophthalmic ultrasound: a conference report from SIDUO/WFMB, Copenhagen, Acta Ophthalmologica 1992;69suppl.204:10–15.

[8] D.S. Fong. Postnatal ocular growth and its regulation. Int. Ophthalmol. Clin. 1992;32(1):25–33.

Dr. Anna Polizzi
Eye Clinic
Clinica Oculistica dell'Università
V.le Benedetto XV No. 10
16132 Genova
Italy.

2.3. The Growth of the Eye in Pediatric Aphakia: Reports of Echobiometry During the First Year of Life

S.M. PANARELLO, A. DOLCI, A. POLIZZI, E. PRIOLO,
M. ZINGIRIAN and P. VITTONE

(Genoa, Italy)

Abstract. In this prospective study the authors have evaluated with echobiometry the growth of axial length in 22 eyes of 11 babies (Group 1) who underwent extracapsular surgical procedures for congenital bilateral cataracts within the third month of life. Group 1 was divided into two subgroups: subgroup 1A of 12 eyes of 6 patients with axial length $\geqslant 17.50$ mm and subgroup 1B of 10 eyes of 5 patients with axial length <17.50 mm before the surgery (third month of life). Group 2 consisted of 20 eyes of 10 normal babies, matched for age and sex with Group 1. The data gathered have been statistically analysed (Wilcoxon test and Analysis of Variance). At the end of follow-up (twelve months of age) there was no significant statistical difference between subgroup 1A and control group ($p > 0.5$). However we found that there was a significant statistical difference between subgroup 1B and the other two groups ($p < 0.01$). We conclude that even if the aphakic eye is shorter than the phakic eye at the end of the follow-up (twelve months of age), extracapsular surgery for congenital cataracts does not influence eye growth during the first year of life.

Key words: Echobiometry, aphakic eye, axial length, congenital cataract.

Introduction

The eye of the newborn differs significantly from the adult's one and it is subject to rapid changes during the first year of life [1–3].

Ultrasound biometry results of Grignolo and Rivara [4] and confirmed by Tane [5] show that there is rapid decrease in the dioptic power of the lens by about 10–15 diopters during the first months of life.

The removal of the lens in the newborn's eye produces a strong ametropia.

The aim of our study has been a prospective evaluation of the aphakic eye growth during the first year of life.

J.M. Thijssen, H.C. Fledelius and S. Tane (eds.), Ultrasonography in Ophthalmology 14, 53–57.

Materials and Methods

Twenty-two eyes of eleven babies (between two and three months of age at first examination) affected by congenital bilateral cataracts without complications (i.e. glaucoma, uveitis, retinal detachment) were studied (Group 1). These eleven babies (6 males, 5 females) underwent cataract extracapsular extraction in the third month of life and were fitted with silsoft contact lenses.

As a control group (Group 2) we selected 20 eyes of 10 normal babies (5 males, 5 females) matched for sex and age with the eleven patients (Group 1).

The twenty-two eyes were investigated by Scan Biometry with a Sonomed A 2500 utilising a 10 MHz probe under topical anaesthesia before the surgery (vel = 1548 m/s) and every 30 days after (vel = 1532 m/s) until 12 months of life.

Intraocular pressure was measured and ophthalmoscopy conducted under general anaesthesia before the surgery and every three months after the surgery.

Group 1 was divided into two subgroups: subgroup 1A of 12 eyes of 6 patients with axial length $\geqslant 17.50$ mm and subgroup 1B of 10 eyes of 5 patients with axial length <17.50 mm before the surgery (third month of life) on the basis of the published literature (5) and our control group.

Results

The data gathered have been statistically analysed with Wilcoxon test (transformation rank) and Analysis of Variance (Kruskal-Wallis) test. These are shown in Tables 1–5. The results of the Wilcoxon test showed a significant statistical difference ($p < 0.05$) in the growth of axial length between six and twelve months for the aphakic group (Group 1) compared to the control group (Group 2) (Table 1).

This statistical difference was not significant for males at six months and not significant at 12 months of age ($p > 0.5$).

However, it was very significant for females at six months ($p < 0.01$) and significant ($p < 0.05$) at twelve months of age (Tables 2 and 3).

The Kruskal–Wallis test (Analysis of Variance) showed a significant statis-

Table 1. Mean axial length (AL in mm) and difference ($\Delta\%$) of eye growth between aphakic (Group 1) and control (Group 2) groups.

	AL 3 months	AL 6 months	Δ (%)	AL 12 months	Δ (%)
Group 1	17.00 (1.26)	18.62 (1.19)	9.71 (3.71)	19.93 (0.90)	17.56 (6.07)
($n = 22$ eyes)			$p < 0.01$		$p < 0.05$
Group 2	18.48 (0.46)	19.42 (0.66)	5.07 (2.05)	20.71 (0.74)	12.04 (2.93)
($n = 20$ eyes)					

Table 2. Mean axial length (AL in mm) and difference (Δ%) of eye growth between aphakic (Group 1) and phakic (Group 2) males.

	AL 3 months	AL 6 months	Δ (%)	AL 12 months	Δ (%)
Group 1 (*n* = 12 eyes)	17.34 (1.06)	18.95 (0.89)	9.40 (3.43) $p < 0.05$	20.17 (0.73)	16.53 (4.68) $p < 0.5$
Group 2 (*n* = 10 eyes)	18.71 (0.33)	19.73 (0.65)	5.47 (2.59)	21.22 (0.59)	13.44 (2.63)

Table 3. Mean axial length (AL in mm) and difference (Δ%) of eye growth between aphakic (Group 1) and phakic (Group 2) females.

	AL 3 months	AL 6 months	Δ (%)	AL 12 months	Δ (%)
Group 1 (*n* = 10 eyes)	16.59 (1.36)	18.24 (1.38)	10.07 (3.99) $p < 0.01$	19.64 (0.99)	18.79 (7.21) $p < 0.05$
Group 2 (*n* = 10 eyes)	8.26 (0.46)	19.11 (0.51)	4.68 (1.16)	20.19 (0.47)	10.63 (2.50)

Table 4. Mean axial length (AL in mm) and difference (Δ%) of eye growth between aphakic (Subgroup 1A and 1B) and control (Group 2) groups.

	AL 3 months	AL 6 months	Δ (%)	AL 12 months	Δ (%)
Subgroup 1A (*n* = 12 eyes)	17.99 (0.61)	19.36 (0.67)	7.65 (2.86) $p < 0.05$	20.30 (0.73)	12.21 (2.66) $p > 0.5$
Subgroup 1B (*n* = 10 eyes)	15.80 (0.67)	17.74 (0.70)	12.18 (3.03) $p < 0.01$	19.49 (0.88)	23.26 (3.60) $p < 0.01$
Group 2 (*n* = 20 eyes)	18.48 (0.46)	19.42 (0.66)	5.07 (2.05)	20.71 (0.74)	12.04 (2.93)

Table 5. Mean axial length (in mm) and difference (Δ%) of anterior chamber (ACD) and posterior segment (PS) growth between aphakic (Group 1) and control (Group 2) groups.

	ACD 3 months	ACD 12 months	Δ (%)	PS 3 months	PS 12 months	Δ (%)
Group 1 (*n* = 22 eyes)	2.52 (0.36)	2.95 (0.45)	19.37 (9.45) $p < 0.005$	14.45 (1.28)	16.80 (0.75)	17.08 (8.73) $p < 0.001$
Group 2 (*n* = 20 eyes)	3.05 (0.52)	3.29 (0.23)	10.69 (6.04)	15.79 (0.81)	17.54 (0.72)	11.21 (4.33)

tical difference between the three groups [subgroup 1A and 1B and the control group (Table 4)].

The axial length recorded at the first examination shows an inverse relationship with eye growth (Fig. 1).

Regarding the mean growth of the posterior segment there was a signifi-

56

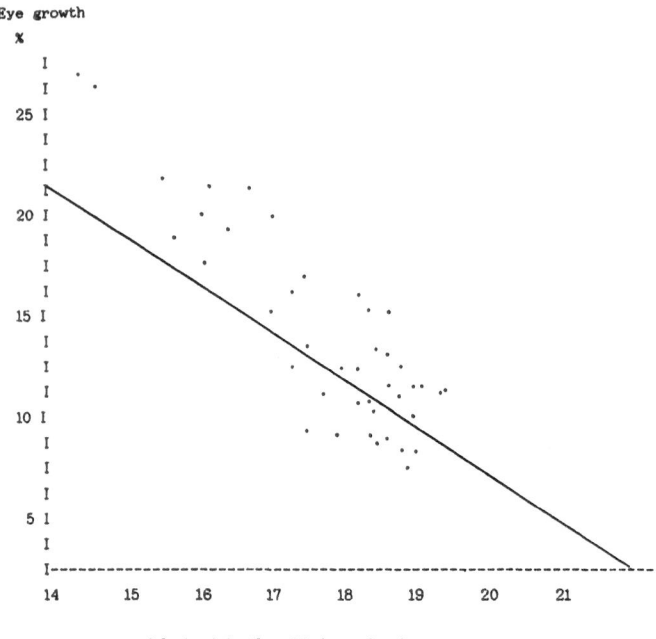

Eye growth
%

A.L. (mm.) in the third month of age

Figure 1. Correlation between eye growth in % and A.L. in the third month of age (Group 1 and Control Group)

cant statistical difference between Group 1 (subgroup 1A and 1B) and the control group at the end of the follow-up (Table 5).

Discussion

Our results showed:
1. The aphakic eyes had greater mean growth by twelve months of age and this was significantly statistically different ($p < 0.05$).
2. This significant statistical difference was primarily determined by the female component of the group ($p < 0.01$).
3. Subgroup 1A (aphakic eyes with axial length $\geqslant 17.50$ mm at the first examination = three months of age) had growth not significantly statistically different from the control group, at the end of the follow-up ($p > 0.5$).
4. Subgroup 1B (aphakic eyes with mean axial length = 15.80 mm at the first examination = three months of age) had the greatest mean growth of the three groups (subgroup 1A and 1B and control group) with significant statistical difference ($p < 0.01$).
5. The aphakic eye of subgroup 1A had a mean axial length of 20.30 mm at twelve months of age, still shorter than the phakic eye grour mean axial length of 20.71 mm (Table 4).

A study by Niederreiter *et al.* (1987) of 2 cases affected by congenital cataract showed there was no significant statistical difference between phakic and aphakic eyes regarding growth.

Our data confirm this for subgroup 1A which was not significantly statistically different from the control group at the end of the follow-up ($p > 0.5$).

However we found that there was a significant statistical difference between subgroup 1B and the other two groups ($p < 0.01$).

The mean axial length growth of subgroup 1A at the end of the follow-up (9 months after surgery) was slightly less than that of the control group (20.30 mm vs 20.71 mm).

This datum accorded with an experimental study by Wilson *et al.* (1987) which showed that monkeys which had undergone lensectomy between 8 and 26 months had aphakic eyes shorter than the unoperated eye. A study by Tigges *et al.* (1990) of newborn rhesus monkeys also demonstrated aphakic eyes being shorter than eyes of age matched controls.

We conclude that even if the aphakic eye is shorter than the phakic eye at the end of the follow-up, extracapsular surgery for congenital cataracts does not influence eye growth during the first year of life.

References

[1] Y. Delmarcelle, J. Francois and F. Goes. Biometrie oculaire clinique (oculometrie). Paris: Masson, 1976.

[2] J.S. Larsen. Sagittal growth of the eye. Acta Ophthalmol. Kbh. 1971;49:239–262, 427, 441–453, 873–886.

[3] J. Francois and F. Goes. Ocular biometry. Doc. Ophthalmol. Proc. Series 1981;29:135–164.

[4] A. Grignolo and A. Rivara. Observations biometriques sur l'oeil des enfants nés à terme et des prématurés au cours de la première annee. Ann. Oculist. 1968;201:817–826.

[5] S. Tane and J. Kohno. Ultrasonic biometry of the sagittal growth of eyes in children. Doc. Ophthalmol. Proc. Series 1984;38:277–293.

[6] P. Niederreiter, U.M. Klemen and J. Leitner. Ultrasonic biometry in childhood. Klin Monatsbl Augenheilkd 1987;191(5):355–357.

[7] J.R. Wilson, A. Fernandes, C.V. Chandler, M. Tigges, R.G. Boothe and J.A. Gammon. Abnormal development of the axial length of aphakic monkey eyes. Invest. Ophthalmol. Vis. Sci. 1987;28:2096–2099.

[8] M. Tigges, J. Tigges, A. Fernandes, H.M. Eggers and J.A. Gammon. Postnatal axial eye elongation in normal and visually deprived rhesus monkeys. Invest. Ophthalmol. Vis. Sci. 1990;31(6):1035–1046.

Simona M. Panarello,
Department of Ophthalmology
Scientific Institute G. Gaslini
Largo G. Gaslini, 5
16148 Genova
Italy

2.4. Ophthalmic Ultrasound as Used in Taiwan Republic of China

A survey with emphasis on glaucoma and myopia

POR T. HUNG, LUKE LONG-KWANG LIN, and YU-CHIH HOU,
(Taipei, Taiwan, ROC)

Abstract. Modern development of ocular sonographic techniques has contributed greatly to the clinical management of ocular disease and to the research into pathogenetic mechanisms as well. In Taiwan, our main interest concerning ophthalmic ultrasound is for the study of glaucoma and myopia with emphasis on biometry aspects, besides the clinical routine diagnostic applications.

Key words: Glaucoma, myopia, ultrasound.

Introduction

Taiwan is a heavily populated island with 20 million Chinese and less than 300.000 of Polynesian branch. The geriatric part of the population has now increased to more than 7%. Due to the strong competition within education, the 3 million school children have to study more than 10 hours everyday to qualify for college and university entrance examinations, and myopia frequency has increased suprisingly over the last decades.

In this communication, ultrasonographic studies of relevance for the characteristic ophthalmic problems of Taiwan such as angle-closure glaucoma and myopia will be emphasized. Mention will be given also of other clinical applications of ultrasound techniques.

Glaucoma Studies in Adults

Glaucoma in the Chinese is predominantly primary angle-closure glaucoma (PACG) [1]. Similar high prevalences are found in the Eskimos as well as in Mongoloid or other Asians [2]. The clinical estimation of the share of PACG of all glaucoma types is about 75 to 94% in mainland China, 79% in Singapore Chinese, 78% in Taiwan, 86% in Greenland Eskimos, and 55% in India [2]. Contrarily, PACG probably occurs in less than 0.2% of those aged over 40 in most Caucasian Studies, where primary open angle glaucoma (POAG) constitutes 75 to 90% of the glaucomas [2].

Early detection of glaucoma to prevent irreversible visual function loss is

J M Thyssen, H C Fledelius and S Tane (eds), Ultrasonography in Ophthalmology 14, 58–62

Table 1. Lens/axial length ratio in primary angle closure glaucoma

	No. of eyes	PACG	Control
Markowitz *et al.*	44	1.87–2.39	<1.91
Panek *et al.*	47	2.27	–
Hung *et al.*	69	2.12–2.33	1.84–2.01

Table 2. ACD/anterior segment depth factor, cf. text

	No. of Eyes	Range
PACG	69	3.05–3.42
Control	60	3.92–4.25

important. However, the established methods for early detection of POAG such as nerve fiber layer or/and disc study, or automated perimetry for functional examination, are not relevant for most PACG. Instead, non-invasive ultrasonographic techniques for ocular analysis may provide valuable statistical information and practical guidelines.

PACG is characterized by a relatively small cornea and a shallow anterior chamber, as part of a 'hyperopic' small anterior segment. Following the pioneer work of Törnquist in 1956 [3], Lowe [4] made extensive studies on biometry aspects of PACG in the early 1970s. He emphasized important points such as shorter axial length, shallower anterior chamber, and a relative forward position of the lens in PACG. Our studies by Haag-Streit No. 2 pachymeters in 1980 [5] and ultrasonography in 1988 [6] confirmed his studies and further pointed out the importance of the lens thickness in PACG. After ultrasound biometry in PACG patients, in 1985 Markowitz and Morin [7] pointed to the ratio between lens thickness and axial length (lens thickness/axial length factor). Their mean normal value was 1.91 ± 0.44 while for PACG in different age groups the range was 1.87–2.39.

In 1990, Panek *et al.* [8] supported that such a lens thickness/ocular axial length ratio might be a useful predictor of PACG. Our own recent biometric study by ultrasonography [9] included 69 patients with PACG, 56 with POAG, 63 with cataract, and 60 normal subjects. We concluded that an ACD ratio factor (anterior chamber depth/total anterior segment depth) is probably even more sensitive for PACG detection (Tables 1 and 2).

Congenital Glaucoma

The detection and follow up of congenital glaucoma is usually based on the clinical symptoms and ocular signs, intraocular pressure (IOP) measurement, and optic nerve examination. IOP measurement is difficult in small children and is also influenced by the general anesthesia or other hypnotics that are used [10]. This makes the non-invasive biometry not influenced by medication

Table 3. Asymmetry of axial length in children without and with congenital glaucoma (CG)

Difference mm	No. of caes	
	Normal	CG
0.1–0.5	11	0
0.5–1.0	0	2
>1.0	0	5

Table 4. Nation-wide myopia survey 1985 covering ages 12–18 years

		Junior High age 12–15	Senior High age 15–18
No. of eyes		1572	1748
Hyperopia	>+2.0	13(0.8%)	10(0.6%)
(Diopter)	≤+2.0	255(16.2%)	78(4.5%)
Emmetropia		427(27.2%)	211(12.1%)
Myopia	≤−3.0	607(38.6%)	688(38.1%)
(Diopter)	−3.0 ~ ≤−6.0	234(14.9%)	568(32.5%)
	>−6.0	36(2.3%)	213(12.2%)

an important tool for follow-up. Sampaolesi reported as ultrasonic features the elongation of axial length, a relatively thin lens, and a deep anterior chamber. We confirmed Sampaolesi's observations. Further we pointed out that a difference between axial length in the two eyes is valuable as an indicator since most of the congenital glaucomas are in a period of natural growth also, and age norms are hard to give. In most cases a side difference of axial length in congenital glaucoma will reflect a difference in degree and onset of IOP elevation (Table 3).

The recent development of high frequency polymer transducers of 50 to 100 MHz with a resolution of 20 to 60 μm and a depth penetration of 4 mm for cross sectional ultrasonic biometry, by Pavlin et al. [11], is another promising tool for the glaucoma investigations as well as for other aspects including anterior segment morphology.

Myopia Studies

The national-wide survey of myopia among school-children in Taiwan by Lin in 1985 [12, 13] showed a myopia prevalence in 6th grade primary school-children aged 11 to 12 of 39% including 9% of −3.0D or higher myopia. The myopia figures increased to 60% at age 14 to 15 (9th grade at junior high school) including 21% of −3.0D or higher myopia. At the last year of high school, age 17 to 18, the myopia rate reached nearly 82%, and even up to 90% in some schools [10] (Table 4). Fledelius and Goldschmidt considered

Table 5. Emmetropic axial lengths in Taiwan school children at the age of 7–15 years, cross-sectional results

Age (years)	Male eyes $n = 1379$			Female eyes $n = 1046$		
	No.	Mean AL	SD	No	Mean AL	SD
7	95	22.80	0.82	65	22.48	0.81
8	53	22.96	0.73	54	22.56	0.75
9	66	23.28	0.79	27	23.21	0.62
10	238	23.45	0.82	245	22.86	0.75
11	292	23.41	0.82	210	22.89	0.72
12	259	23.35	0.82	160	23.10	0.87
13	175	23.28	0.68	116	22.69	0.75
14	113	23.66	1.16	127	23.06	0.62
15	88	23.27	0.66	42	22.94	0.83
7–15 y., total		23.34	0.84		22.88	0.76

such figures from Taiwan an epidemic of significant teen-age myopia, including many cases around 3–6 diopters [14].

Ultrasonographic studies were carried out (a) in emmetropic eyes of age 16 to 19 for basic axial length data, (b) as correlation studies on myopia and axial length elongation, and (c) as longitudinal three years follow up to clarify the relationship of axial length change and myopia development [15].

We obtained the mean axial length of emmetropic eyes at age 16 to 19 to be 23.92 ± 0.75 mm for males and 23.11 ± 0.72 mm for females, in a binomial pattern [15]. For the younger age group, the details are shown in Table 5.

In an investigation by Lin in 1986 [15] including 6502 eyes from subjects aged 16 to 19, with a refraction range from more than −10 diopters (in 34 eyes) to more than +5 diopters (in 10 eyes) the correlation between refraction and axial length was high ($r = -0.74$), with a regression line of AL = 23.78–0.39 × D. In a 3 year longitudinal study on 368 male and 454 female junior high school children from age 13 to 16 there was no corneal curvature change while axial length elongation was closely related to refractive change toward myopia [15].

Myopia is a global problem. Sonographic approaches by biometric, biomicroscopic, Doppler or other new designs for future studies of myopia appear promising.

Miscellaneous Sonographic Applications in Our Clinic

Red eye is still an important sign in our daily practice. For differentiation between active hyperemia produced by inflammation and mechanical orbital congestion imaging by ultrasound is often useful.

With the increasing population of geriatric subjects in general, the cataract

62

problem in our country is becoming just as important as in the developing countries. Intraocular lens implantation is now the method of choice for optical rehabilitation, as based on IOL power calculation by ultrasound. Further, the phacoemulsification technique is based on the ultrasound principle.

Finally we should mention that ultrasonography is also well established and widely applied for the diagnosis of intraocular or orbital lesions in general.

Supported by Grant No.: DOH83-HR-320, National Institute of Health, National Health Department, Republic of China.

References

[1] P T Hung Aetiology and mechanism of primary angle-closure glaucoma, Asia-Pacific J Ophthalmol 1990,2 82

[2] N Congdon, F Wang, and J M Tielsch Issues in the epidemiology and population-based screening of primary angle-closure glaucoma, Survey Ophthalmol 1992,36 411

[3] R Tornquist Chamber depth in primary acute glaucoma, Brit J Ophthalmol 1956,40 421

[4] R F Lowe Primary angle closure glaucoma A review of ocular biometry, Australian J Ophthalmol 1977,5 9

[5] M Y Chang and P T Hung Anterior chamber depth in angle-closure glaucoma, Transaction of Ophthalmogical Society of Republic of China 1980,19 76

[6] J T Shum, P T Hung, and C S Lin Angle closure glaucoma and cataract – a biometrical study, Transaction of Ophthalmological Society of the Republic of China 1988,27 177

[7] S N Markowitz and J D Morin The ratio of lens thickness to axial length for biometric standardization in angle-closure glaucoma, Amer J Ophthalmol 1985,99 400

[8] W C Panek, R E Christensen, D A Lee et al Biometric variables in patients with occludable anterior chamber angles, Amer J Ophthalmol 1990,110 185

[9] Y C Hou, P T Hung, T C Ho et al A new proposal for early detection of primary angle-closure glaucoma by biometric study formula, Invest Ophthalmol Vis Sci (Suppl) 1993,34 1191

[10] P T Hung Ultrasound and glaucoma, J Clinical Ophthalmol (Taipei) 1987,5 119

[11] C J Pavlin, Eng, P Harasiewiczk et al Clinical use of ultrasound biomicroscopy, Ophthalmology 1991,98 287

[12] L K Lin Epidemiological study on myopia among school children, Ph D Thesis, Gradual Institute of Clinical Medicine, College of Medicine, National Taiwan University, 1985

[13] L L K Lin, C J Chen, P T Hung et al Nation-wide survey of myopia among school children in Taiwan 1986, Acta Ophthalmol Suppl 1988,185 34,Vol 66

[14] H C Fledelius and E Goldschmidt Myopia Workshop, Chapter 1 Epidemiology, Acta Ophthalmol Suppl 1988,185 11,Vol 66

[15] L L K Lin, L F Hung, and Y F Shih et al Correlation of optical components with ocular refraction among teenagers in Taipei, Acta Ophthalmol Suppl 1988,185 34,Vol 66

Por T Hung, M D
Department of Ophthalmology
Taiwan University Hospital
#7, Chung-Shan South Road
Taipei, ROC 100
Taiwan

2.5. Axial Length Measurement in Silicone-Oil-Treated Eyes

ATSUSHI SAWADA, TAKAYUKI NAGATOMO,
KEIKO KITAMURA and NOBUHISO NAO-I

(Miyazaki Japan)

Abstract. Axial length measurement for IOL power calculation is troublesome in silicone-oil injected eyes. The sound velocity of silicone-oil is necessary for axial length calculation in such eyes. Using a specially designed chamber the velocity of our clinically used silicone-oil at 38 °C was measured to be 964 m/s. It was almost two thirds of that of saline solution. In clinical cases the result was applicable. Axial length in the silicone-oil injected eye is to be corrected for sound velocity of silicone-oil for the vitreous compartment.

Key words: Axial length measurement, ultrasound biometry, silicone-oil.

Introduction

Implant of gas, silicone oil, or other substances into the vitreous has been used as an adjunct to vitreoretinal surgery. To ultrasonography in eyes treated with these materials special attention should be paid, for several reasons.

First, because the reflection of ultrasound from the surfaces of these substances in the eye is extremely strong, several kinds of errors in imaging are met.

Second, the ultrasound velocity of the various materials is quite different from that of the normal vitreous. So in case of silicone-oil, for instance, the vitreous length is displayed much longer than the real distance.

Such erroneous elongation of the vitreous length in ultrasonograms has been noticed by many. Recently we had a case, in which an IOL implant was planned to be done after the removal of silicone-oil in the vitreous. Sound velocity of the used silicone-oil was measured and the real vitreous length was calculated.

J.M. Thijssen, H.C. Fledelius and S. Tane (eds.), Ultrasonography in Ophthalmology 14, 63–68.
© *1995 Kluwer Academic Publishers, Dordrecht.*

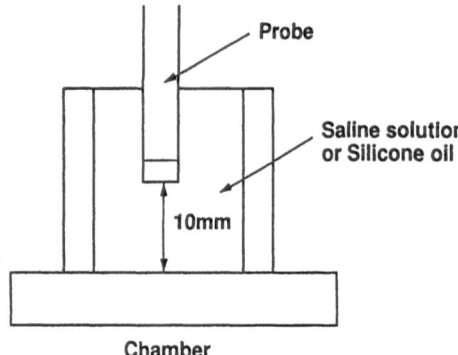

Figure 1. The model in which the sound velocity of silicone-oil can be compared with that of saline solution and calculated.

Materials and Methods

In the eye into which silicone-oil had been previously injected into the vitreous for vitreoretinal disorders, the axial length for IOL power calculation could not be measured with the ordinary automated instruments. A correction of sound velocity within the vitreous cavity was required. So we measured the sound velocity in the relevant silicone-oil (Koken, 1000 cSt) using the specially designed chamber shown in Fig. 1. A chamber of acrylics was made, into which either a 0.9% saline solution or silicone-oil could be put. The ultrasonic A-mode probe was held perpendicular to the bottom and at 1 cm distance from the bottom. The frequency of the used probe was 10 MHz. The temperature of the chamber was kept at 37 °C. In case of silicone-oil the distance from the probe to the bottom in A-mode echogram was measured and compared with that in saline solution.

To ascertain whether the sound velocity determined in the silicone-oil was reliable, the model shown in Fig. 2 was used. In the model, a sheet of cellophane separated the saline solution and silicone-oil. The distance from the probe to the cellophane membrane, and that from the membrane to the bottom was set at 5 mm and 20 mm, respectively.

Based on the ratio of the sound velocity between saline solution and silicone-oil, the distance from the probe to the cellophane membrane and that from the cellophane membrane to the bottom were calculated. For subsequent clinical application the calculated sound velocity of silicone-oil was used.

Results

In the A-scan echogram of the experiment using the chamber shown in Fig. 1. the apparent distance for 10.0 mm in the physiologic saline solution with the sound velocity of 1530 m/s, was 16.0 mm (Fig. 3). In the case of silicone-

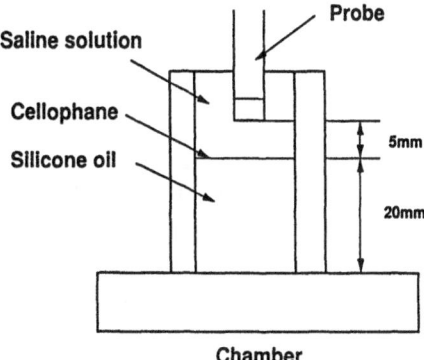

Figure 2. The model in which the calculated sound velocity of silicone-oil was subsequently controlled.

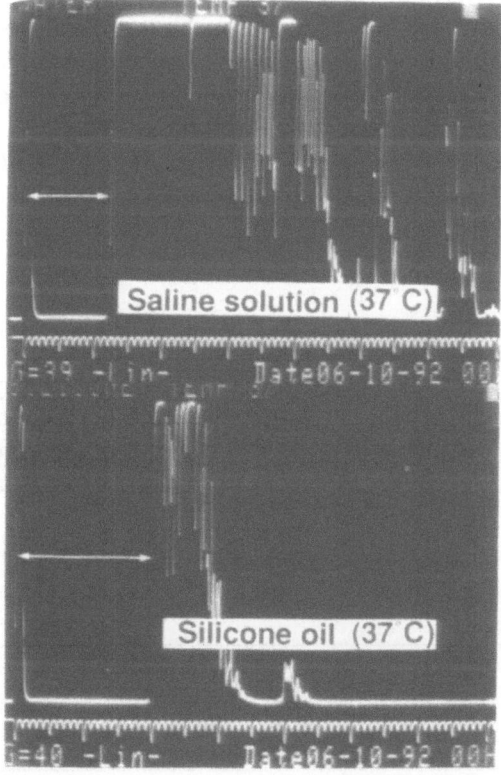

Figure 3. A-mode echograms of saline solution and silicone-oil in the model shown as Fig. 1. Echo spikes distance (horizontal white arrow) corresponding to 10 mm.

oil an apparent echo distance of 25.4 mm was shown. The ultrasonic velocity was calculated to be 964 m/s.

In the second chamber (Fig. 2) the calculated values were as follows. Saline solution: Calculated value 5.3 mm; actually measured value 5.0 mm. Silicone-oil: 19.7 and 20 mm, respectively.

The discrepancy between the calculated and the actually measured might be due to flexion of the cellophane membrane. All considered, the value of the sound velocity of the silicone-oil used in the study seemed to be fairly precise and therefore useful in clinical application. The clinical results will be described.

Two Case Stories

The first case was a 48-year-old man, who had vitrectomy, lensectomy, intraocular laser coagulation, encircling band and silicone-oil tamponade for a huge rhegmatogenous retinal detachment October 1991. In May 1992 as lens opacity had progressed, IOL implantation was planned after the removal of silicone-oil. The axial length was measured using the automatic instrument as usual oculometry, but the instrument would not work. On A- and B-scan echograms the eye ball was displayed much too large. To get the real axial length of the eye, the sound velocity of silicone-oil was required.

The echo distance of the anterior chamber and the vitreous on the manual A-mode echogram was measured three times. With the sound velocity of saline solution of 1530 m/s and that of silicone-oil of 964 m/s, the axial length was calculated using the following formula (Araki, 1961).

$$L \text{ (axial length)} = \frac{1}{d \times s} (d_1 s_1 + d_2 s_2)$$

where s is sound velocity of saline solution (1530 m/s), s_1 is sound velocity in the anterior chamber (1530 m/s), s_2 is sound velocity in the vitreous (964 m/s), d is echo distance of 1 cm in the saline solution, d_1 is echo distance of the anterior chamber and d_2 is echo distance of the vitreous.

Echo distance of the anterior chamber and the vitreous, and the calculated axial lengths were as follows.

	Anterior chamber (= aqueous)		Vitreous (= silicone-oil)	Calculated axial length
1st	6.2		51.2	24.0
2nd	6.0		51.3	24.0
3rd	5.5		51.4	23.7
		Average		23.9

Three weeks after the removal of silicone oil, the axial length was measured on the A-mode echograms. The calculated axial length was 24.1 mm, which was close to the axial length estimated before the silicone-oil removal.

In an additional case the axial length before and after the removal of silicone oil was measured. The axial length before the removal was calculated to be 24.5 mm. After the removal it was measured to be 24.7 mm. The results were satisfactory.

Discussion

Apparent elongation of the vitreous length in ultrasonography in eyes with silicone-oil implant has been noticed by many.

Verbeek et al. (1981) described various conditions after silicone-oil treatment. Among them the abnormal axial eye length could be explained by the sound velocity difference, and the real dimensions could be obtained if 2/3 of the measured length was taken.

Clemens et al. (1984) pointed out that the vitreous cavity after silicone oil was greatly prolonged in A-scan ultrasonography, and disclosed a 50% echographic prolongation of the vitreous cavity due to the delay of sound velocity in silicone-oil.

Komatsu et al. (1985) also noticed the elongation of the axial length in the ultrasonograms as an acoustic character of the silicone oil.

Yokogawa et al. (1986) noticed that the apparent elongation of the vitreous was approximately 1.5 times and explained it due to the difference of the sound velocity between the not treated vitreous and silicone-oil.

Torii et al. (1987) mentioned that axial length, especially vitreous length displayed in ultrasonography, was longer than its true length in eyes after silicone oil injection

Therefore it could be easily understood that the axial length of the silicone-oil injected eyes should be given not as measured but using the corrected value of sound velocity of silicone-oil for the vitreous.

The sound velocity of silicone-oil was reported by several.

Verbeek et al. (1981) reported that the sound velocity of silicone-oil was 982 ± 1 m/s at 35 °C, while Clemens et al. (1984) measured the sound velocity of silicone-oil at 20 °C to be 1,010 m/s.

Apparently, the sound velocity of the silicone-oil in clinical cases is not constant. Therefore we measured the sound velocity of the silicone-oil actually used in our cases. The calculated value of the silicone-oil using the specially designed chamber was 964 m/s at 37 °C. It was almost two thirds of the velocity of saline solution and coincided with the above results reported by others. The axial length in the silicone-oil injected eyes should be calculated on the base of the corrected sound velocity of silicone-oil.

68

Acknowledgement

This study was supported in part by a grant-in-aid for scientific research (01570978) from the Japanese Ministry of Education.

References

Araki, M. Studies on reflective elements of human eye by ultrasonic wave, (1st report) accuracy of the measurement of ocular axial length by ultrasonic echography, Rinsho Ganka 1961;15:111–119.

Clemens, S. and Kroll, P. Ultrasonic findings after treatment of retinal detachment by intravitreal silicone instillation. Am. J. Ophthalmol. 1984;98:369–373.

Komatsu, A., Ohhashi, K., Iguchi, T. and Kogakura, H. Experimental study of ultrasonic image display, Folia Ophthalmol. Jpn. 1985;36:1770–1777.

Torii, H., Chihara, E. and Sawada, A. Echographic images of the eye after silicone injection and its removal. First Congress of Asian Federation of Societies for Ultrasound in Medicine and Biology, Tokyo June 22–25, 1987.

Verbeek, A.M., Bayer, A.L. and Thijssen, J.M. Echographic diagnosis after intro-ocular silicone oil injection, in J.M. Thijssen and A.M. Verbeek (eds.), Docum. Ophthalmol. Proc. Series, Vol. 29, Dr. W. Junk Publishers, The Hague, 1981, pp. 59–66.

Yokogawa, Y., Usukura, H. and Tanabe, J. Ultrasonography of silicone oil injected into the vitreous, Jpn. Rev. Clin. Ophthalmol. 1986;80:1251–1255.

Department of Ophthalmology
Miyazaki Medical College
5200 Kihara
Kiyotake, Miyazaki 889-16
Japan

2.6 The Ratio Axial Eye Length/Corneal Curvature Radius and IOL Calculation

HANS C. FLEDELIUS and MARIANNE FICH

(Central Hospital, Hillerød, Denmark)

Abstract. Before changing to the Catrefract calculation program for intraocular lens prediction after cataract surgery we took guidance from combined use of the Binkhorst and the SRK2 formulas. In a period with frequent discrepancies between the two we analysed a good fit and a poor fit sample, each counting 30 subjects. Oculometric 'harmony' between axial length and corneal curvature radius was the main feature of the good fit group, as given by AL:Crad ratios of 2.8–3.05. All poor fit eyes were outside this range, predominantly to the high side. It seems as if conventional prediction formulas cannot safely foresee refractive outcome in eyes with a correlation between AL and Crad away from near-to-norm. Subsequently we examined a larger sample ($n = 598$). Low ratios (<2.8) were found in 6%, high ratios (>3.05) in 25%. It still remains to be proven whether a skew ratio should be regarded an extra parameter, of its own right, to be considered in IOL prediction, at least in selected patients.

Key words: Intraocular lens prediction, Binkhorst, SRK2, Catrefract, cataract surgery, ultrasound oculometry, keratometry, axial eye length, ratio axial length, corneal curvature radius

Introduction

In a previous follow-up study after cataract surgery with anterior chamber intraocular lens (IOL) insertion visual and refractive results were analysed (Fledelius *et al.* 1987). Adding an evaluation of SRK-formula IOL predictions and comparing with those obtained from our basic choice till then, the Binkhorst formula, subsequently we included both formulas as routine in our councelling before surgery. When SRK 2 appeared we changed to the updated version.

The usual guidance from a fair fit between prediction results was challenged during part of 1989. We suddenly experienced an accumulation of patients where predictions differed markedly. An analysis was initiated with

J.M. Thijssen, H.C. Fledelius and S. Tane (eds.), Ultrasonography in Ophthalmology 14, 69–74.
© 1995 *Kluwer Academic Publishers, Dordrecht.*

the aim of possibly detecting oculometric features likely to cause difficulty regarding safe choice of IOL dioptric power.

The present study has two parts:

(a) A comparison of oculometric parameters in two groups of cataract patients, one with a good fit (GF) and one with poor fit (PF) between the above-mentioned prediction methods (Fich and Fledelius 1991).

(b) Subsequently, the trends of the above study have been elaborated epidemiologically in a larger sample of cataract patients, with emphasis on what we originally labelled as 'oculometric disharmony'. This designation was chosen for skew values of the ratio between axial eye length and corneal curvature radius (AL:Crad).

Material and Methods

The comparison between good fit and poor fit patients comprised groups with 30 subjects in each. The criteria were
(a) only one posterior chamber IOL type (the biconvex Rayner 2 Superflex; manufacturers' A-constant 118.5, the corresponding standard value for post-operative IOL position being 4.5 mm behind corneal vertex),
and (b) a discrepancy between Binkhorst and SRK emmetropia predictions of less than 1 D and above 1.6 D, respectively.

Consecutive patients during part of 1989 fulfilling the criteria made up the samples. All had extracapsular cataract surgery. Age ranged from 20 to 90 years; median age was 76 and 77 years in the two groups.

In the GF group prediction differences grouped around zero.

Originally, the PF group had one more case. Differing from the rest of the group by having a plus sign when subtracting the individual SRK emmetropia prediction from that obtained by the Binkhorst formula, it was omitted from the analysis due to its skewing effects, on range values, statistical calculations etc. Otherwise, in the poor-fit group all differences had a negative sign (−4.11 to −1.6 D).

Supplementary study: Now routinely employing the Danish developed Catrefract IOL prediction program (Olsen et al. 1991) we recently performed an 'epidemiological' analysis based on the oculometry parameters kept in the database of the programme. The investigation comprised 598 consecutive cataract patients from 1991–92, all with intended ECCE surgery, but with various IOL brands inserted. The aim was to describe the distribution of the AL:Crad ratios in an unselected population of cataract patients, and in particular to identify those with a – probably – higher risk of IOL prediction failure, as suggested from the results of the initial good/poor-fit study (a).

Results

The main results of the primary study (a) are condensed in Fig. 1 showing the ranges of AL and Crad measurements and of the ratio between the two

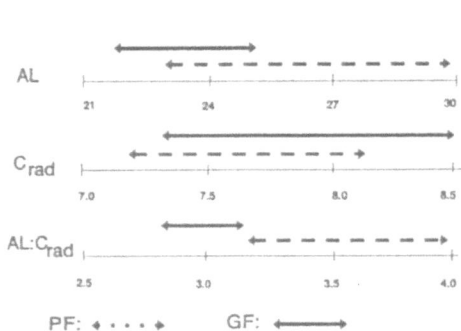

Figure 1 Ranges are shown for axial length, corneal curvature radius, and the ratio AL - Crad in the good fit and the poor fit sample, *cf* text

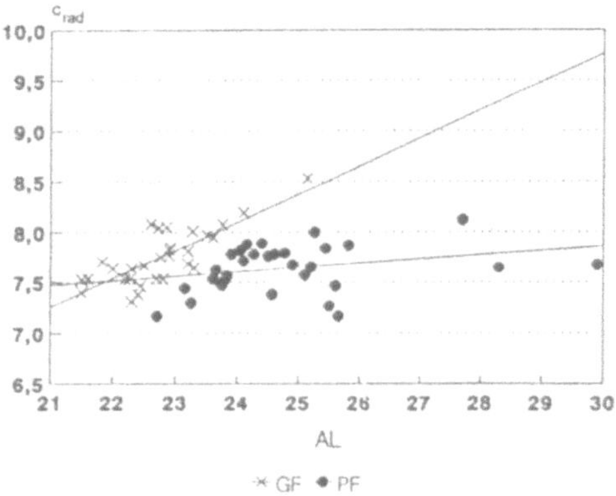

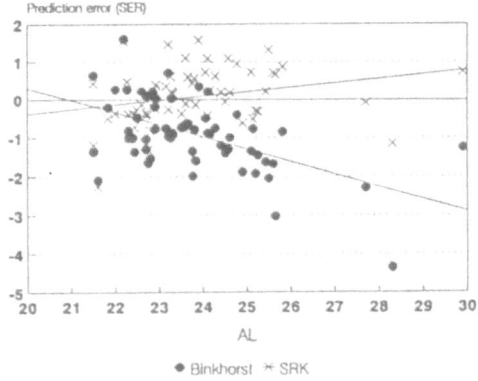

Figure 2 The association between axial length and corneal curvature radius in the two samples (good fit and poor fit) shown by scattergrams and regression lines

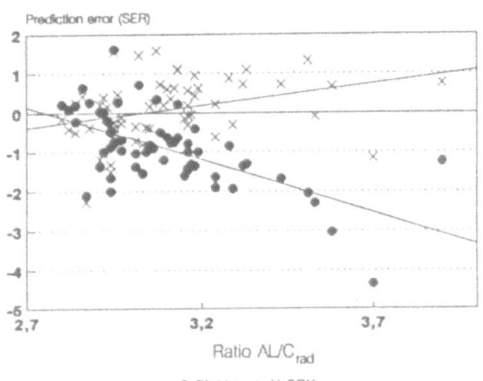

Figure 3 The association between prediction error (in D , spherical equivalent), by Binkhorst and SRK2 and axial length measurements, with all 60 subjects pooled (GF + PF)

Figure 4 As Fig 3, except AL Crad ratio on x-axis

parameters (AL:Crad, bottom). While the two separate parameters showed a certain overlapping, there was full separation between good fit and poor fit groups considering the combined parameter, the ratio.

Table 1 gives the figures in more detail. The median values of the three parameters at top can be added: AL 22.7 mm, Crad 7.69 mm, and AL:Crad ratio 2.94 in the group with a good fit between emmetropia predictions by

Table 1. Mean values and (SD), and ranges, in the two groups under comparison, of the parameters under study

	Good fit n = 30	Poor fit n = 30
Axial length (mm)	22.8 (0.79) 21.5–25.1	24.9 (1.54) 22.7–29.9
Crad (mm)	7.75 (0.28) 7.31–8.53	7.66 (0.25) 7.17–8.12
AL:Crad	2.94 (0.07) 2.80–3.05	3.26 (0.23) 3.06–3.90
Binkh. minus SRK2 predict value (D)	−0.29 (0.52) −1.0 to 0.8	−2.24 (0.68) −4.1 to -1.61
Binkhorst prediction error (D)	−0.55 (0.85) −2.1 to 1.61	−1.29 (0.91) −4.4 to 0.35
SRK2 prediction error (D)	−0.28 (0.78) −2.3 to 1.6	0.43 (0.60) −1.2 to 1.57

Table 2. Correlation between prediction error by Binkhorst and SRK2 and axial length, corneal curvature radius, and the ratio AL:Crad, as given by the Spearman correlation coefficient (rS) calculated on the pooled group (GF + PF), $n = 60$)

	Binkhorst prediction error	SRK2 prediction error
Axial length	−0.447	0.358
Crad	0.246 (n.s.)	−0.154 (n.s.)
AL:Crad ratio	−0.546	0.448

the two methods, and 24.5 mm, 7.64 mm, and 3.18, respectively, in those with a poor fit.

Fig. 2 shows the regression lines calculated between AL and Crad, with the former as the independent parameter. The good fit group showed a strong correlation, as given by an rS-value of 0.74 ($y = 0.279X + 1.398$). In contrast, the poor fit group regression line was almost horizontal, and with a correlation coefficient (rS) of only 0.305.

Figs. 3 and 4 roughly show the eventual prediction errors by Binkhorst and SRK2 over the full oculometric distribution, i.e. with the two samples, each of 30 subjects, combined to one.

In Table 2, again after pooling all 60 patients, the correlation values are given concerning the actual prediction errors by the two methods.

Finally, Fig. 5 depicts the distribution of AL and Crad values in the subsequent study comprising 598 subjects. Contrary to the very selected sampling in the above investigation (a) it is considered epidemiologically valid for a cataract population. Axial lengths showed a range of 20.3–

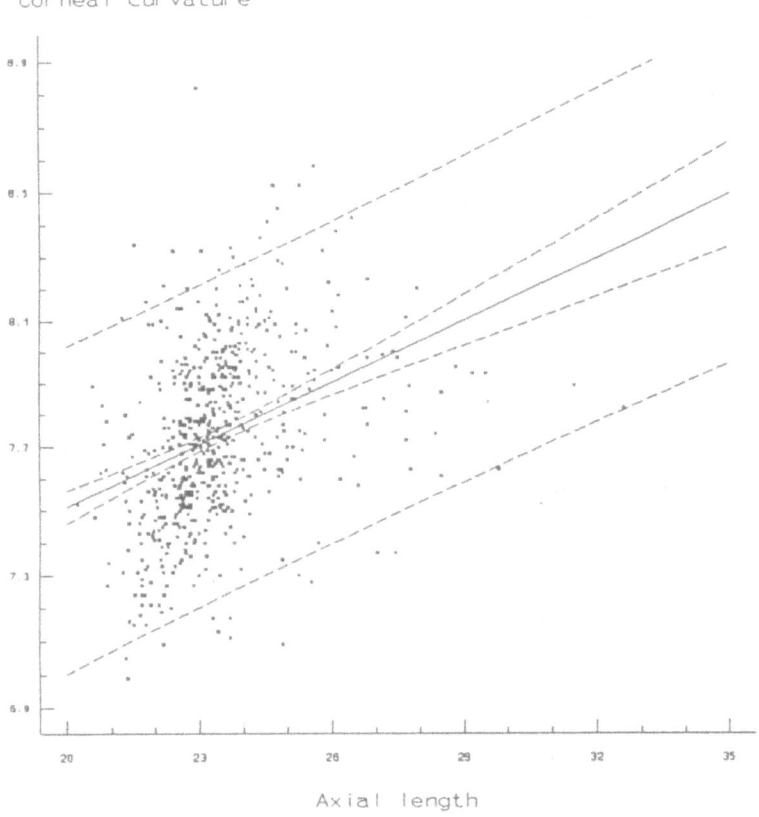

Corneal curvature

Axial length

Figure 5. Oculometric presentation of an unselected cataract population (*n* = 598, *cf.* text), given by AL and Crad values. Regression line and ±2 SD are shown.

32.6 mm, mean value and (SD) 23.44 (1.49); corneal curvature radius 6.99–8.82 mm, mean values and (SD) 7.73 (0.27). The parametric correlation coefficient between AL and Crad was 0.35. The AL:Crad ratio ranged from 2.58 to 4.19, mean value and (SD) 3.03 (0.18). With reference to the near-to-norm range of 2.8–3.05, as given by the primary study, in the large sample 6% had ratios below 2.8 and 25% above 3.05.

Discussion

The paper having been prepared for the 1991 Copenhagen WFUMB/SIDUO sessions (Fich and Fledelius) and subsequently published (1993) only a short discussion will be presented here.

It is usually forwarded that IOL prediction is accurate in the average size eye, and that problems are met especially in the very short and the very long eyes. As judged from the present investigation primarily this statement might be based on subgroups of short and long eyes where the orderly correlation between AL and Crad is absent (labelled as oculometric disharmony in our initial presentation). In particular, this was met in long eyes without compensatory correlational flattening of corneal curvature, but theoretically a short eye with a non-steep cornea is another possibility. In the primary poor fit group one such eye occurred showing an AL-Crad ratio of 2.62.

This atypical eye was excluded from calculations (cf. Material) but the subsequent analysis (b) of a larger cataract sample showed that the actual combination, to the low side, of main optical components is not infrequent. About 6% had an AL:Crad ration below the lower value of the good fit group (range 2.8–3.05). The other tail, above 3.05, was found in about 25%.

So far, the independent importance of the ratio has been demonstrated only the one way round. However, the importance was suggested also in a previous study, with a different approach, from the same clinic (Fledelius *et al.* 1987).

The importance the other way round remains to be analysed. Will specific IOL prediction features be disclosed when doing follow-up on samples comprising subjects with skew oculometric ratios? At the moment we are doing a pilot study to elucidate the item, acknowledging that our primary observation might be accidental.

As conclusion: When analysing refractive outcome after IOL surgery in the future it is recommended to include the AL:Crad ratio as an extra parameter, even though AL and Crad as separate parameters appear weighted duly already. An empirical correction factor might result herefrom, to indicate a skew ratio of AL:Crad as a warning, or a guide, to the cataract surgeon prior to selecting IOL power for the individual patient.

References

Fledelius, H.C., Alsbirk, P.H. and Goldschmidt, E. Intraocular lens calculation. An evaluation of Binkhorst and SRK estimates, Acta Ophthalmol. (Copenh) 1987;65:579–84.

Olsen, T.K., Thim, K. and Corydon, L. Accuracy of the newer generation intraocular lens power calculation formulas in long and short eyes. J. Cataract Refract. Surg. 1991;17:187–93.

Fich, M. and Fledelius, H.C. Intraocular lens prediction and skew ratio between axial length and corneal curvature radius. Paper prepared for the Copenhagen 1991 WFUMB/SIDUO conference. Revised for Acta Ophthalmol. (Copenh) 1993;71:408–10.

Rigshospitalet, University Eye Clinic E2061
Blegdamsvej 9
DK-2100 Copenhagen Ø, Denmark

2.7. Intraindividual Difference of Calculated Lens Power in Patients with Different Degrees of Anisometropia and Clear Lens

DANIELE DORO, LORETTA BERGAMO, ENRICO
MONTOVANI and ELISABETTA MILIZIA

(Padua, Italy)

Abstract. Cycloplegic retinoscopy and echobiometry was performed in 55 subjects with anisometropia (up to 14 D), all with clear media. Lens powers (as calculated by Holladay's IOL-formula; range 15.8–23.9 D) contributed to refractive side difference only by anisometropia >3 D. The other way round: the anisometropia actually present could be estimated with fair precision from keratometry + axial length differences, a finding of possible importance when clinically assessing eyes with opaque media.

Key words: Anisometropia, lens power, intraindividual difference, axial length measurement, keratometry, retinoscopy.

Introduction

According to Gullstrand's normal eye, lens power is 20.5 D [6]. In the following literature mean lens power in diopters calculated from ultrasound measured axial length and keratometry is reported 23.72 D [4], 22.27 ± 2.15 D [1] and 18.00 D [5]. More precisely, Gordon *et al.* [5] found that lens power ranges from 16.7 to 21.3 D in adult eyes without statistically significant intraindividual difference, according to their SRK I modified regression formula used for intraocular lens power calculation [2].

Actually the interindividual variability of lens power is a limiting factor for the calculation of the total refraction of an eye from axial length and corneal power measurements [3].

The aims of our study were (1) to verify intraindividual difference of calculated lens power in patients with varying degree of anisometropia and clear media and (2) to check the ability of ultrasonic biometry combined with keratometry in predicting anisometropia.

Patients and Methods

We enrolled 55 patients (mean age 29 years; range 10–52 years); inclusion criteria were absence of ocular or systemic disease, clear media, corrected or natural visual acuity greater than 20/30, corneal astigmatism less than 2.0 D.

Refraction was obtained by cycloplegic (Tropicamide 0.5% and Phenyl-

J.M. Thijssen, H.C. Fledelius and S. Tane (eds.), Ultrasonography in Ophthalmology 14, 75–79.
© *1995 Kluwer Academic Publishers, Dordrecht.*

Refraction was obtained by cycloplegic (Tropicamide 0.5% and Phenyl-ephrine 10% twice in five minutes) streak retinoscopy, confirmed by subjec-tive distance reading. Mean K readings were obtained with a calibrated Haag Streit keratometer. Axial length measurements were performed with a 10 MHz contact water-filled probe (Coopervision Ultrascan Digital IV B^{TM}) and for each eye at least two axial length measurements within ±0.1 mm difference were averaged.

To simplify the calculation of lens power, we used Holladay's formula [7] with an arbitrary 0.37 mm surgeon's factor (corresponding to 116.5 SRK A-constant); intraocular lens power needed to restore the cycloplegic refrac-tion was considered equal to the cristalline (lens) power. Lens power in eyes with different refraction (±1 D; between −1 and −5.5 D; between +1 and +7 D) was studied.

Patients were divided into three groups with cycloplegic anisometropia: (a) smaller than 1 D, (b) between 1 and 3 D and (c) greater than 3 D. Intraindividual lens power difference in the three groups and between groups was respectively studied by means of paired t-test (difference from average equal to 0 D) and Mann-Whitney test.

Conversely, assuming lens power equal in the two eyes, as 1 mm of axial length difference has been reported to correspond to 2.77 D [8], for each patient anisometropia (Delta) was calculated from algebraic addition of axial length (converted into dioptres by a factor 2.77) and mean K-reading differ-ences of the two eyes. The used formula was:

$$\text{Delta} = 2.77 * (AL_{RE} - AL_{LE}) + (K_{RE} - K_{LE})$$

where AL and K indicate axial length and mean K-readings of right ($_{RE}$) and left ($_{LE}$) eye.

For each patient the Delta value was compared to the anisometropia as evaluated with cycloplegic retinoscopy as the "golden standard". Intraindivi-dual difference in the three groups and between groups was studied by means of paired t-test and Mann–Whitney test respectively.

Results

The mean cycloplegic refraction in the 110 eyes was −1.84 ± 3.38 D (range −15 ÷ +7 D); mean axial length was 24.27 ± 1.48 mm (range 20.37 − 29.44 mm); mean keratometry was 42.90 ± 1.35 D (range 38 − 45.25 D). Mean cycloplegic anisometropia in the 55 patients was 1.54 ± 2.48 D (range 0 − 14 D).

In the 110 eyes mean lens power (Holladay's formula) was 19.54 ± 1.56 D (range 15.84 − 23.94 D). Three subgroups were evaluated separately. In 34 eyes with refraction within ±1 D mean lens power was 19.80 ± 1.46 D (range 17.27 − 23.22 D); in 28 eyes with refraction between −1 and −5.5 D mean lens power was 19.59 ± 1.49 (range 15.84 − 22.91 D); in 6 eyes with refraction between +1 and +7 D mean lens power was 19.64 ± 1.28 D

Table 1. Lens power (D) according to Holladay's formula* in all eyes and in subgroups with different cycloplegic refraction

	Mean	t±S.D.	Range
All 110 eyes	19.54	1.56	15.84–23.94
11 eyes (over +1 D)	19.44	1.21	17.55–21.26
37 eyes (±1 D)	19.77	1.41	17.27–23.23
50 eyes (− 1 − −5.5 D)	19.31	1.65	15.84–23.94
12 eyes (over −5.5 D)	19.93	1.93	17.55–22.92

*SF = 0.37 corresponding to SRK A-constant = 116.5.

Table 2. Intraindividual difference of calculated lens power (D) according to Holladay's formula* in subjects with varying degrees of anisometropia

	Mean	±S.D.	Range	p^*
All patients (55)	0.72	0.71	0.01–2.60	0.162 n.s.
(a) Anisometropia <1 D (34)	0.40	0.27	0.01–1.22	0.751 n.s.
(b) Anisometropia 1–3 D (11)	0.84	0.67	0.18–2.50	0.343 n.s.
(c) Anisometropia >3 D (10)	1.77	0.92	0.54–2.61	0.014 sign.
Intergroups Mann-Whitney test:				
(a) vs. (b)	$z = -2.56$		$p = 0.01$	
(a) vs. (c)	$z = -3.61$		$p = 0.0003$	
(b) vs. (c)	$z = -2.27$		$p = 0.023$	

*SF = 0.37 corresponding to SRK A-constant = 116.5.
**Paired t-test against difference equal to 0 D.

(range $17.55 - 20.97$ D). No statistically significant difference was noted between these three groups (Mann–Whitney test) (Table 1).

Mean intraindividual lens power difference in the 55 patients was 0.72 ± 0.71 D (range 0.01–2.60 D) without a statistically significant difference from the assumed average equal to 0 D (paired t-test; $p = 0.162$). In the three groups with different degree of anisometropia, mean intraindividual lens power difference was respectively: 0.40 ± 0.27 D (range $0.01 - 1.22$ D) in the 34 patients with anisometropia smaller than 1 D (group a), 0.84 ± 0.67 D (range $0.18 - 2.5$) in the 11 patients with anisometropia between 1 and 3 D (group b) and 1.77 ± 0.92 (range $0.54 - 2.6$ D) in the 10 patients with anisometropia greater than 3 D (group c). A statistically significant difference from zero D was found only in the group c (paired t-test; $p = 0.014$).

Comparing all three groups, Mann-Whitney test evidenced a statistically significant difference in intraindividual lens power difference: $p = 0.01$ in group a) vs. group b), $p = 0.0003$ in group a) vs. group c) and $p = 0.023$ in group b) vs. group c) (Table 2).

Mean absolute difference in diopters between anisometropia evaluated by cycloplegic retinoscopy (golden standard) and by calculation from echobiometry and keratometry (Delta) in all 55 patients was 0.51 ± 0.5 D (range

Table 3 Absolute difference between anisometropia evaluated with cycloplegic retinoscopy and as calculated from echobiometry and keratometry in patients with varying degrees of anisometropia

	Mean	±S D	Range
All patients (55)	0 51	0 5	0 00–1 92
(a) Anisometropia <1 D (34)	0 29	0 17	0 01–0 63
(b) Anisometropia 1–3 D (11)	0 72	0 59	0 15–1 76
(c) Anisometropia >3 D (10)	1 09	0 65	0 27–1 92
Intergroups Mann-Whitney test			
(a) vs (b)	z = −1 75		p = 0 079 (n s)
(a) vs (c)	z = −3 52		p = <0 001
(b) vs (c)	z = -1 49		p = n s

*Paired t-test against difference equal to 0 D

Table 4 Percentage of cases with different absolute difference between anisometropia evaluated with cycloplegic retinoscopy and echobiometry and keratometry in patients with varying aniso-metropia

	<0 5 D	<1 0 D	<1 5 D	<2 0 D
All patients (55)	69 1%	83 6%	92 7%	100 0%
(a) Anisometropia <1 D (34)	88 2%	100 0%	100 00%	100 00%
(b) Anisometropia 1–3 D (11)	41 7%	66 7%	91 7%	100 00%
(c) Anisometropia >3 D (10)	33 3%	44 4%	65 7%	100 0%

$0 - 1.92$ D). In group a) ($n = 34$) the absolute difference was 0.29 ± 0.17 D, with all cases within 1 D error. In group b) ($n = 11$) the absolute difference was 0.72 ± 0.59 D, with 91.7% of cases within 1.5 D error. In group c) ($n = 10$) the absolute difference was 1.09 ± 0.65 D, with all cases within an error of 2 D.

Mann–Whitney test evidenced a statistically significant difference between golden standard anisometropia and Delta anisometropia only in group a) (anisometropia less than 1 D) vs. group c) (anisometropia greater than 3 D) ($p < 0.001$) (Tables 3 and 4).

Conclusions

Our results enables us to give the following statements:

1. Mean lens power is virtually identical in eyes with different refraction. There is no obvious association with refractive value.
2. Intraindividual difference in lens power increases with increasing aniso-metropia (from average 0.4 D with anisometropia smaller than 1 D to average 1.7 D with anisometropia greater than 3 D) according to Holla-day's formula.
3. Intraindividual lens power difference is statistically significant only when

anisometropia is greater than 3 D. Thus we can confirm the finding of Gordon *et al.* (1985) of no statistically significant intraindividual lens power difference [5] only when anisometropia is below 3 D.

4. Calculation of anisometropia by ultrasonic biometry combined with keratometry (assuming 0 D as the intraindividual difference of lens power) is more reliable if anisometropia is within 1 D than if above 3 D (100% of cases within 1 D vs. 2 D error); however a 0.50 D error must be considered possible even with correct axial length measurement and K-readings [9].

5. The refraction of an eye with opaque media and/or small rigid pupil can be calculated if refraction of the fellow eye, bilateral K-readings and axial lengths are known. The accuracy of the calculation will depend on degree of anisometropia.

6. Obviously our original method of calculating anisometropia is time consuming but may be useful when, for clinical or medico-legal purposes estimation of refraction is required in an eye with hazy media or a small pupil where retinoscopy or autorefractometry cannot be performed.

References

[1] F. Daxecker and C. Marth. Correlation analysis of emmetropic and ametropic eyes. Fortschr. Ophthalmol. 1985;82(1):94–97.

[2] P.B. Donzis, P.R. Kastl, and R.A. Gordon. An intraocular lens formula for short, normal and long eyes. CLAO J. 1985;11:95–98.

[3] D. Doro, P. Borsetto, G. Sato, and L. Carturan. Is ultrasonic biometry associated with keratometry reliable for evaluating refractive errors in eyes with transparent media? In: Ultrasonography in Ophthalmology – 11, J.M. Thijssen (ed.), Kluwer Academic Publ., Dordrecht NL, 1988;321–325.

[4] H. Gernet and H. Ostholt. Augenseitige Optik. Ein neues Gebiet der Klinischen Okulometrie. Ophthalmologica 1973;166:120–143.

[5] R. Gordon and P. Donzis. Refractive Development of the Human Eye. Arch Ophthal. 1985;103:785–789.

[6] A. Gullstrand. Handbuch der physiologischen Optik. 3. Aufl, L Voss, Hamburg Leipzig 1909;1:295–296,300–301.

[7] J.T. Holladay, K.H. Musgrove, T.C. Praeger, J.W. Lewis, T.Y. Chandler, and R.S. Ruitz.A three-part system for refining intraocular lens power calculation. J Cataract Refract. Surg. 1988;14:17–24.

[8] Y. Le Grand. Optique physiologique. Xeme ed., Edition de la Revue d'Optique, Paris, 1952.

[9] J.R. McEwan, R.K. Massengill, and S.D. Friedel. Effect of keratometer and axial length measurement errors on primary implant power calculation. J. Cataract Refract. Surg. 16(1):61–70.

Clinica Oculistica
Università di Padova
Via Giustiniani 2
I35128 Padova
Italy

2.8. Changes in the Thickness of the Lens During Imagination: An Echographic Study

G. IACCARINO,** G. CENNAMO,* N. ROSA,*
G. ALFIERI,*** A. PASQUARIELLO* and V. RUGGIERI***

(*Eye Department, II University Hospital, Naples, **Eye Department,
I University Hospital, Naples, ***Clinical Psychophysiology Dept,
University "La Sapienza", Rome, Italy)

Abstract. Several authors have pointed out a correlation between perception and imagination. In particular some authors suggested that during imagination not only the brain, but also other structures are involved. It is possible that the eye too is involved in this process. For this reason we decided to study the role of the lens during the mental process of imagination: we examined with standardized echography the lenses of 10 emmetropic subjects. The lenses were measured by ultrasound to verify changes in thickness when some tests were submitted to the patients.

Key words: Lens thickness, imagination, standardized echography.

Introduction

Neuropsychologists have suggested a correlation between perception and imagination [1–3, 5].

Our hypothesis is that even the most peripheral visual components are involved during imagination. Storey and Rabie [6] measured a thickening of the lens during accomodation.

On this background we tried to establish if there is any correlation between imagination of objects located close to the patient or far away, and changes in the thickness of the lens.

Material and Methods

To test this hypothesis we performed an echobiometric evaluation of the lens in 10 patients to detect any changes during the mental imagination of objects located close to or far from the patient. We measured the lens thickness with standardized A Scan utilizing the immersion scleral shells with Mini-A by Biophysic Medical according to K.C. Ossoinig [4].

All the patients were emmetropic with an age ranging from 20 to 30 years.

Before performing the test we explained the method to the patients, without explaining the purpose of this test.

J M Thijssen, H C Fledelius and S Tane (eds) Ultrasonography in Ophthalmology 14 80–82

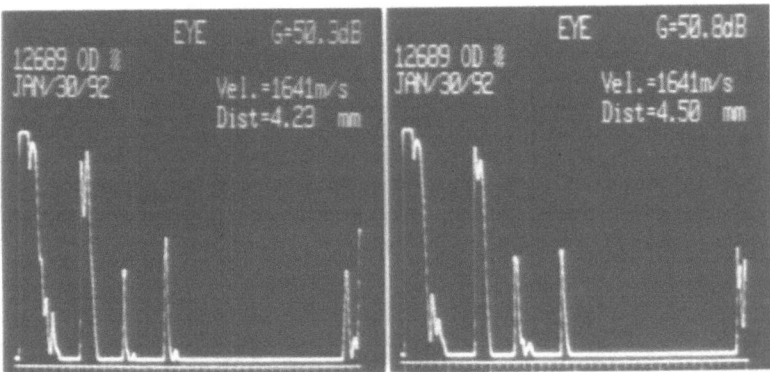

Figure 1. Lens thickness of a patient during the imagination of an object located far away (e.g. a boat on the horizon), left, and of the same patient during the imagination of reading a book, right.

Each patient, in supine position, received a topical anesthesia and the immersion scleral shell was inserted between the lids and filled with saline solution. The other eye was occluded. After reaching a state of relaxation, the first measurement was performed.

Then the following imaginative stimuli were explained to the subject:

(1) Imagine an object located far away (e.g. a boat on the horizon).

(2) Imagine the same object coming close to you.

(3) Imagine the same object moving back towards the horizon.

(4) Imagine to read a book and reading a specific word.

The patient was instructed to raise his hand when he found that the mental image was clear and in that moment we performed the measurement of the lens (Fig. 1)

After this imaginative phase we started the perceptive phase: we took the patch from the other eye and the patient had to visualize a word written on a piece of paper 15 cm from the eye (near perception). Subsequently the patient was asked to look at a small object located on the ceiling, 4 meters from the patient (far perception).

The measurements were performed on the non fixing eye.

Results

The results are shown in Table 1.

We found a significant difference in the lens thickness ($p < 0.02$) during the imagination of objects located far away compared to close to the patient, mainly in the left eye.

Table 1. In the horizontal row the different sizes of the lens during the different phases of imagination are displayed (A–E), compared to real perception in the far and near vision situation (F and G). A = measurements of the lens during the relaxing phase. B = measurements of the lens during the imagination of an object located far away (e.g. a boat on the horizon). C = measurements of the lens during the imagination of the same object coming close to the patient. D = measurements of the lens during the imagination of the same object moving back towards the horizon. E = measurements of the lens during the imagination of reading a book and reading a specific word. F = measurements of the lens during far perception. G = measurements of the lens during near perception.

	Right eye							Left eye						
	A	B	C	D	E	F	G	A	B	C	D	E	F	G
1	4.27	4.14	4.27	4.11	4.36	4.33	3.97	4.42	4.27	4.23	4.20	4.30	4.50	4.06
2	3.94	3.81	3.97	3.91	4.00	3.97	3.81	3.94	4.14	4.23	4.00	4.33	4.20	4.07
3	4.00	4.03	4.11	4.06	4.14	4.42	4.06	4.11	4.17	4.39	4.27	4.17	4.23	4.20
4	3.77	3.94	3.87	3.87	4.00	4.30	3.77	4.00	4.04	4.04	3.97	4.04	4.63	3.77
5	3.15	3.45	3.25	3.35	3.45	3.94	3.25	3.64	3.41	3.58	3.41	3.48	4.10	3.51
6	3.94	4.50	4.20	3.91	4.23	4.07	4.04	4.23	4.17	4.27	4.14	4.23	4.33	4.10
7	4.00	3.77	3.91	3.94	4.07	4.14	3.91	3.77	4.00	4.04	4.00	4.10	4.46	3.77
8	3.49	3.44	3.51	3.60	3.60	3.60	3.23	3.23	3.32	3.58	3.40	3.61	3.64	3.16
9	3.70	3.79	3.82	3.82	3.90	3.55	3.39	3.70	3.74	3.87	3.73	3.94	3.60	3.33
10	4.40	4.14	4.23	4.10	4.50	4.43	4.17	4.20	4.20	4.27	4.07	4.27	4.50	4.07

Discussion

Our data suggest the presence of accommodation during imagination ($p < 0.05$).

The accommodation is more evident in the left eye. This finding could be explained by the eye dominance. The other explanation could be that the test has always been performed first on the right eye and then on the left eye. In this way the subject was more active in imagination with better results.

References

[1] J.S. Antrobus, J.S. Antrobus and J.L. Singer. Eye movement accompanying daydreaming, visual imagery and thought suppression. J. of Abnormal and Social Psychology. 1964;69(3):244–252.
[2] M.J. Farah. The neurological basis of mental imagery: a componential analysis. Cognition 1984;18:245–277.
[3] M.J. Farah. Is visual imagery really visual, overlooked evidence from neuropsychology. Psychological Review 1988;95(3):307–317.
[4] K.C. Ossoinig. Standardized echography: basic principles, clinical applications and results. Int. Ophth. Clin. 1979;19(4).
[5] V. Ruggieri. On the hypothesized physiological correspondence between perceptual and imagery processes. Perceptual and Motor Skills. 1991;73:827–830.
[6] J.K. Storey and E.P. Rebie. Biometry of the eye during accomodation. In J.S. Hilmann and M.M. Le May (eds.), Ophthalm. Ultrasonography. Dr. W. Junk Publ. 1983, 295–301.

2.9 A Biomechanical Model for the Mechanism of Accommodation

A.P.A. BEERS and G.L. VAN DER HEIJDE

(*Amsterdam, The Netherlands*)

Abstract. The changes in lens thickness during far-to-near and near-to-far accommodation were measured in 17 healthy young subjects using continuous ultrasonographic biometry. With the use of a biomechanical model information about the visco-elastic properties of the elements of the accommodative mechanism can be obtained.

Key words: Ultrasonography, accommodation, presbyopia, biomechanics, model.

Introduction

Information about the biomechanical properties of the tissues involved in accommodation is important to understand the physiology of accommodation and the changes that cause, for example, presbyopia.

Knowledge on this subject in humans originates mainly from in vitro studies and is limited to the elasticity of these tissues [1–5].

Using continuous ultrasonographic biometry we are able to measure the change in axial lens thickness during accommodation. The dynamics of the response measured in this way enclose information about the elastic as well as the viscous properties of the elements of the mechanism of accommodation. With the use of a biomechanical model this information can be extracted.

Material and Methods

Accommodation is stimulated in one eye by a blur stimulus and measured in the fellow eye by continuous biometry.

The subject is in supine position and two targets are positioned at different distances from the fixating eye. One target is illuminated by a beam of light that is projected via a mirror. In a darkened room the subject only sees the illuminated target. A small rotational movement of less than 5 ms duration by the mirror changes the direction of the beam of light to the other target.

J.M. Thijssen, H.C. Fledelius and S. Tane (eds.), Ultrasonography in Ophthalmology 14, 83–88.
© 1995 *Kluwer Academic Publishers, Dordrecht.*

Thus the fixating eye suddenly sees a blurred target. An eye movement does not have to be made because the fixating eye is aligned with the two targets.

The accommodation response is recorded from the fellow eye by A-scan ultrasonography [6]. To enable undisturbed measurements of accommodation during miosis and vergence eye movements a small 10 MHz transducer with a narrow beam (3 mm) is used, and is mounted in a cup that is fixed on the limbal conjunctiva by suction through 25 small holes in the rim of the cup.

The ultrasound beam is reflected by the cornea, the anterior and posterior surfaces of the lens and the retina. After a time delay following the moment that the anterior lens echo exceeds a threshold level, the transit time is linearly transformed to a voltage until the posterior lens echo exceeds a threshold level. The signal is 50 Hz low pass analog filtered and sampled at 100 Hz by a personal computer with 12 bit A/D conversion. The data are then 8 Hz low pass digitally filtered and calibrated using 1640 m/s as the velocity of sound in the lens. The accuracy of the measurements is $\pm 2 \mu m$ [7].

Experiments were performed on 17 healthy subjects, aged 18–25 years, with a visual acuity of 1.0 or better in both eyes. The stimulus was presented in the far-to-near (FN) direction, followed by the same stimulus in the near-to-far (NF) direction after a random period of time of ± 5 sec. This was repeated 5 times.

A simple mechanical model of the accommodative mechanism was designed to describe the responses (Fig. 1). The model is based on the anatomy and physiology of the accommodative mechanism and on the resemblance of the responses to the output of a first order system. The accommodative mechanism consists of four passive elements: the choroid, the peripheral and axial zonules and the lens, and an active element: the ciliary muscle. The elastic choroid and zonules are each replaced by a spring. The lens is replaced by a spring that represents the capsule, and a parallel dashpot that represents the damping action of cytoplasm movement in the lens fibres during accommodation. Because the ciliary muscle behaves like a twitch skeletal muscle with tetanization [8], it is assumed that its action is fast compared to the changes of the lens. Thus it can be replaced by a force that acts at the axial end of the peripheral zonule and changes the position of the ciliary ring with a step. The angles between the acting forces are small and are ignored.

In this model the change in lens equatorial radius exhibits first order dynamics. To be able to compare the model with the experimental data, the measured changes in axial lens thickness are transformed to relative changes in equatorial radius. For this purpose it is assumed that the lens can be described by two half ellipsoids connected in the frontal plane through the equator, and that lens volume remains constant during accommodation. With this assumption the relative change in equatorial lens radius will be proportional to the square root of the relative change in axial lens thickness.

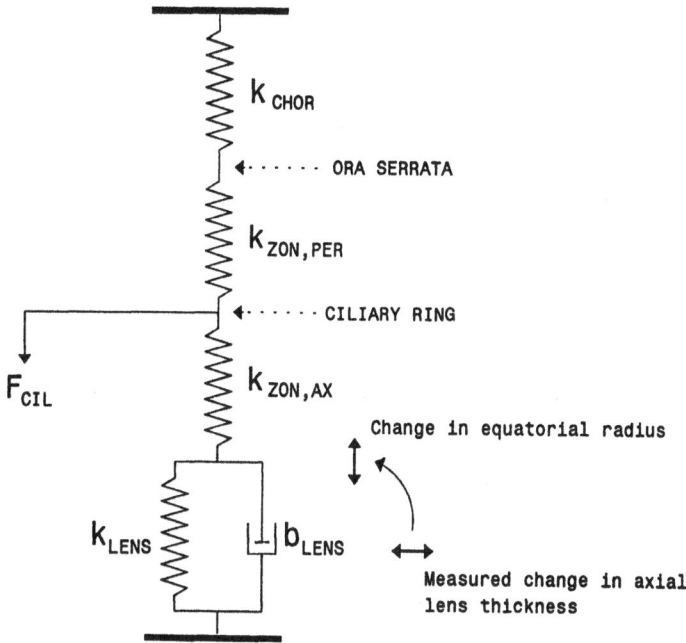

Figure 1. Mechanical model. Spring constants are indicated by k, damping coefficient by b and ciliary muscle force by F_{CIL}.

All responses were fitted separately with this first order model and step input. Fitting was done by a nonlinear regression procedure that obtains least squares estimates of three parameters using the Marquardt search algorithm. The three parameters were: response latency, time constant and amplitude. Goodness-of-fit was evaluated by the correlation coefficient between response and model and by the ratio of the residual sum of squares to response amplitude.

Results

Fig. 2 shows the accommodation responses in FN and NF directions. Fig. 3 gives examples of the responses and their fits using the model. Table 1 gives for each subject the average time constant estimates and goodness-of-fit parameters for FN and NF accommodation.

The data show, firstly, that the accommodation responses can be accurately described by the step response of the first order model, except for the beginning of the NF response (see Fig. 3). Secondly they show that the NF response is completed faster than the FN response.

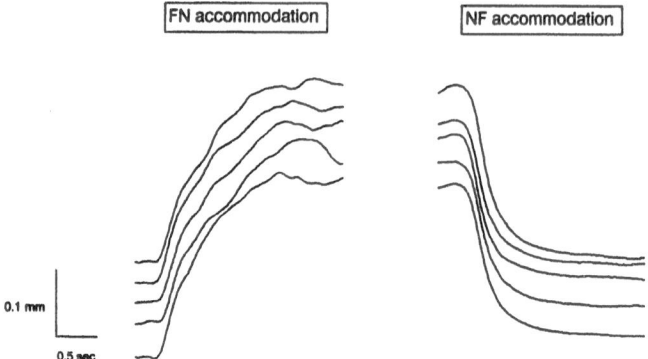

Figure 2. Accommodation responses. Stimulus is presented at $t = 0$ sec. Traces represent the measured change in axial lens thickness.

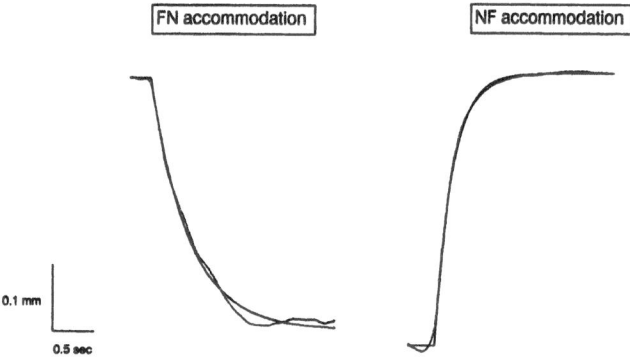

Figure 3. Fitting the first order model. Dotted line represents the response transformed to change in equatorial lens radius. Solid line represents the fitted model.

Discussion

Apparently FN and NF accommodation are not simply the same processes in opposite directions. This can be expected from what we know about the physiology of accommodation and the different dynamics of ciliary muscle contraction and relaxation.

During FN accommodation the ciliary muscle contracts, thus pulling on the peripheral zonules and choroid and moving the ciliary ring inward. Because ciliary muscle contraction is fast compared to the whole response, the ciliary ring will be moved almost like a step to its new position. This allows the lens to round up as result of the molding force of the lens capsule. During NF accommodation the ciliary muscle relaxes. This allows the peripheral zonule and choroid to pull at the axial zonule and the lens equator to flatten the lens.

Table 1. Average time constant estimates (Tau) in ms. R^2 is the squared correlation coefficient; $Rel\chi^2$ is the ratio of the residual sum of squares to response amplitude.

Subject	FN accommodation			NF accommodation		
	Tau FN	R^2	$Rel\chi^2$	Tau NF	R^2	$Rel\chi^2$
1	166	0.962	0.203	264	0.995	0.019
2	268	0.976	0.118	154	0.990	0.055
3	343	0.988	0.050	160	0.990	0.050
4	784	0.999	0.008	211	0.994	0.041
5	574	0.987	0.046	171	0.994	0.030
6	574	0.985	0.075	157	0.990	0.067
7	621	0.997	0.013	337	0.989	0.054
8	260	0.919	0.221	207	0.978	0.065
9	381	0.996	0.020	250	0.998	0.015
10	563	0.991	0.040	214	0.993	0.036
11	315	0.991	0.040	158	0.992	0.047
12	481	0.989	0.064	217	0.996	0.025
13	548	0.995	0.026	215	0.995	0.031
14	310	0.998	0.015	251	0.995	0.032
15	479	0.995	0.023	122	0.987	0.059
16	299	0.990	0.058	200	0.998	0.015
17	680	0.999	0.004	209	0.998	0.010

Thus, even though all elements of the accommodative mechanism must play a role in the total response, it is still possible to distinguish dominance of one or more elements at certain time intervals and in different directions of the response.

Firstly ciliary muscle dynamics are fast compared to the whole accommodation response and therefore dominate only the beginning of the response. The rest of the response is dominated by the passive elements: choroid, zonules and lens. Because ciliary muscle contraction is faster than relaxation, the beginning of the FN response is abrupt, while the beginning of the NF response is more gradual.

Secondly, during FN accommodation the lens behaves almost like a free body, and consequently the FN response is dominated by the properties of the lens. Figure 4 shows the simplified mechanical model for FN accommodation.

Thirdly during NF accommodation the lens as well as the zonules and choroid play a substantial role (Fig. 4, right). The influence of the zonule and choroid spring constants results in a smaller time constant than that of FN accommodation and explains why NF accommodation is completed faster.

We conclude that, with the use of continuous ultrasonography and the mechanical models presented, information about the visco-elastic properties of the lens, zonules and choroid can be obtained. This information is however mainly 'relative', in the sense that changes in the visco-elastic pro-

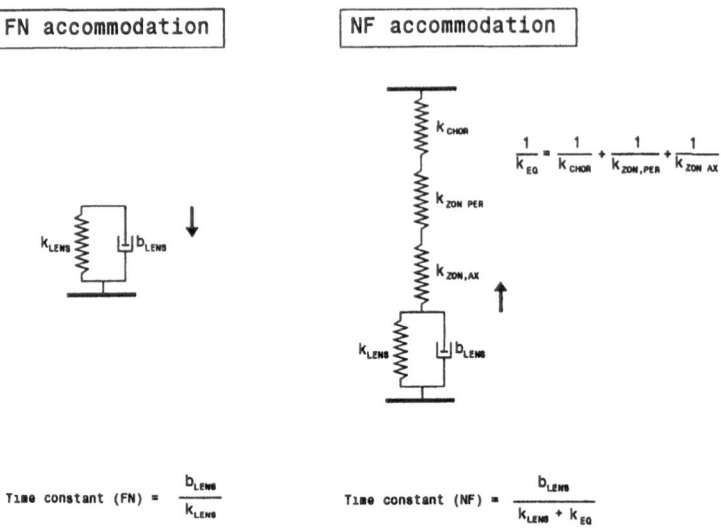

Figure 4 Passive elements determining the main part of the accommodation response Arrows indicate the direction of change of the lens equator, k = spring constant and b = damping coefficient The time constants of the change in equatorial radius are given for FN (left) and NF accommodation (right)

perties of the elements with respect to each other can be evaluated. This may be especially helpful in determining the changes that give rise to presbyopia when the accommodation dynamics in different age groups are analyzed.

References

[1] R F Fisher Elastic constants of the human lens capsule J Physiol 1969,201 1–19

[2] R F Fisher The elastic constants of the human lens J Physiol 1971,212 147–180

[3] R F Fisher Presbyopia and the changes with age in the human crystalline lens J Physiol 1973,228 765–779

[4] R F Fisher The ciliary body in accommodation Trans Ophthalmol Soc UK 1986,105 208–219

[5] G W H M Van Alphen and W P Graebel Elasticity of tissues involved in accommodation Vision Res 1991,31(7/8) 1417–1438

[6] F R De Vries, G L Van der Heijde and H G Goovaerts System for continuous high-resolution measurement of distances in the eye J Biomed Eng 1987,9 32–37

[7] G L Van der Heijde and J Weber Accommodation used to determine ultrasound velocity in the human lens Optom Vis Sci 1989,66(12) 830–833

[8] R Suzuki Neuronal influence on the mechanical activity of the ciliary muscle Br J Pharmacol 1983,78 591–597

Department of Medical Physics,
Free University,
Van der Boechorststraat 7, 1081 BT Amsterdam,
The Netherlands

2.10 Biometry with Mini A-Scan Instrument

W. HAUFF and A. KUCHAR
(*Vienna, Austria*)

Abstract. A description is given of the new Mini A scan equipment (Biophysic/Alcon). For axial length measurement an accuracy of 0.1 mm is achievable. The echo peaks can be frozen on the screen and intraocular distances are displayed on the screen. With the contact method a two gates measurement is performed. By the immersion technique all five relevant echo peaks are captured by electronical gates automatically. In combination with a keyboard intraocular lens power can be calculated directly on the screen of the Mini A instrument. Advantages and disadvantages of immersion and contact techniques are discussed.

Key words: A-scan oculometry, ultrasound biometry, contact technique, immersion technique.

Introduction

The most common use of echography in the eye is the measurement of axial length for intraocular lens calculation. But also for diagnostic purposes such as pseudoexophthalmus, microphthalmus, nanophthalmus, phtisis bulbi, congenital glaucoma or leucocoria the use of biometry is of great clinical value. As a result there has been a continual improvement of instrumentation and examination techniques, and various machines are used in routine examination today.

One of the best equipped and newly fashioned instruments is the Mini A-scan unit. This digitalized A-scan unit is designed for standardized echography for diagnostic purposes as well as for A-scan biometry.

There are two different techniques for measuring the axial length with an A-scan unit, the contact method and the immersion technique. Both are practicable with the Mini A-scan unit.

J.M. Thijssen, H.C. Fledelius and S. Tane (eds.), Ultrasonography in Ophthalmology 14, 89–92.
© 1995 *Kluwer Academic Publishers, Dordrecht.*

Contact Technique

In the contact technique the probe is placed directly on the cornea. This can be performed by holding the probe with the hand or by applanation. In case of a hand-held technique, the patient is usually reclined or supine; performing the applanation method the patient is normally seated in an upright position.

When the phakic eye is measured correctly, four spikes appear in the echogram, in addition to the initial spike. In case the probe is placed on the cornea the initial spike represents the corneal surface followed by spikes of the anterior and posterior lens surface and the retinal peak. A fourth spike originating from the sclera appears just behind the retinal spike.

Using the contact method measuring the axial length on a frozen echogram of the Mini A-scan the two gates appearing on the screen are shifted to the initial echo presenting the corneal spike and to the retinal spike. The equipment assumes an average sound velocity of 1550 m/sec for measuring the total axial length but this value can be changed from 1000 m/sec to 1700 m/sec by 1 m/sec steps.

The examination of phakic and pseudophakic eyes is slightly different. In the phakic eye, a sound velocity of 1532 m/sec is used, whereas in the pseudophakic eye sound velocities of 1546 m/sec or 1550 m/sec are recommended. Another alternative velocity for the pseudophakic eye is 1532 m/sec adding 0.2 mm to the final result.

All of these values assume, however, that the lens implant is polymethylmethacrylat (PMMA). Lower velocities are required for silicone implants.

In the pseudophakic eye the extremely high implant spike is normally followed by a chain of multiple signals (artefacts) along the vitreous baseline. These multiple signals are caused by reverberations occuring between the sound probe and the surface of the implanted lens. The examiner must identify these artificial spikes in order to avoid misinterpreting them as the retinal spike. Such mistakes are most easily made in short eyes, in which the multiple signals may be superimposed on the retinal spike. Decreasing system sensitivity while observing the screen, the disappearence of the reverberation signals and the persistence of the high retinal spike can be documented.

The primary sources of error using the contact technique include corneal compression, fluid meniscus between the tip of the probe and cornea and misalignment of the sound beam. Corneal compression results in a shortened axial length measurement. A gentle on-and off technique is recommended to avoid corneal indentation. In our experience it is more difficult to control compression of the cornea with the use of a hand-held technique than when using the applanation technique.

Immersion Technique

Using an immersion technique for axial length measurement, the patient will be examined in a supine position. A small plastic cylinder, a so-called scleral shell, is inserted between the lids after topical anesthetic eye drops. The cylinder is filled with methylcellulose or/and physiological saline solution.

Beginning at high system sensitivity, the examiner directs the sound beam perpendicular to the cornea, the anterior and posterior lens surfaces, the retina and the sclera. High spikes are displayed from these interfaces at high gain setting; then the decibel level is reduced for improved resolution.

Pressing the foot switch of the Mini A-scan unit you can freeze the picture and the measurement is taken on a frozen echogram at lowered system sensitivity. Chosen the five gates biometry the program automatically identifies an immersion technique and the five relevant echo spikes of the intraocular surfaces are captured. By activating one gate, you can correct each gate position.

On top of the screen intraocular distances and the total axial length are displayed. Automatically the instrument takes the correct sound velocities for different intraocular tissues into consideration, for the cornea 1620 m/sec, for the anterior chamber and vitreous 1532 m/sec and 1641 m/sec for the lens.

When the total axial length of the examined eye is determined, you can easily change to the calculation program of the Ophthascan Mini A-scan, with a choice between four calculation formulas: BINKHORSTII, HOLLADAY, SRK-II and SRK-T.

On the screen appears a proposal for lens implantation. Keratometer readings and the aimed postoperative refraction can be changed quickly. In the calculation program, 10 different anterior or posterior chamber lenses are determined. If desired, the surgeon can easily change to another lens type, simultaneously modifying the A-constant, Holladays surgeon factor, or the expected postoperative anterior chamber depth.

For the single lens type you can also document the results of calculation with all four formulas in the machine.

Conclusions

The primary advantage of the immersion technique over the contact method is that corneal compression does not occur during the examination. This is of particular importance in patients with a short axial length (less than 22.0 mm), where small errors in measurement can lead to significant error in postoperative refraction.

In addition, the display of a separate corneal spike makes it easier to determine when the sound beam is properly aligned along the optical axis.

If a posterior staphyloma is present and the macula lies on a slope the tendency for most examiners is to accept the longest measurement displayed, which may be at the base of the staphyloma, away from the macular area. To obtain the best possible measurement in high myopic eyes, an immersion technique is recommended. By obtaining high spikes from the cornea, anterior and posterior lens surfaces, the examiner can be reasonably certain, that the sound beam is directed toward the macular region. This is in spite of the fact, that a high quality retinal spike cannot be displayed. Looking at the historical background, the immersion technique came first and may yet see a well observed comeback.

2nd University Eye Clinic
Vienna, Austria

2.11. Accuracy of the Modified IOL Power Formulas for Emmetropia

H. JOHN SHAMMAS

(*Los Angeles, CA, U.S.A.*)

Abstract. Five modern IOL power formulas for emmetropia were evaluated. They included the Shammas, SRK-T, Holladay, Hoffer-Q and Binkhorst II formulas. In 230 consecutive extracapsular cataract extractions with in-the-bag insertion of a plano convex posterior chamber lens, the accuracy of all formulas exceeded 95% (within ±1.0 diopter). The difference between all formulas were compared in the short, medium and long eyes, as well as in the presence of flat and steep corneas.

Key words: Intraocular lens prediction formulas.

Intraocular lens (IOL) power calculations have become an integral part of the preoperative cataract evaluation. During the past decade, formulas used for such calculations have evolved to a high level of accuracy. We herein reviewed our results in 230 consecutive cases using the Shammas formula [1], and comparing the results to four other popular formulas, the SRK-T [2], Holladay [3], Hoffer-Q [4] and Binkhorst II [5] formulas.

Material and Methods

We reviewed the post-operative results in 230 consecutive cases of extracapsular cataract and implant surgery where the final visual acuity was 20/40 or better. All lenses used were plano-convex posterior chamber lenses, Model SK62CP from Cilco, Inc., with 10° angled loops. The axial length was measured with the Kretz 7200 MA standardized A-Scan, using an immersion technique [6]. The K readings were taken with a Bausch and Lomb Keratometer. All post-operative K readings were within ±0.50 diopter of the preoperative readings.

Five popular formulas were used to calculate the IOL power for emmetropia. They included the Shammas, SRK-T, Holladay, Hoffer-Q and Binkhorst II formulas. A specific constant was calculated for each formula. These values were established by reviewing the results of twenty surgeries

J.M. Thijssen, H.C. Fledelius and S. Tane (eds.), Ultrasonography in Ophthalmology 14. 93–99.

on eyes with an axial length ranging between 23.0 and 24.0 mm, and K readings ranging between 43.0 and 44.0 diopters. The constant was adjusted for each formula until the final refraction equaled the predicted refraction in each eye. The values were then averaged to obtain the personalized constant for each formula. The following constants were obtained:

an anterior chamber depth constant (ACD) of:
- · 3.90 in Shammas formula
- · 4.46 in Binkhorst II formula
- · 4.50 in Hoffer-Q formula
- an A constant of 117.3 for the SRK-T formula
- an S factor of 0.74 for the Holladay formula.

Results

The difference between the final and predicted refractions was tabulated for each eye with each of the five formulas. The final refraction was within ±0.50 diopter of the predicted values in 73.9% with the Hoffer-Q formula and 77.0% with the Shammas formula (Table 1). The difference between all the percentages is not statistically significant ($p > 0.10$). The final refraction was within ±1.0 diopter of the predicted values in 94.8% with the SRK-T formula and 97.0% with the Holladay formula. The difference between all the percentages is not statistically significant. Table 2 shows the absolute error and the range of errors with each formula.

The accuracy of the formulas in the short, (less than 23.0 mm), average

Table 1. Difference between the final and predicted refraction in the 230 consecutive cases of ECCE surgery.

	≤0.50 diopter	≤1.0 diopter
Shammas formula	177 (77.0%)	220 (95.7%)
SRK-T formula	172 (74.8%)	218 (94.8%)
Holladay formula	175 (76.1%)	223 (97.0%)
Hoffer-Q formula	170 (73.9%)	219 (95.2%)
Binkhorst II formula	176 (76.5%)	220 (95.7%)

Table 2. Average errors obtained with the IOL power formulas in the 230 consecutive cases of ECCE surgery.

	Mean absolute error in diopters	Range of errors in diopters
Shammas formula	0.52 ± 0.37	+1.3 to −1.6
SRK-T formula	0.54 ± 0.39	+1.4 to −1.7
Holladay formula	0.52 ± 0.39	+1.4 to −1.6
Hoffer-Q formula	0.54 ± 0.39	+1.4 to −1.6
Binkhorst II formula	0.52 ± 0.38	+1.3 to −1.6

Table 3. Accuracy within ±0.50 diopter of the different formulas in the short, average and long eyes.

Formula	Axial length		
	Less than 23 mm (*n* = 70)	23–24 mm (*n* = 97)	Over 24 mm (*n* = 63)
Shammas	48 (68.6%)	77 (79.4%)	52 (82.5%)
SRK-T	49 (70.0%)	77 (79.4%)	46 (73.0%)
Holladay	49 (70.0%)	77 (79.4%)	49 (77.8%)
Hoffer-Q	47 (67.1%)	76 (78.3%)	47 (74.6%)
Binkhorst II	48 (68.6%)	77 (79.4%)	50 (79.4%)

Table 4. Accuracy within ±1.0 diopter of the different formulas in the short, average and long eyes.

Formula	Axial length		
	Less than 23 mm (*n* = 70)	23–24 mm (*n* = 97)	Over 24 mm (*n* = 63)
Shammas	64 (91.4%)	94 (96.9%)	62 (98.4%)
SRK-T	62 (88.6%)	95 (97.9%)	61 (96.8%)
Holladay	65 (92.9%)	96 (99.0%)	62 (98.4%)
Hoffer-Q	64 (91.4%)	94 (96.9%)	61(96.8%)
Binkhorst II	64 (91.4%)	94 (96.9%)	62 (98.4%)

(23.0 to 24.0 mm) and long (over 24.0 mm) eyes is shown in Tables 3 and 4. The accuracy was the highest when the axial length exceeded 23.0 mm and slightly worse when the axial length was below 23.0 mm.

Discussion

Formulas for IOL power calculations have evolved from the original formulas of the 1970's to the present formulas. In 1982, we reported on our results with Colenbrander's formula and we noted that stronger power lenses were implanted in short eyes and weaker power lenses in long eyes [7]; we then introduced our modification of Colenbrander's formula [1] by changing the axial length (L) to L − 0.1 (L − 23). This fudge factor increases the axial length by 0.1 mm for each 1 mm shorter than 23 mm, thus closing the gap in our cases between the calculations and the final refractions in short and long eyes.

A few years later, Binkhorst adjusted his formula [5], by changing the post-operative anterior chamber depth; this was based on a positive correlation noted by Binkhorst between the post-operative anterior chamber depth and the axial length. In the presence of a posterior chamber lens, the estimated post-operative anterior chamber depth is decreased by 0.17 mm for

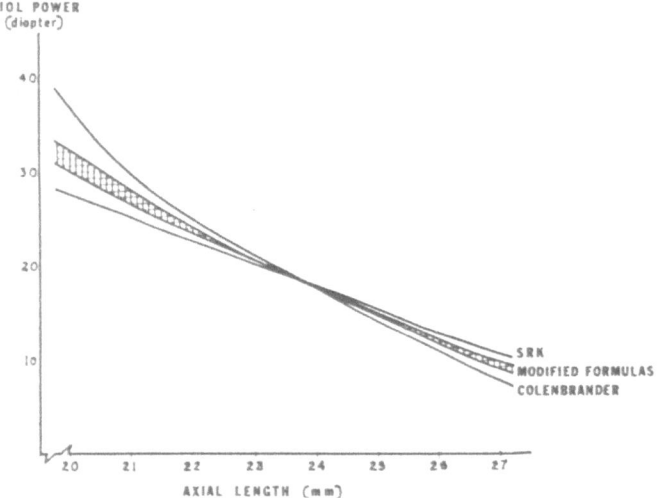

Figure 1. (Shammas): Power for emmetropia obtained with the modified formulas compared to the original Colenbrander and SRK formulas. All calculations are made with an average corneal curvature of 43.50 D. Axial length varies from 21.0 mm to 26.0 mm.

each millimeter the axial length is shorter than 23.45 mm, and increased by 0.17 mm for each millimeter the axial length is longer than 23.45 mm.

In 1988, Holladay [3] introduced his modification of the theoretical formula based on a three-part system that includes, (1) data screening criteria to identify improbable axial length and keratometry measurements, (2) a more accurate post-operative anterior chamber depth estimate that increases the accuracy in short, medium, and long eyes, and (3) a personalized surgeon factor that adjusts for any consistent bias in the surgeon's formula.

In 1990, Retzlaff, Sanders and Kraff [2] introduced the SRK-T formula. Contrary to the original SRK and SRK-II equations, the SRK-T is a theoretical formula based on Fyodorov's formula, and used empirical regression methodology for optimization of the post-operative anterior chamber depth, prediction of the retinal thickness correction factor, and of the corneal refractive index.

The Hoffer-Q formula [4] is a further modification of Hoffer's formula, introduced in 1992. It also adjusts the post-operative anterior chamber depth in short and long eyes.

All these modified formulas change the anterior chamber depth or the axial length to correct for inaccuracies in the short and long eyes. Figure 1 shows that their results fall in between the results of the original theoretic (Colenbrander) and regression (SRK) formulas.

Variations between the formulas still exist, especially in the short and long eyes. They are related to changes in the corneal curvature. Figure 2 shows that in a 21 mm eye, the formulas differ by almost two diopters in the

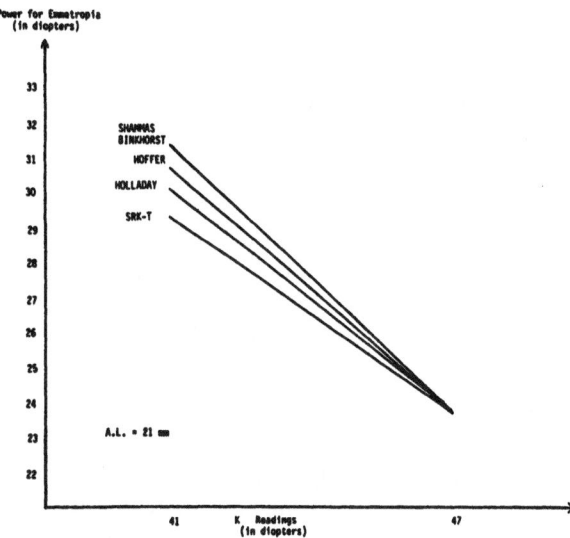

Figure 2. (Shammas): Power for emmetropia obtained with the different modified formulas in the short 21 mm eyes. The corneal curvature varies from a flat 41.0 D to a steep 47.0 D.

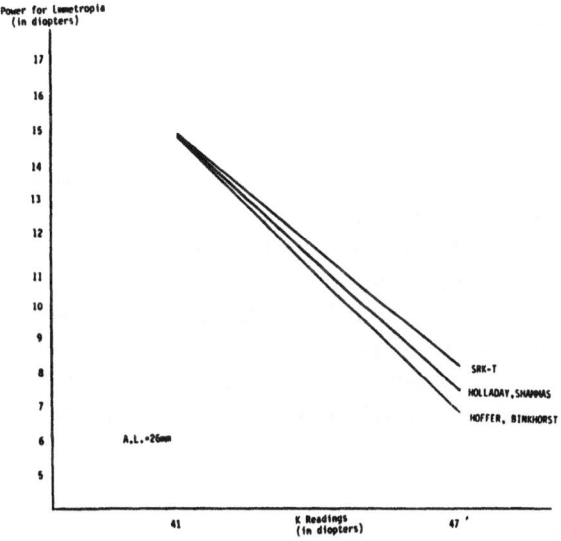

Figure 3. (Shammas): Power for emmetropia obtained with the different modified formulas in the long 26 mm eyes. The corneal curvature varies from a flat 41.0 D to a steep 47.0 D.

unusual short eyes with flat corneas (4.1 diopters) and they differ by less than 0.50 diopter in the most commonly encountered short eyes with steeper corneas (47 diopters). Similarly, in the long eyes (Fig. 3), the formulas differ by almost 1.5 diopters in the unusual long eyes with steep corneas (47 diopters) and differ by less than 0.5 diopter in the most common long eyes with a flat cornea (4.1 diopters).

In our study, all the formulas yielded excellent results with an accuracy (within ±1.0 diopter) of over 95%. It is important to note that in our series, the constants have been optimized in a smaller series of 20 cases with average axial length and average corneal curvature. We thus obtain a personalized anterior chamber constant for each of the Shammas, Hoffer-Q, and Binkhorst formulas, as well as a personalized A constant for the SRK-T formula and S factor for the Holladay formula. A personalized constant is important to accommodate any consistent shift that might affect IOL power calculations, namely the surgical technique, the biometer used, the implant's style and manufacturer.

In our study, we used a more advanced surgical technique with in-the-bag placement of all intraocular implants and minimal variation in the corneal curvature. Most importantly, the high accuracy in our cases is due to a more accurate measurement of the axial length using an immersion technique [6]. With this technique, the ultrasound probe is immersed in a scleral cup, placed on the eye, and kept 5 to 10 mm away from the cornea. Contrary to the contact technique where the probe touches the cornea, there is no possibility of corneal compression with our method. Also, the non-focused beam in our ultrasound unit allows for better alignment within the optical axis of the eye. These factors decrease the margin of error in axial length measurement; a 1 mm error affects the final refraction by approximately 2.5 diopters in an average eye, and increases to over 3.0 diopters in a short eye.

There is no fool-proof method to avoid an error in an axial length measurement [8]. Bilateral axial length measurements should be performed by the ophthalmologist or a certified technician. Consistency is very important; variations in the ultrasound probe design, in the sound velocity, or in the technique can cause up to 0.5 mm difference in measurement. Prior to surgery, the surgeon should, personally, review the pictures of the measurement and correlate the results with the clinical data. It is then, and only then, that a potential error in IOL power calculation can be avoided.

References

[1] H J F Shammas The fudged formula for intraocular lens power calculations Am Intraocular Implant Soc J 1982,8 350–352
[2] J Retzlaff, D R Sanders and M C Kraff Development of the SRK/T intraocular lens implant power calculation formula J Cat Refract 1990,Surg 16 333–340
[3] J T Holladay, T C Praeger, T Y Chandler and K H Musgrove A three-part system for refining intraocular lens power calculations J Cat Refract Surg 1988,14 17–24
[4] K J Hoffer The Hoffer-Q formula In print
[5] R D Binkhorst Intraocular lens power calculation manual A guide to the author's TICC-40 Programs 3rd Ed , 1984 New York, R D Binkhorst

[6] H.J. Shammas. Atlas of ophthalmic ultrasonography and biometry, pp 273–308. The C.V. Mosby Co., St. Louis, 1984.
[7] H.J.F. Shammas. Axial length measurement and its relation to intraocular lens power calculations. Amer. Intraocular Impl. Soc. J. 1982;8:346–349.
[8] J.J. Shammas. The 9 diopter surprise revisited. J. Cat. Refract. Surg. 1988;14:580.

H. John Shammas, M.D.
Department of Ophthalmology
USC School of Medicine
Los Angeles
California, U.S.A.

2.12. Ultrasonographic Evaluation of Axial Length Changes Following Scleral Buckling Surgery

KAZUIKO TOYOTA, YUKO YAMAKURA and
SACHIKO HOMMURA

(Ibaraki, Japan)

Abstract. In order to assess postoperative refractive changes, the influences of two different scleral buckling surgical techniques on the refractive ocular media and on the axial eye length were studied. Buckling with a circling element induces a significant enlargement of the eye length and a corresponding negative sperical refraction change.

Key words: Refractive change, axial length change, echographic biometry, scleral buckling surgery.

Introduction

Refractive changes are one of the most common postoperative complications of scleral buckling surgery [1–3, 5]. It is considered that the quantity and quality of these refractive changes depend on the surgical technique [2, 5], because the eyeball shape modification following the surgical procedure could lead to the optical changes of the eye [2–5]. However, conflicting results concerning postoperative refractive changes have been reported in different scleral buckling procedures, and in literature there is only little information about refractive and axial length changes after scleral buckling using lamellar scleral dissection.

We conducted this study in order to analyse the influences of two different scleral buckling techniques on refractive elements and axial length of the eyes operated on for rhegmatogenous retinal detachment.

Patients and Methods

In the present study, we prospectively analysed the axial length changes following scleral buckling surgery and their relationship to the clinically observed refractive changes in 37 patients (38 eyes) operated on for rhegmatogenous retinal detachment from 1990 to 1992 at The University of Tsukuba Hospital. All patients gave informed consent prior to the start of this study.

Preoperative examinations were done at the moment of admission and at

J M Thijssen, H C Fledelius and S Tane (eds), Ultrasonography in Ophthalmology 14, 100–103

the time of 2 weeks, 3 months and one year or more postoperatively. The comparative studies of the data from admission and after one year follow-up were done. All examinations for both refraction and axial length were performed under cyclopegia.

For measurement of axial length, we used a 10 MHz non-immersed contact hand-held A-scan transducer connected to the Ultrascan Digital B System IV from CooperVision-Alcon Co. Axial length datum for each eye was a result of the average value of five measurements. The '+' sign omitted before the axial length mean values have the meaning of increased axial length.

To provide a uniform basis for these comparative studies, spherical and cylindrical powers were considered separately, and all positive cylindrical powers were converted to minus cylindrical ones. Conventionally, the '−' (negative) sign appearing before the refractive mean values has the meaning of changes in the direction of decreased plus or increased minus spherical power or changes in the direction of increased minus cylindrical power; the '+' sign has just the opposite meaning for both spherical and cylindrical power changes.

According to the surgical technique, we divided the operated eyes in two groups. Group A, in which only 'silicone implant elements' were used, and Group B in which 'silicone implant elements plus silicone circling elements' were used. In both groups, the scleral buckling elements used were from the MIRA Series of solid silicone components. They included silicone rubbers, silicone circling bands and double tantalum clips. Episcleral exoplants and radial element implants were not included in this study. Diathermy was applied to the undermined sclera in all patients, and mattress sutures of polyester fibers were used to close the scleral flap and to secure the circling element in place. No patients with retinal detachment of the macula were included in this study. Subretinal fluid drainage and intraocular injection of physiologic solution were performed in some patients.

The examinations of the fellow eyes were performed not only to statistically control the results, but also possibly to distinguish between the small inherent errors associated with the ultrasonographic repeatability and the small real changes due to the surgical procedure itself. The axial length changes and the refractive ones were statistically analyzed by the paired (2-tail) Student's t-test.

Results

Of the 38 eyes, 14 eyes were the left and 22 eyes were the right ones. Both eyes were involved in one patient. Twenty three eyes were from males and 15 eyes were from females. The patient's mean age was 45.2 years; it ranged from 15 to 73 years, with a peak around the sixth decade.

In buckling without a circling element (18 eyes, 47%), the postoperative axial length changes (0.04 ± 0.3 mm) (mean $\pm$ SD) and spherical power changes (0.01 ± 0.6 D) (mean $\pm$ SD) were not statistically significant (n.s.).

In buckling with a circling element (20 eyes, 53%), the axial length was increased by 0.6 ± 0.2 mm (mean $\pm$ SD, $p = 0.0001$) and the induced spherical power changes were -2.2 ± 0.9 D (mean $\pm$ SD, $p = 0.0001$). Despite the marked scleral indentation in some patients, there were no patients with axial length decrease by this technique.

Next, we measured the changes in cylindrical power for both techniques. Group A showed -0.2 ± 0.6 D (mean $\pm$ SD, $p =$ n.s.), and group B -0.3 ± 0.8 D (mean $\pm$ SD, $p = 0.08$) of cylindrical power changes.

The spherical equivalent change was -0.1 ± 0.5D (mean $\pm$ SD, $p =$ n.s.) for Group A and -2.3 ± 0.9 D (mean $\pm$ SD, $p = 0.0001$) for Group B. All patients who underwent the Group B technique showed a clear tendency to decrease the plus or increase the minus spherical power.

The control group composed by the fellow eyes did not show any statistically significant changes from the preoperative values for refraction and axial length.

Discussion

In order to compare our results to a known model, we took the Gullstrand's schematic eye (G.S.E.) for an optical comparison. From the G.S.E., we know that 1.0 mm of axial length increase results in about -2.6 D of induced spherical changes [3]. Supposing a change in axial length of zero mm in buckling without a circling element and of 0.6 mm in buckling with a circling element, and supposing that the corneal, anterior chamber and lens parameters are constant as with the G.S.E., we can expect about zero and -1.6 D of spherical change, respectively. In our study we had a postoperative mean spherical change around zero and a mean spherical equivalent change by -0.1 D in buckling without a circling element that were not statistically significant. In buckling with a circling element, we had -2.2 D of mean spherical changes and -2.3 D of mean spherical equivalent changes which means values above those expected from the model eye.

Considering the amount of spherical and cylindrical changes and the difference between the expected refractive changes according to the G.S.E. and the real ones obtained from the studied eyes, our results strongly suggest that the main part of the induced refractive change can be explained by the axial length change. Possibly optical changes of the anterior segment can explain the difference observed between the model eye and the studied eyes, especially when buckling with a circling element technique was used. This means that changes of corneal curvature or anterior chamber depth or lens thickness or a combination of these factors can be responsible for part of the postoperative observed changes.

In conclusion, an axial length increase is expected after scleral buckling with a circling element technique, and the postoperatively induced refractive changes associated to the axial length increase were in the direction of decreased plus or increased minus spherical power [4, 5]. Despite the high scleral indentation induced by circling elements in some operated eyes, neither axial length decrease nor hyperopization tendency was observed, in contrast to a previous report [3], where axial length decrease and hyperopization were induced by high indentation. Probably the differences in results could be explained by the used techniques.

Acknowledgments

Dr. Kazuiko Toyota is a recipient of a scholarship from the Ministry of Education, Culture and Science of Japan (University of Tsukuba: No. 905251). The authors thank Dr. Tsuboi and Dr. Spyridon Lazaratos for English review.

References

[1] S.S. Gruposo. Visual results after scleral buckling with silicone implant. In C.L. Schepens and C.D.J. Regan (eds), Controversial aspects of the management of retinal detachment. Boston: Little Brown and Co., 1965; 354–363

[2] H.N. Jacklin. Refraction changes after surgical treatment of retinal detachment. Southern Medical Journal 1971;64:148–150.

[3] M.L. Rubin. The induction of refractive errors by retinal detachment surgery. Trans. Am. Ophthalmol. Soc. 1975;73:453–490.

[4] J.S. Larsen and P. Syrdalen. Ultrasonographic study on changes in axial eye dimensions after encircling procedure in retinal detachment surgery. Acta Ophthal. 1979;57:337–343.

[5] K. Toyota, Y. Yamakura and S. Hommura. Refractive changes after scleral buckling surgery. In K. Shimizu (ed), Current Aspects in Ophthalmology. Amsterdam: Elsevier Science Publishers B.V. 1992;2:1120–1122

Department of Ophthalmology
Institute of Clinical Medicine
University of Tsukuba
Tsukuba, Ibaraki 305, Japan

3.1. Intraocular Inflammation and Combined Annular Choroidal and Retinal Detachment

G. CENNAMO, N. ROSA, G. DE CRECCHIO and
M.C. ALFIERI

(*Naples, Italy*)

Abstract. The presence of a choroidal detachment combined with a retinal detachment sometimes can be misdiagnosed. The presence of cells in the anterior chamber, opacities of the lens, or vitreal haze may add trouble in the evaluation of the fundus, which is already difficult to examine due to the presence of the double detachment.

Performing an examination with standardized echography is crucial in deciding the management of this disease. A case report that proves the usefulness of echography is discussed.

Key words: Retinal detachment, choroidal detachment, standardized echography.

Introduction

The combination of retinal and choroidal detachment is more frequent in the 7th decade of life, and in 37% of the cases it is present in high myopic eyes [1]. Sometimes there is an increase in myopia due to a swelling of the lens, which is caused by the detachment of the ciliary body [2].

Low IOP and uveitis are almost always present.

Sometimes, the presence of cells in the anterior chamber, a lens not perfectly clear, or a vitreal haze can add trouble in the evaluation of the fundus, which is already more difficult due to the presence of the double detachment.

After the diagnosis of combined retinal and choroidal detachment, it is very important to decide how to perform the surgery.

Most of the authors agree that choroidal detachment is a prognostic worsening factor for anatomical and functional recovery of the retinal detachment. This is mostly due to the hypotonic eye that is more difficult to manage. For this reason the surgery should be postponed till after a therapy with steroids and cycloplegia [3].

J M Thijssen, H C Fledelius and S Tane (eds), Ultrasonography in Ophthalmology 14, 105–108

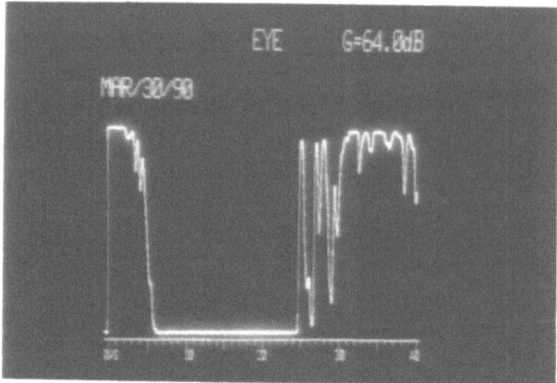

Figure 1. Standardized A Scan showing a 100% high spike from the detached retina, followed by a double spike from the detached choroid.

Standardized echography [4] is crucial in making a diagnosis of choroidal detachment in the presence of retina detachment and to evaluate its extension and location. Moreover, it allows to better evaluate the regression after steroid therapy. In this way, it is possible to decide the best moment to perform surgery.

Case Report

A 68 years old white male was referred to our eye clinic for a decrease in visual acuity in his left eye.

The examination of the right eye showed an uncorrected V.A. of 20/400 that improved to 20/30 with a −11 D.

The IOP was 15 mm Hg, the fundus examination showed myopic degenerations without retinal detachment. The left eye examination showed an uncorrected V.A. of 20/400, that improved to 20/200 with a sph. −7.

The cornea presented some wrinkles and few deposits at the Descemet membrane, Tyndall was +++, IOP = 4 mm Hg. The fundus examination showed a total retinal detachment with a tear in the superior/nasal quadrant.

The echographic examination of the left eye, performed with standardized echography, showed a total retinal detachment with a combined peripheral annular choroidal detachment (Figs. 1–3). After 5 days of therapy with steroids and cycloplegia, the Tyndall was negative, and the pressure raised to 10 mm Hg.

The retinal detachment was still present, but the echographic examination showed an almost complete recovery of the choroidal detachment.

The patient underwent a retinal detachment surgery, so far he is doing well.

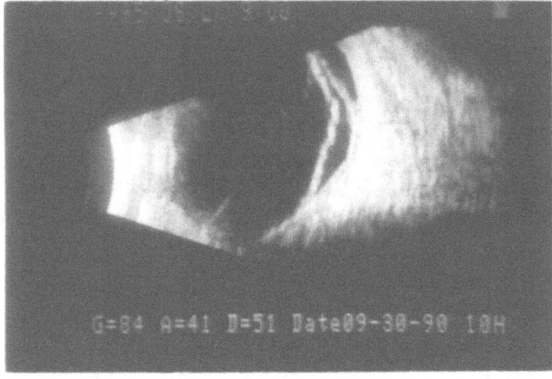

Figure 2 Contact B Scan in a longitudinal scan showing the retinal detachment and the anterior location of the choroidal detachment

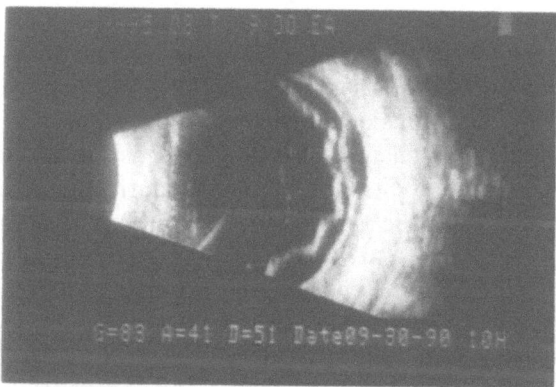

Figure 3 Same eye of Fig 2 in a transversal scan showing the anterior choroidal detachment

Discussion

We should suspect a choroidal detachment when we find a patient with retinal detachment and very low IOP [5].

In case of retinal detachment, the decrease in blood flow in the posterior ciliary artery can decrease the aqueous humour production. This will produce a decrease in the IOP with a massive fluid exudation in the choroidal layer.

This fluid in the choriocapillary will reach the suprachoroidal space through medium and large choroidal vessels.

In this way a ciliochoroidal detachment will be observed with a further reduction in the aqueous production and further decrease in the IOP.

Another hypothesis is that the hypotension could be the result of a toxic effect on the ciliary body from an inflammatory reaction in case of retinal detachment [6–7].

For example, it has been proven that hystamin is produced for the contact between vitreous and pigmented epithelium. Maybe this is the reason of the anterior uveal reaction.

The recovery of choroidal detachment and increase of IOP after steroids is another proof of the inflammatory mechanism involved in the choroideal detachment.

Conclusions

Some authers [1] believe that the best results in the retinal detachment surgery in these cases, have been achieved if the surgery has been performed one week from the onset of CD. They suggest to perform surgery, even if after the medical treatment the CD is still present.

In our opinion, we believe that the patient should undergo a surgery when
(1) The choroidal detachment disappears, and however not after 15 days from its onset.
(2) After 1 week of therapy if this did not produce any improvement.
In these cases we would not have any gain in proceeding with the therapy, but the possibility of a functional recovery will be reduced.

For these reasons, standardized echography is crucial not only in the diagnosis of these kind of diseases, but mainly during the follow-up because it allows us to decide the best period to perform the surgery.

References

[1] S. Okinami and R. Nagayama. Retinal detachment combined with choroidal detachment as a preoperative complication. 1. Clinical features. Acta Soc. Ophthalmol. Jpn. 1984;88:795–799.
[2] R. Weekers. Le decollement cilio choroidien. J. Fr. Ophthalmol. 1979;2(3):217–224.
[3] G. de Crecchio, R. Sgrosso, M.C. Alfieri and B. Matursi. Distaco anulare di coroide associato a distacco di retina. Ann. Ott. e Clin. Ocul. 1988;8:801–806.
[4] K.C. Ossoinig. Standardized echography: basic principles, clinical applications and results. Int. Ophth. Clin. 1979;19(4).
[5] W.H. Jarret. Reghmatogenous retinal detachment complicated by severe intraocular inflammation, hypotony, and choroidal detachment. Trans. Am. Ophthalmol. Soc. 1988;79:664–683.
[6] F. Gottlieb. Combined choroidal and retinal detachment. Arch. Ophthalmol. 1972;88:481–486.
[7] P.A. Graham. Unusual evolution of retinal detachments. Trans. Ophthalmol. Soc. UK. 1969;81:820–829.

Eye Department
University Federico II
Naples, Italy

3.2. Echographic Study of Severe Vogt–Koyanagi–Harada Syndrome with Bullous Retinal Detachment

JO FUKIYAMA, YOSUKE FUTAMAI, SHUJI NAKAZAKI,
NOBUHISA NAO-I, and ATSUSHI SAWADA

(Miyazaki, Japan)

Abstract. Two patients with Vogt–Koyanagi–Harada (VKH) syndrome who had bullous retinal detachment were examined with standardized echography. Diffuse choroidal thickening underlying the detached retina was observed in both cases. In one case, choroidal detachment was found under the inferior bullous retinal detachment. Resolution of the retinal detachment and choroidal thickening were noted by high dose systemic corticosteroid therapy. Standardized echography was useful to detect the choroidal condition in the acute phase of VKH syndrome and also to monitor the response to therapy.

Key words: Echography, Vogt–Koyanagi–Harada syndrome, retinal detachment, choroidal detachment, choroidal thickening

Introduction

The Vogt–Koyanagi–Harada syndrome is a bilateral panuveitis associated with neurologic and cutaneous findings. The most characteristic ocular findings are serous retinal detachment of the posterior pole in the acute phase and sunset glow fundus in the convolescent stage. By using the technique described by Ossoinig [1], we performed echographic examination on VKH patients with bullous retinal detachment and found it to be very useful to make the diagnosis and to follow-up.

Case Reports

Case 1
A 59-year-old man was referred to us on May 24, 1990 with a complaint of metamorphopsia and blurred vision. Two days prior to the initial visit he consulted a local physician who found posterior pole changes of both fundi. He had no previous history of trauma and ocular surgery. His past and family history were non-contributory.

On examination, best-corrected visual acuity was R.E.:20/200, and L.E.

J.M. Thijssen, H.C. Fledelius and S. Tane (eds.), Ultrasonography in Ophthalmology 14, 109–112.

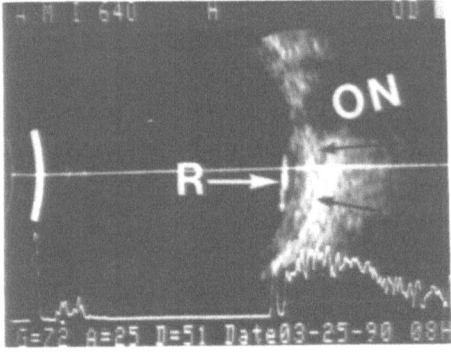 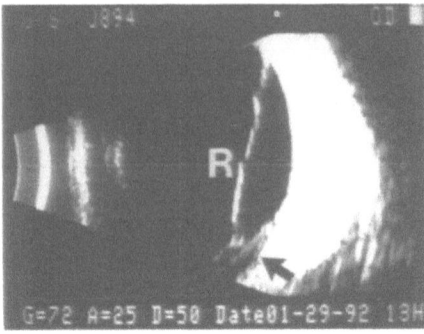

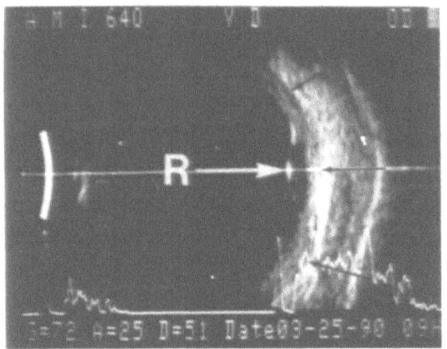 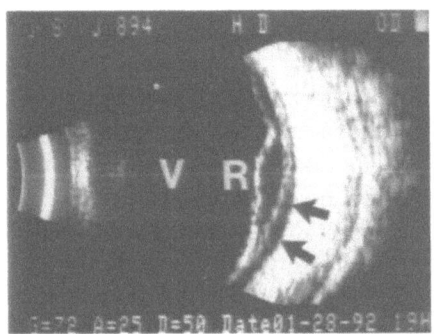

Figure 1 Top, Contact B-mode echogram demonstrating shallow serous retinal detachment of the posterior pole (R, white arrow) and diffuse choroidal thickening (black arrows) ON, optic nerve Bottom, Localized small bullous retinal detachment (R, white arrow) with diffuse choroidal thickening (black arrows) present in the temporal midperiphery

Figure 2 Top, Transverse section of the inferior bullous retinal detachment (R) and choroidal detachment (black arrow) Bottom, More peripheral section showing the same findings Choroidal detachment is evident (black arrows), R, retinal detachment, V, vitrous cavity

20/80. Pupils, ocular motility, and external eye were normal. On slit-lamp examination, there were a few cells in the anterior chamber but none in the anterior vitreous in both eyes. The IOP was within normal limits. Fundus examination of both fundi disclosed serous retinal detachment of the posterior pole as well as a localized small bullous retinal detachment in the temporal midperiphery. The results of the fluorescein angiography mimicked the diagnosis of VKH syndrome. On contact B-mode echography, irregular serous retinal detachment and diffuse choroidal thickening were easily identified. The choroidal thickening was most marked at the posterior pole and thinned out towards the periphery (Fig. 1). Lumbar paracentesis disclosed pleocytosis of the cerebrospinal fluid which confirmed the diagnosis. With high dose systemic corticosteroid therapy, both the retinal detachment and choroidal thickening resolved rapidly, which was easily identified by echography.

Case 2

A 55-year-old woman was referred to us on Jan. 28, 1992 with complaints of right decreased vision and left phthisis. She experienced headache and left ocular pain on Oct. 10, 1991 and consulted a local physician who diagnosed left uveitis and treated her with steroids and antibiotics. However, she developed secondary glaucoma in her left eye and uveitis occured in the contralateral right eye, accompanied by headache and tinnitus on Jan. 17, 1992. VKH syndrome was suspected by the results of fluorescein angiography. The left eye became hypotonic and the right visual acuity declined in spite of the steroid therapy which prompted referral. Although she had no history of ocular surgery or trauma, she had hypertension, left ventricular hypertrophy, and osteoporosis (compression fracture of the lumbar vertebra). Her family history was noncontributory.

On examination, best-corrected visual acuity was R.E.:20/80 and L.E.:LP only. The left pupil was irregular in shape and showed no reaction to light. Ocular motility and external eye were normal. On slit-lamp examination, anterior chamber and also anterior vitreous inflammation was present in the right eye. The left globe was phthitic. Granulomatous anterior uveitis with exudation was present in the left eye. The IOP was R.E.:15 mmHg and L.E.:0 Hg. Visualization of the left fundus was impossible because of the cataract and posterior synechia.

Funduscopic examination of the right eye disclosed multicentric extensive shallow serous retinal detachment with large bullous detachment inferiorly. Echographic examination disclosed shallow retinal detachments and diffuse choroidal thickening in the right eye, and shortened axial eye length with moderate vitrous opacity in the left eye. Peripheral ciliochoroidal detachment was found under the inferior bullus retinal detachment (Fig. 2). The thickened choroid showed medium reflectivity on standardized A-scan. Intravenous steroid pulse therapy performed for three days which was followed by oral tapering administration. The bullous retinal detachment was resistant to the therapy but gradual resolution of the detachment occurred. Later she developed complicated cataract in her right eye and underwent cataract extraction without IOL insertion. Postoperatively, her right visual acuity retured to 20/20 and typical sunset glow fundus with macular pigment clumping was clearly seen by funduscopic examination.

Discussion

The typical serous retinal detachment of the VKH syndrome is shallow and confined to the posterior pole, usually in the macula and around the optic nerve head.

The two patients we described herein had bullous retinal detachment in the mid- and far periphery, in addition to the serous detachment of the posterior pole.

In case 1, a localized small bullous retinal detachment was present superotemporal midperiphery and in case 2, a large bullous retinal detachment was present inferiorly. On echographic examination, we are able to detect the diffuse choroidal thickening underlying the detached retina. Thickened choroid showed medium reflectivity on standardized A-scan. In case 2, peripheral ciliochoroidal detachment revealed under the inferior bullous retinal detachment.

Ultrasonographic findings of VKH syndrome appeared on the literature recently. In 1982, Benson reported the B-mode echograms of VKH syndrome in the review of posterior scleritis [2]. He stated the reflectivity difference of the sclero-choroidal layers between these diseases.

In 1990, Forster et al. reported the detailed echographic features of the VKH syndrome [3]. They reported the findings of contact B-mode echography with standardized A-mode echograms. In 1991, Rubsamen et al. showed echogram of a case with diffuse choroidal thickening and a large bullous retinal detachment [4].

Forster et al. stated that the thickening was most marked near the optic nerve head and thinned-out towards the periphery [3, 5]. We found the same finding in case 1, but did not find it in case 2. We found in another VKH patient, that the choroidal thickening was most marked in the superotemporal macula under the detached retina and not adjacent to the optic nerve head. We did not find the scleral and episcleral involvement that Forster et al. had mentioned.

In the past few decades, fluorescein angiography has been the most useful ancilliary test in the diagnosis and following-up the VKH patients. We believe standardised echography will be a diagnostic adjunct of VKH syndrome, because it enables us to detect the sclero-choroidal condition in the acute phase of this syndrome.

References

Benson, W.E. Posterior Scleritis. Surv. Ophthalmol. 1988;32:297–316.

Forster, D.J., Cano, M.R., Green, R.L. and Rao, N.A. Echographic features of the Vogt–Koyanagi–Harada syndrome. Arch. Ophthalmol. 1990;108:1421–1426.

Forster, D.J, Green, R.L. and Rao, N.A. Unilateral manifestation of the Vogt–Koyanagi–Harada syndrome in a 7-year-old child. Am. J. Ophthalmol. 1991;111:380–382.

Ossoinig, K.C. Standardized echography: basic principles, clinical applications and results. Int. Ophthalmol. 1979;19:127–210.

Rubsamen, P.E. and Gass, J.D.M. Vogt–Koyanagi–Harada Syndrome. Clinical course, therapy, and long-term visual outcome. Arch. Ophthalmol. 1991;109:682–687.

Dept. of Ophthalmology, Miyazaki Medical College
5200 Kihara, Kiyotake-cho, Miyazaki-Gun,
Miyazaki 889–16 Japan

3.3. Ultrasonographic Features of Various Ocular Disorders Using Experimental Rabbit Models

RITSUKO YAMADA, AKIRA KOMATSU, SADANAO TANE
and KOHJI OHASHI
(Kawasaki, Japan)

Abstract. We have investigated acoustic properties of various ocular disorders using experimental rabbit models to clarify the pathological features displayed in echograms. Experimental vitreous hemorrhage was induced by the injection of whole blood. Retinal detachment was established by a dissection of the retina. Uveitis was induced by the injection and booster of chicken albumin. Ocular hypotony was induced by paracentesis. Intravitreal tamponage was performed by injecting silicone oil, sulfur hexafluoride or sodium hyaluronate. Sensitivity graded tomography revealed that vitreous hemorrhage or detached retina disappeared at 12 to 24 dB reduction of the gain sensitivity. Following to the intravitreal tamponage of silicone oil after simple vitrectomy, axial length appeared elongated. Spikes at the anterior surface of silicone oil did not disappear at 30 dB of reduction. Immediately after the injection of sodium hyaluronate, multiple spikes complex of air bubbles were presented on the A-mode and they were disappeared at four days. After the injection of sulfur hexafluoride, A-mode images showed a strong reduction of the posterior pole echo, and the rear wall echo disappeared at 30 dB of attenuation on B-mode. These features of experimental ocular disorders were similar to those of humen eyes.

Key words: Echography, vitreous hemorrhage, retinal detachment, ocular hypotony, uveitis, silicone oil, sodium hyaluronate, sulfur hexafluoride, intravitreal tamponade.

Introduction

The ultrasonic assessment of intraocular diseases is clinically as reliable as direct visualization and in cases of opaque media, it may provide the only rational basis for surgical judgment. The indications for diagnostic echography are including vitreous hemorrhage, retinal detachment, uveitis, intraocular tumor and so on. Echography has its potentials in the diagnosis and observation of the course of diseases and in the examination before vitrec-

J.M. Thijssen, H.C. Fledelius and S. Tane (eds.), Ultrasonography in Ophthalmology 14, 113–120.
© 1995 *Kluwer Academic Publishers, Dordrecht.*

tomy. Moreover, orbital echography, as well as CT scan, is an efficient and reliable diagnostic tool for the evaluation of soft orbital tissues.

In this study, the acoustic properties of various ocular disorders were investigated using experimental rabbit models, to reveal pathological features of echography.

Material and Methods

Animals. Sixteen eyes of sixteen adult colored rabbits (body weight 1.8–3.3 kg) were used to perform the echography.

Methods. Under sodium pentobarbital anesthesia with the intraperitoneal injection, echographic examinations of eyes were performed and employed to observe the course of various experimental ocular disorders, such as vitreous hemorrhage, retinal detachment, uveitis, ocular hypotony and eyes after intravitreal injections of silicone oil, sulfur hexafluoride or sodium hyaluronate.

A. Echographic Technique
A-mode and B-mode scans were examined using a PZT focused transducer of 10 MHz or 15 MHz attached to the St. Marianna's high-resolution ophthalmic ultrasonic diagnostic equipment model ZD-252; and the ultrasound equipment of General's ZD-101 and a 15-MHz transducer.

Experimental Models of Various Ocular Disorders
1. *Experimental Vitreous Hemorrhage.* Autogenous whole blood obtained from auricular vein without anticoagulant was injected (0.3–0.4 ml) through pars plana into the vitreous cavity of a rabbit (No. 1).

2. *Experimental Retinal Detachment.* An incision was made using a 27 gauge needle from pars plana to the posterior pole and a dissection was carried down into the retina, then induced a retinal detachment in rabbits (No. 2 and 4).

3. *Experimental Uveitis.* Chicken albumin (5 ml) was injected into rabbit footpad, and boosted two weeks later. After a week, 0.1 ml of chicken albumin was injected through pars plana into the vitreous cavity. Experimental uveitis was established in a rabbit (No. 8) by hyperimmunity of fourth injection with chicken albumin.

4. *Experimental Ocular Hypotony.* Ocular hypotony was induced in rabbits by paracentesis and aspiration of 0.4 ml of aqueous humor.

5. *Internal Tamponade after Simple Vitrectomy.* Intravitreal tamponade of silicone oil was performed by injecting 0.5 ml of silicone oil (Koken, Tokyo).

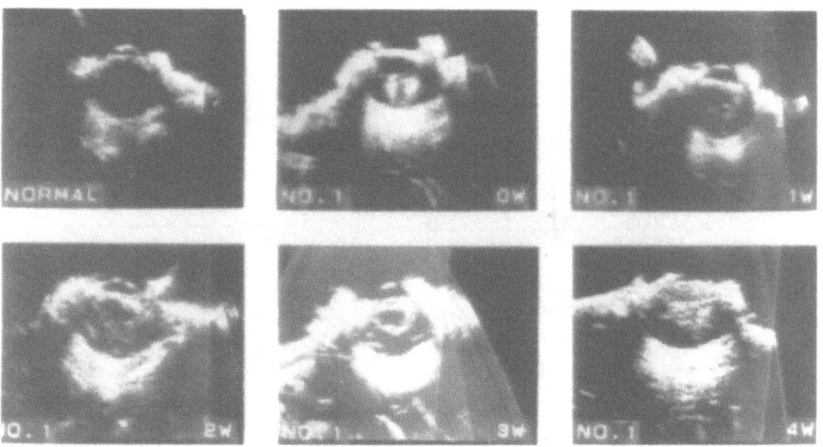

Figure 1 Echograms of experimental vitreous hemorrhage immediately, at one week, two weeks, three weeks and four weeks after the injection of autogenous blood

Intravitreal tamponades of sulfur hexafluoride and sodium hyaluronate tamponade were made by the intravitreal injections with 0.2 ml of sulfur hexafluoride (SF$_6$, Asahi garasu, Tokyo) and 0.4 ml of sodium hyaluronate (Pharmacia, Sweden), respectively.

Results

1. *Experimental Vitreous Hemorrhage*. Fig. 1 shows B-mode images at one, two, three and four weeks after the injection of autogenous blood, and Fig. 2 displays images using the sensitivity graded tomography on the A-mode. Massive shadows were present immediately after the injection, and diffuse scattering echoes were seen after one or two weeks, then funnel-shaped proliferative vitreoretinopathy (PVR) and incomplete posterior vitreous detachment (PVD) were shown after four weeks (Fig. 1). Twelve dB of the gain reduction eliminated the display of the vitreous hemorrhage on the A scan (Fig. 2). Membranous echoes of an incomplete PVD disappeared by 12 dB of reduction of the gain.

2. *Experimental Retinal Detachment*. The echo peaks of detached retina disappeared by 24 to 30 dB of reduction. After one week, hemorrhage was observed ophthalmologically and echographically in the vitreous cavity.

3. *Experimental Uveitis*. Thickening of choroid was observed at two weeks after hyperimmunity of the fourth injection, choroidal detachment appeared at three weeks and retinal detachment at four weeks (Fig. 3). Echo peaks

116

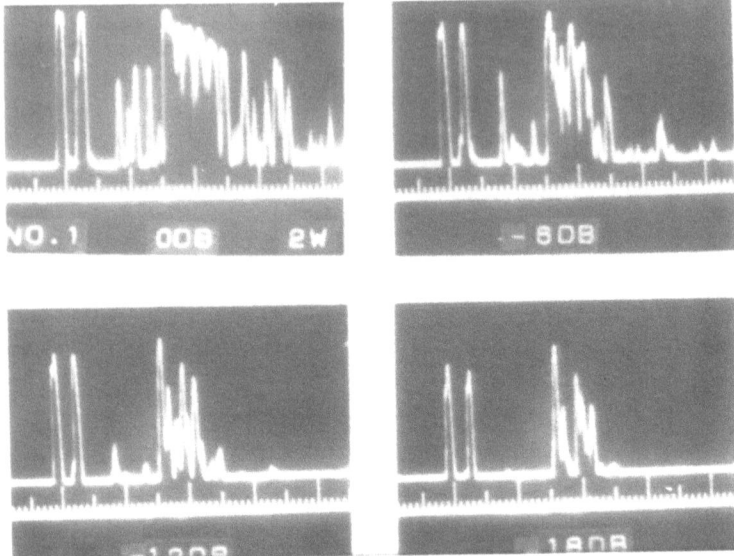

Figure 2 Findings of sensitivity graded tomography of experimental vitreous hemorrhage at two weeks after the injection of autogenous blood

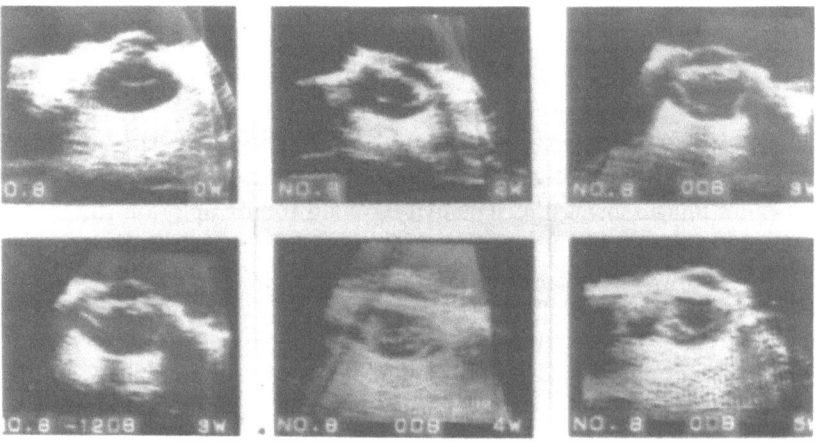

Figure 3 Findings of experimental uveitis immediately after, at two weeks, three weeks and four weeks after the fourth injection

of the detached retina disappeared by 24 dB of reduction. Figure 4 shows findings of sensitivity graded tomography on the A-mode.

4. *Experimental Ocular Hypotony.* Substratificated choroidal thickening was

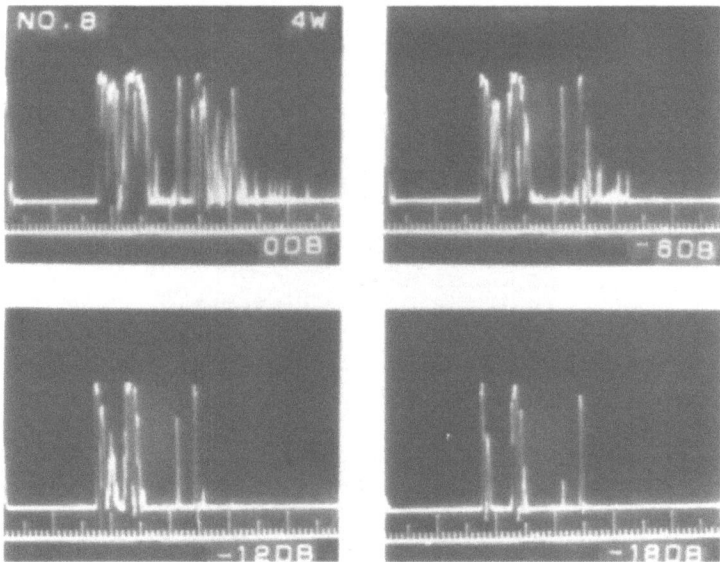

Figure 4. Sensitivity graded tomograms on the A-mode of experimental uveitis after four weeks.

observed in the rear wall. Figure 5 present the features of sensitivity graded tomography at three days. Images of thickening choroid and choroidal detachment did not disappear by 24 dB of the reduction.

5. *Internal tamponade after simple vitrectomy*:
a. *Silicone oil*. Moderate amplitude of spikes of air bubbles were shown on the A-mode immediately after the injection, and were decreased after four days; moreover an image of axial length was elongated. Spikes at the anterior surface of silicone oil did not disappear by greater than 30 dB of the reduction of sensitivity. Attenuation of the rear ocular wall and massive scattered echoes observed on the B-mode image (Fig. 6).

b. *Sodium hyaluronate*. A well-circumscribed shadow was seen in the vitreous cavity on the B-mode. Multiple spikes complex of air bubble echo were shown immediately after injection, and they did not disappear at more than 30 dB of the gain reduction. These images were not detectable at four days after the injection. An eye treated with intravitreal sodium hyaluronate did not show acoustic properties such as excavation of retrobulbar area, or elongation of axial length.

c. *Sulfur Hexafluoride*. Immediately after the injection, the vitreous cavity was filled with sulfur hexafluoride and air bubbles, and ill-defined shadows from rear wall were seen at 0 dB on B scan. Moderate amplitude of spikes and attenuation of posterior polar echo were observed. Characteristic acoustic properties were detectable at 30 dB of the reduction of sensitivity, i.e. disap-

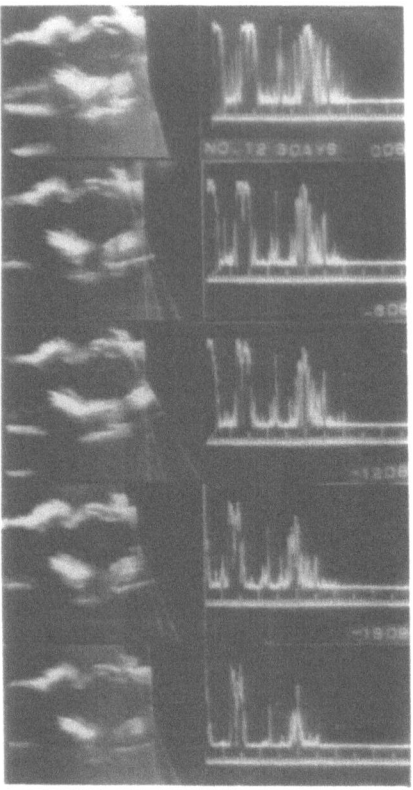

Figure 5. Images of sensitivity graded tomography of experimental hypotony after three days.

disappearance of posterior polar echoes on the B-mode, and choroidal membrane's and scleral echoes on the A-mode. After a week, sound of sulfur hexafluoride and air bubbles were attenuated, and posterior polar echoes were detectable. On the tenth day, high spikes were detectable on the A-mode by 12 dB of the reduction of sensitivity, however, they disappeared by 24 dB of reduction of sensitivity.

Discussion

Scott [1], Andoh [2] and Yamanaka *et al.* [3] have reported that internal tamponade is an important treatment for proliferative vitreoretinopathy (PVR) and retinal detachment complicated with giant tear or macular hole; and it is accepted as one of the commonly used techniques.

In this study, we prepared an experimental model of vitreous hemorrhage and retinal detachment using an eye of rabbits and performed the sensitivity graded tomography. As a result, echoes of vitreous hemorrhage disappeared

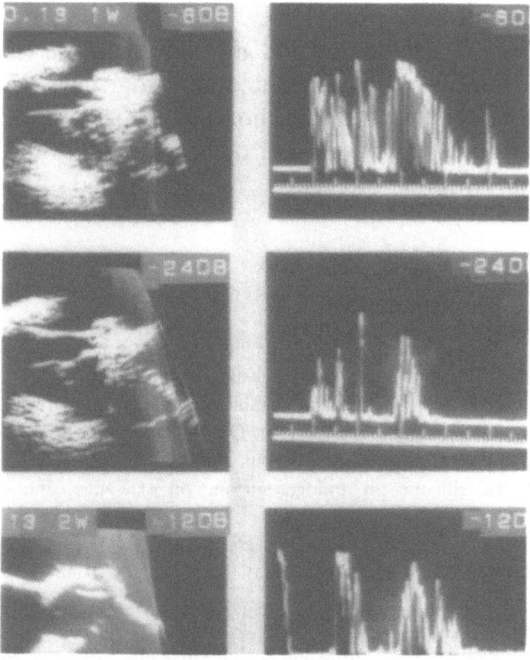

Figure 6 An eye treated with silicone oil at one and two weeks

by 12 dB of reduction on of sensitivity, and the echo of detached retina disappeared by 24 dB reduction of sensitivity. This result was coincident with a report that Tane [4, 5] has described in human eyes. Tane [5] has pointed out that images of vitreous hemorrhage were attenuated as the time proceeds, followed by disappearing of acoustic barrier due to hemolysis and diffusion of blood. Experimental uveitis induced by chicken albumin showed choroidal detachment at three weeks after the fourth injection, and secondary retinal detachment at five weeks. Ocular hypotony by paracentesis revealed thickening and detachment of choroid. Hiromori *et al.* [6] have reported that thickening of choroid may be induced by dilatation of choroidal vessels and filling of red blood cells in the vascular cavity. It was considered that pathogenesis of choroidal changes had to be investigated as a next project. Verbeek *et al.* [7] and Hayashi *et al.* [8, 9] have reported about acoustic properties of eyes injected with silicone oil. Verbeek *et al.* have described that eyes injected silicone oil revealed specific features as follows:

1. Abnormal axial eye length on A-mode echograms and distortion of the B-mode images can easily be explained by the sound velocity.
2. Low posterior polar echoes can be understood from the high attenuation of ultrasound in silicone oil. These findings of eye injected silicone oil are coincident with our results.

Eyes treated with intravitreal sulfur hexafluoride set forth the attenuation and disappearing of rear wall echoes. The ultrasound was absorbed and attenuated by sulfur hexafluoride and air bubbles. These features related to sodium hyaluronate were not detectable after four days. Eyes treated with intravitreal sodium hyaluronate injection did not show the specific acoustic properties like silicone oil or sulfur hexafluoride, due to the similar velocity of sound in the vitreous (1532 m/sec at 37 °C) and sodium hyaluronate (1538 m/sec at 35 °C).

References

[1] J.D. Scott, A rationale for the use of the liquid silicone in retinal detachment surgery, XXIII: 433–437, Concilium Ophthalmologicum, Kyoto, 1978.
[2] F. Andoh, Y. Miyake et al. Vitrectomy combined with intravitreal silicone oil injection for intractable retinal detachment. Jpn. J. Clin. Ophthalmol. 1981;75:1576–1583.
[3] A. Yamanaka, T. Ikeuti et al. Internal tamponade after vitrectomy. Comparative study of the results of gas, silicone oil and gas-silicone oil exchange. Jpn J Clin Ophthalmol, 1984;38:69–74.
[4] S. Tane. The studies on the ultrasonic diagnosis in ophthalmology. (report 4). The quantitative ultrasono-tomography on intravitreal hemorrhage. Acta Soc Ophthalmol Jpn, 1972;76:1318–1325.
[5] S. Tane. Image diagnosis in ophthalmology. Kanehara Publishers, Tokyo, Japan.
[6] T. Hiromori, M. Yamauti et al. Ultrasonic findings in ocular hypotony, Jpn. J. Clin. Ophthalmol. 1972;38:565–568.
[7] A.M. Verbeek, A.L. Bayer and J.M. Thijssen. Echographic diagnosis after silicone oil injection. Docum Ophthalmol Proc Series, (J.M. Thijssen and A.M. Verbeed, eds.), Vol. 29: Dr. W. Junk Publishers, The Hague, 1981:59–66.
[8] E. Hayashi, Y. Takao et al. An experimental study of ultrasonic characteristic of intravitreally injected sodium hyaluronate, Folia Ophthalmol. Japonica 1984;35:118–123.
[9] H. Hayashi, K. Oshima et al. Use of ultrasonography in the management of eyes following vitrectomy, Jpn. J. Clin. Ophthalmol. 1983;37:631–637.

Department of Ophthalmology
St. Marianna University School of Medicine
2-16-1, Sugao, Miyamae-ku
Kawasaki-city, 216, Japan.

3.4. Investigation on the Accuracy of Measurement Parameters for the Diagnosis of Cataract by Ultrasonic Tissue Characterization

TSUYOSHI SHIINA, ANDREAS BUDI, MASAYASU ITO,
YASUO SUGATA and YUKIO YAMAMOTO
(Tokyo, Japan)

Abstract. It is well known that in soft tissues, the attenuation coefficient measured in dB/cm approximately increases linearly with frequency. The slope of this linear function, denoted by β, has been shown to be a good indicator of tissue state. So far we have tried to measure the attenuation coefficient of a lens from echo signal and have shown the possibility of quantitative description of cataract. However, it was also found that the measurement error increased when the amplitude ratio of anterior and posterior echoes decreased. This measurement error is attributable to the deviation of the beam from the lens center, the displacement from the focus of the beam to the lens, and the declination from the lens axis. Therefore, in order to assess the relationship between measurement error and the amplitude ratio, we have been conducting a series of experiments using the lens phantom of polyhydroxyethylmetacrylate(HOYA). As a result, it was shown that if the normalized amplitude ratio of anterior and posterior echoes was larger than 0.5, the measurement errors can be neglected. To evaluate the reliability of this result, we measured the attenuation coefficient of cataractous and normal lenses as a function of amplitude ratio and compared these with the result of the lens phantom experiments.

Key words: Ultrasound attenuation, eye lens, cataract, ultrasonic tissue characterization.

Introduction

Quantitative ultrasonic tissue characterization is attracting increased attention as a means of discriminating normal tissue from diseased tissue [1]. Among a number of parameters which can be used for this purpose, attenuation has received wide attention. The frequency dependence of ultrasonic attenuation can be used for quantitative tissue characterization. The relationship between the attenuation coefficient and frequency is generally expressed as [2]

$$\alpha(f) = \beta f^n \tag{1}$$

J.M. Thijssen, H.C. Fledelius and S. Tane (eds.), Ultrasonography in Ophthalmology 14, 121–129.
© 1995 *Kluwer Academic Publishers, Dordrecht.*

where f = frequency; $\alpha(f)$ = frequency dependent attenuation; β, n = attenuation parameters to characterize the tissue, which are experimentally determined

It is commonly assumed that the value of n for soft tissues is very close to unity. Although attenuation of acoustic energy during propagation is a complex phenomenon, this assumption is satisfied for the biological soft tissues. The following two mechanisms are primarily responsible for the attenuation:

1. The scattering of energy out of the acoustic pathway
2. Absorption, in which acoustic energy is transformed into thermal energy.

The two mechanisms interact in biological tissue to produce a net acoustic attenuation which has an approximately linear frequency dependence over the frequency range of typical ultrasound equipment. While some mechanisms have been proposed for this behavior, no definitive explanation yet exists.

The slope of this linear loss function β, has been observed to correlate with the disease condition of soft tissue: cirrhotic livers produce larger β values than normal [3], and infarcted regions of myocardial muscle's β values increase with the amount of collagen tissue present [4]. Similar characteristic is expected for the attenuation coefficient of crystalline lens. Thus, we have tried to measure the attenuation coefficient of the lens from echo signals and have shown the possibility of quantitative description of cataract. It was also found that the measured value of attenuation depended on the way of irradiating the ultrasonic-beam to the lens. Therefore, in order to get reliable data, it is important to evaluate how the measured attenuation values depend on the incidence angle of the beam, displacement from focal zone and deviation of the beam from the lens center.

In this work, we examined these problems by experiment, using the lens phantom of polyhydroxyethylmetacrylate(HOYA). As a result, it was shown that the ratio of the amplitude of echoes from two, i.e., anterior and posterior, surfaces proved to be a good criterion for suppressing measurement errors. To evaluate the reliability of this result, we measured the attenuation coefficient of cataracts and normal lens as a function of amplitude ratio and compared the results with those of the lens phantom experiments.

Methods

Experiments were carried out by using a phantom lens made of polyhydroxyethylmetacrylate(HOYA), where the ultrasonic characteristics and shape conditions are approximating the crystalline lens. Those characteristics and shape conditions are listed in Table 1.

A block diagram of the experimental setup is shown in Fig. 1. The A mode transducer (Optiscan 2H01, San-ei) with a center frequency 10 MHz and with a $2 \sim 2.5$ cm focal region was fixed on the XYZ stage (which allows the transducer to move in x, y and z directions with high accuracy) and

Table 1 Specifications of the employed lens phantom

	Sound speed	Density	Diameter	Anterior radius of curvature	Posterior radius of curvature
Phantom	1680 m/s	1 3 g/cm^3	9 6 mm	8 2 mm	7 7 mm

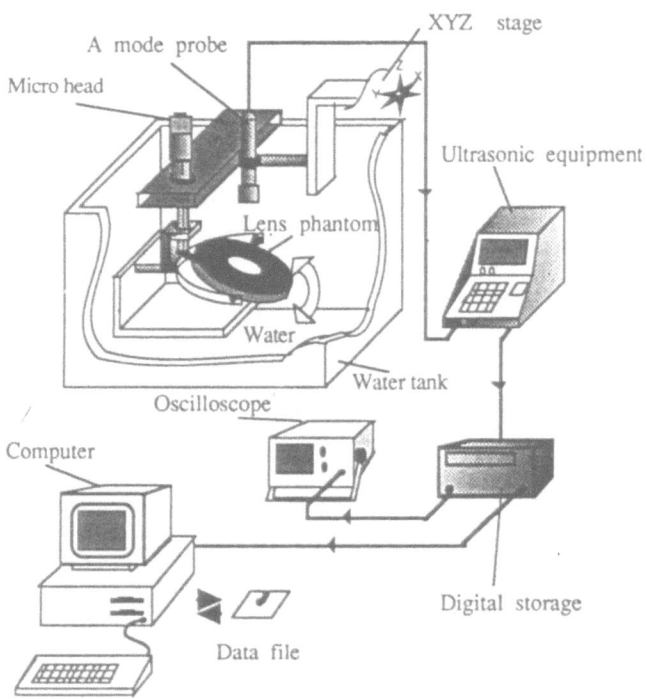

Figure 1 Block diagram of experiment setup

placed at the top of a degassed water tank. The lens phantom was set on a rotatable stand with a radius direction of the lens phantom as an axis, and located in the focal region of the transducer. As reference to coordinates, the center of the lens phantom is considered to be the origin.

The received echoes were stored in a digital storage with an interval 1/60 second. The sampling rate was 50 MHz, and the A-D converter was used in 10 bit full scale mode. The stored waveform was processed by a personal computer (NEC 9801RX) using Fast Fourier Transform (FFT) technique, where the 128 stored sample points were used. The average attenuation coefficient, β was obtained by dividing the slope of the log spectral difference by the roundtrip distance between the anterior and posterior surface. Figure 2 is an example of RF signals reflected from anterior and posterior surfaces of lens phantom. The process of calculating the β is illustrated.

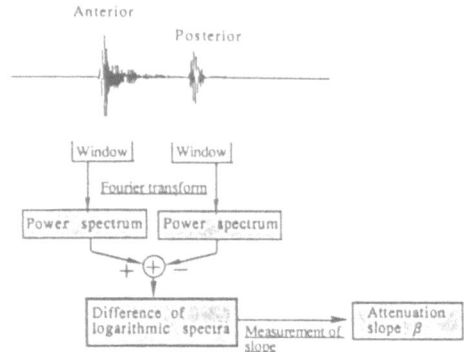

Figure 2. RF signal from the lens phantom.

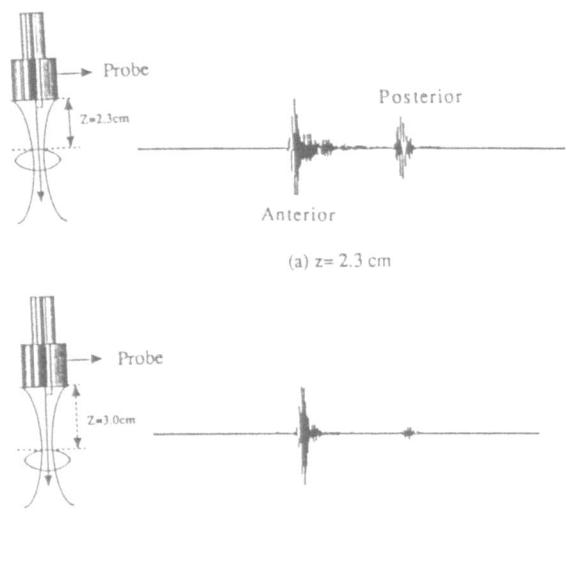

(a) z= 2.3 cm

(b) z= 3.0 cm

Figure 3. RF signals of the lens phantom at the distance from the transducer $z = 2.3$ cm (a) $z = 3.0$ cm (b).

Results and Discussion

(a) *Lens phantoms*
RF signals of the anterior and posterior surfaces at the distance 2.3 cm and 3.0 cm shown in Fig. 3a and 3b respectively. It can be seen clearly from the figures that the echo amplitude ratio of anterior and posterior (posterior echo amplitude–anterior echo amplitude) at distance $Z = 2.3$ cm is larger than at distance $Z = 3.0$ cm. The power spectra and the log spectral differ-

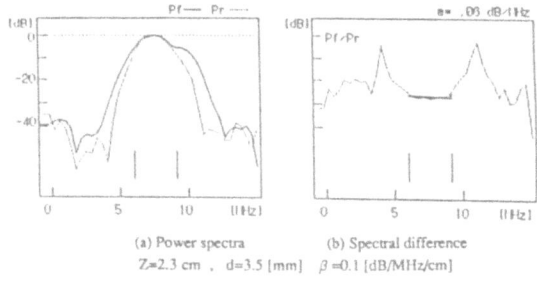

(a) Power spectra   (b) Spectral difference

Z=2.3 cm , d=3.5 [mm] β =0.1 [dB/MHz/cm]

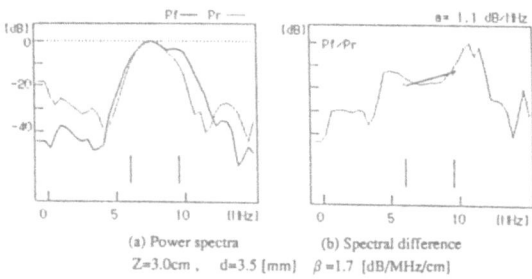

(a) Power spectra   (b) Spectral difference

Z=3.0cm ,   d=3.5 [mm] β =1.7 [dB/MHz/cm]

Figure 4   Measurement of β from the lens phantom

ences of these RF signals are shown in Fig. 4a and 4b respectively. It can be seen from Fig. 4b that when Z = 2.3 cm, β is 0.1 [dB/MHz/cm], but when Z = 3.0 cm, β becomes larger than 1.0 [dB/MHz/cm]. Consequently, in order to get reliable data it is important to take the distance between the observed object and the transducer into account. In Fig. 5, the measurement errors are plotted as a function of distance to the transducer. This figure shows that the measurement error can be neglected when the lens is located at the focal region. Therefore, it is necessary to set the object to be observed at the focal region of the transducer in case of the diagnosis of tissue state using ultrasonic equipment.

Figure 6 shows the relationship between the measurement error and the incidence angle of the beam to the lens phantom. From Fig. 6, it can be seen that the measurement error can be ignored when the absolute incidence angle $|\ \theta\ | \leqslant 1$ degree. However, it is difficult to observe the incidence angle of beam directly in the mobile, living eye. The incidence angle θ can nevertheless be estimated by using the echo amplitude ratio of anterior and posterior as an indicator. The relationship between the normalized echo amplitude ratio and absolute incidence angle is shown in Fig. 7.

Figure 8 shows the relationship between the measurement error and the displacement of the beam from the lens center. It can be seen from Fig. 8 that appreciable values of the measurement error are encountered when

126

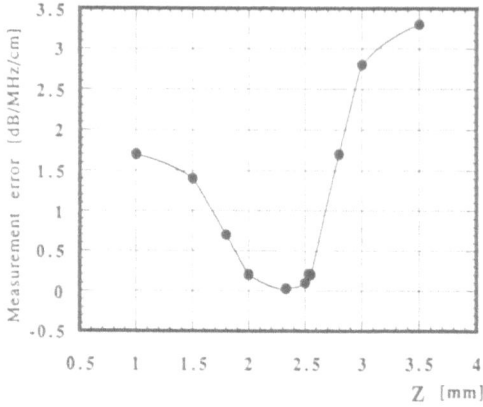

Figure 5 Relation between the measurement error and distance from the transducer to the lens phantom.

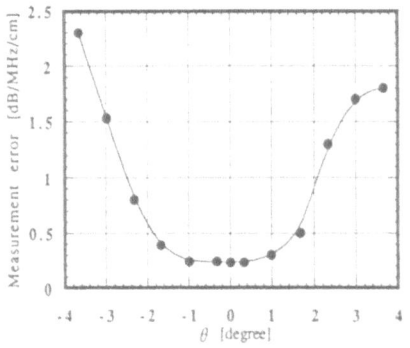

Figure 6. Relation between the measurement error and incident angle of the beam

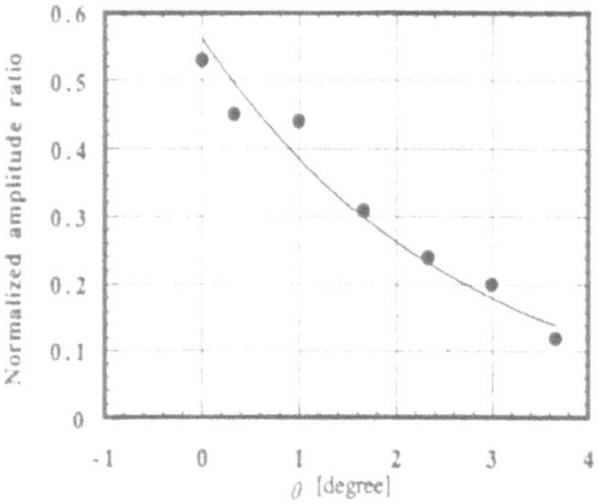

Figure 7 Relation between normalized amplitude ratio and incident angle of the beam.

the deviation of the beam from the lens center $| X | > 0.5$ mm. Thus, the measurement error can be neglected at $| X | \leq 0.4$ mm range.

Figure 9 shows the correlation between the measurement error and the normalized echo amplitude ratio for above three factors of errors: the deviation of the beam from the lens center, the displacement from the focus of the beam to the lens, and the declination from the lens axis. It can be concluded from Fig. 9 that for all cases the measurement error can be ignored when the normalized echo amplitude ratio is larger than 0.5. This result quantitatively verified the validity of an empirical technique which we have employed, i.e., using the normalized echo amplitude ratio as indicator for selecting reliable data under clinical condition.

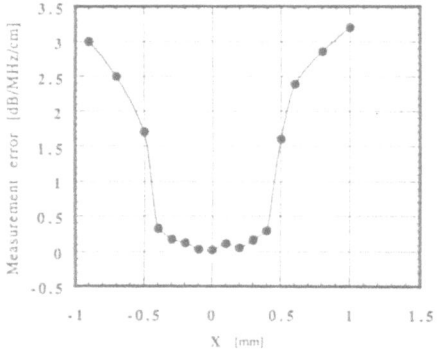

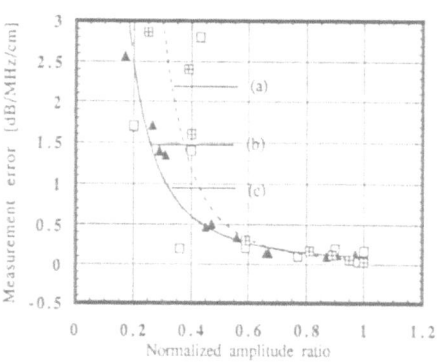

Figure 8 Relation between the measurement error and the deviation of the beam to the lens center.

Figure 9 The correlation between the measurement error and the normalized echo amplitude ratio for the declination from the lens axis (a), the deviation of the beam from the lens center (b), and the displacement from the focus of the beam to the lens (c).

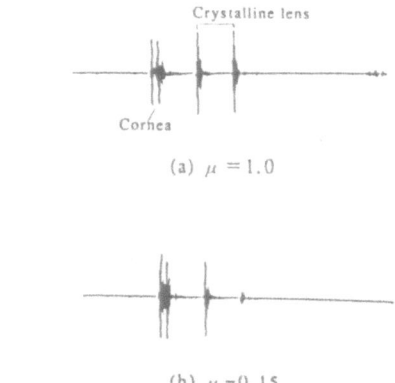

Figure 10 RF signals of normal eye with the normalized echo amplitude ratio $\mu = 1.0$ (a), and $\mu = 0.15$ (b)

(b) *Cataract and Normal Eye*

As has been shown in previous section the echo amplitude ratio proved to be a good criterion for suppressing the measurement error. In order to demonstrate that this technique was capable of minimizing the measurement error under clinical conditions, the value of β for normal eyes and nuclear cataracts were measured.

RF signals of normal eyes with the normalized echo amplitude ratio $\mu = 1.0$, and $\mu = 0.15$ are shown in Fig. 10a and 10b, respectively. The power spectra of the anterior and posterior surfaces are shown in Fig. 11a and the log spectral difference of them and the estimated slope indicated by lines in

128

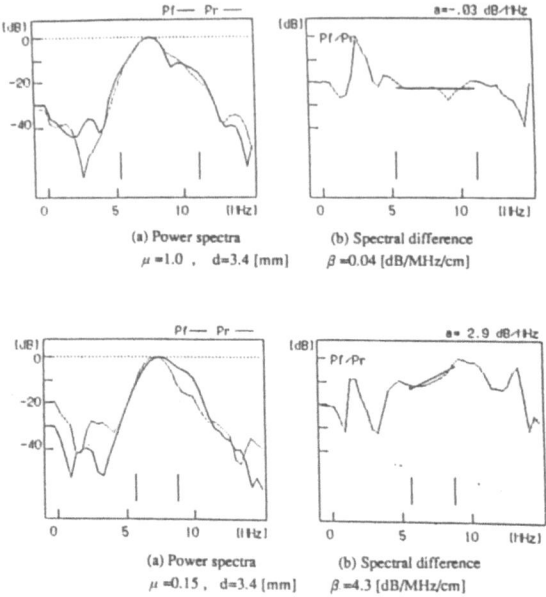

(a) Power spectra
$\mu = 1.0$, $d = 3.4$ [mm]

(b) Spectral difference
$\beta = 0.04$ [dB/MHz/cm]

(a) Power spectra
$\mu = 0.15$, $d = 3.4$ [mm]

(b) Spectral difference
$\beta = 4.3$ [dB/MHz/cm]

Figure 11. Measurement of β for normal eyes.

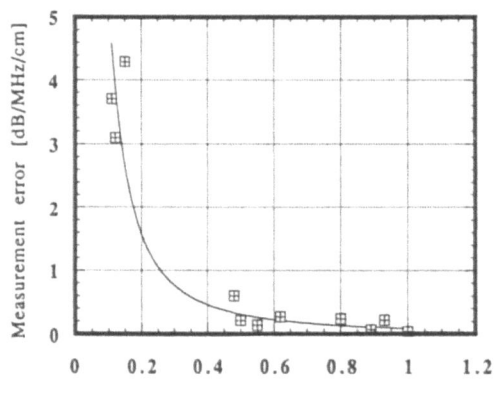

normalized amplitude ratio

Figure 12. Relation between measurement error and normalized amplitude ratio for normal eyes.

Fig. 11b. Analysis of this case showed the value of β to be 0.04 [dB/MHz/cm] when the normalized echo amplitude ratio was $\mu = 1$, and $\beta = 4.3$ [dB/MHz/cm] when $\mu = 0.15$. This is an expected result which indicates that the measurement error increases as the normalized echo amplitude ratio decreases. The relation between the measurement error and the normalized echo amplitude ratio μ is shown in Fig. 12. It can be seen from this figure

129

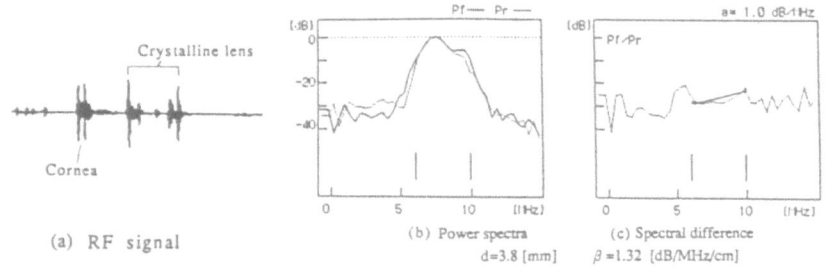

Figure 13 Measurement of β for nuclear cataracts

that the measurement error can be neglected when $\mu > 0.5$. This result was in good agreement with the experimental result using the lens phantom.

Experimental results for a nuclear cataract are shown in Fig. 13. It can be seen clearly that weak echoes were present between the anterior and posterior lens echoes, which were due to the scattering caused by inhomogeneous media. Analyzing RF signals with normalized echo amplitude ratio $\mu > 0.5$, the average value of $\beta = 1.32$ [dB/MHz/cm] is obtained. Nuclear cataract exhibits considerably higher attenuation values than normal eyes, thus it can be concluded that this technique was capable to describe cataracts quantitatively.

Acknowledgment

The authors would like to express a special thanks to Rahman Rahim for his expert and timely typing of the several revisions of this paper.

References

[1] M Linzer and J E Norton Ultrasonic tissue characterization Ann Rev Biophys Bioeng 1982,11 303–329
[2] C R Hill Ultrasonic attenuation and scattering by tissue In de Vlieger *et al* (eds), Handbook of Clinical Ultrasound New York Wiley, 1978, pp 91–98
[3] Kuc, R and K J W Taylor Variation of acoustic attenuation coefficient slope estimates for in vivo liver Ultrasound Men Biol 1982,8 403–412
[4] J G Miller Ultrasonic tissue characterization, an approach based on quantitative backscatter and attenuation In IEEE Ultrasonic Symposium Proceedings, 1983
[5] P A Narayana and J Ophir On the validity of the linear approximation in the parametric measurement of attenuation in tissues, Ultrasound Med Biol 1983,9 357–361
[6] T Shiina *et al* An application in ultrasonic tissue characterization to ophthalmic diagnosis Proc of 14th Annual Int Conf of the IEEE EMB Soc , 1992

Dr Tsuyoshi Shiina
Tokyo University of Agriculture and Technology
Tokyo, Japan

3.5. Staging of Retinopathy of the Premature by Means of Computerized Echography

ALFREDO REIBALDI, TERESIO AVITABILE and
VINCENZO RUSSO
(*Catania, Italy*)

Abstract. In this paper the authors stress the role of echography in the diagnosis of the Retinopathy of the Premature, on the basis of greater knowledge of this pathology, and because today it is possible to have more sophisticated computerized equipment with programs allowing us image processing. Nowadays, the echography is very useful to make diagnosis and to establish the echographical classification of the ROP, while in the past it was only possible by echography to perform differential diagnosis between ROP and other leukokorias. The authors finally show the role of echography in following the eyes after surgical treatment (criopexis, encirclement and vitrectomy).

Key words: Retinopathy of the Premature (ROP), computerized echography, staging.

Introduction

The ROP is a multifactorial pathology that hits the premature newborns. Among the different concomitant causes responsible for this pathology, the low gestational age represents the main cause of ROP. The immature retinal vascularization in newborns shows several concomitant risk factors which complicate the retinal alterations (ROP Study Group, 1988). Our recent study (Scuderi *et al.*, 1990) has pointed out three main risk factors in the ROP etiopathogensis:
– retinal immaturity
– increased synthesis of free radicals
– prenatal and perinatal factors (O2 administration, adult blood transfusions, sepsis, intense light exposition, perinatal asphyxia, congenital cardiopathies, hypothermia, hypocapnia, hypoxia and hyperoxia, hypertension).
Among these factors, the most important seems the hyperoxya, caused by oxygen therapy to which the newborns used to be subjected after birth.
  Terry (1942) hypothesized the toxic effect of oxygen on the immature

J.M. Thijssen, H.C. Fledelius and S. Tane (eds.), *Ultrasonography in Ophthalmology 14*, 130–136.

retina and called in 'retrolental fibroplasia'. Parker in 1951 called it 'retinopathy of the premature' (ROP).

In 1953 Reese, using ophthalmoscopy, made the first classification of ROP, distinguishing an acute and a cicatrizial stage.

Subsequently, recent studies stressed prematurity as an important cause of this disease. In fact, they observed a correlation between the incidence of this disease and gestational age, stressing also severe lesions in prematures whose weight was below 1500 gr.

The improvement of prematures assistance has lead to a growing survival rate of the prematures whose weight was inferior to 1 kg and whose gestational age was very low; 8% in 1950, 35% in 1980 (Phelps 1981), 65% in 1990 (Brown *et al.* 1990). Therefore, new techniques allowed us to observe a higher number of cases and to recognize the disease in its early stage.

Ophthalmic aspects related to prematurity required a more detailed classification. In 1984 an International Committee made up of 23 members met in Baltimore, established definitively the international classification of ROP, which considered two parameters:
– the disease staging,
– the lesion localization.
Regarding staging, they distinguished 5 grades corresponding to the growing severity of the disease:
– Grade I or demarcation line, characterized by a thin and marked whitish line separating the vascularized from the non vascualarized retina.
– Grade II or intraretinal ridge, distinguishable for the presence of a salience growing high and wide.
– Grade III or intraretinal ridge, with fibrovascular extraretinal proliferation. This stage can be subdivided into III A or moderate with small proliferations accumulating along the posterior edge of the ridge to which they adhere; III B or medium showing small aggregates of fibrovascular proliferation which may unite; III C or severe, in which the fibrovascular proliferation is perpendicular to the retina and projects into the vitreous.
– Grave IV in which we found a tractional retinal detachment.
– Grade V or retrolental fibroplasia with such a massive proliferation that the retinal detachment takes the funnel-shape more or less open.

In case of tortous and congestive vessels, the word 'plus' is added to the described grade.

The literature described also the 'rush disease' characterized by a rapid evolution of ROP and by retinal haemorrhages in the posterior sectors.

In the past years, in most cases ROP was recognized only in its advanced or in the cicatricial stage, and then echography was used for differential diagnosis between this pathology and other leukokorias (retinoblastoma, hyperplastic vitreous, etc.).

Recently, thanks to the newest techniques of vitreoretinal surgery, we observed an improvement of the anatomical and functional prognosis of eyes affected by this pathology (Treese 1985); for this reason a preoperative echographical examination might be very useful for the surgeon to obtain some information about the anatomical situation of ocular structures.

In fact, echography played always a fundamental role in all cases with opaque media, and yielding an important contribution both for the diagnosis, and therapy.

The first contributions of echography were due to Gitter (1969), Steindler (1974), Berteny (1980) and Goes (1984), who described the echographical aspects of cicatricial stage diseases, and the differential diagnosis with other leukokorias.

In 1984 Takao et al. described echographical aspects of the rush stage by means of 3-D echography. The latest contributions are from Mazzeo et al. (1984), Shapiro et al. (1985), Jabbour et al. (1987), De Juan et al. (1988), Frazier et al. (1988), Mazzeo et al. (1989), Reibaldi (1990).

In the last years, the early diagnosis, thanks to more diffused use of screening and the more sophisticated equipment, allowed to recognize and to stage acute ROP in its early stage (Reibaldi et al. 1990).

Recently, we assessed the role of the choroid in the pathophysiology of ROP, measuring the retina-choroid thickness and comparing it with the retina-choroid thickness of preterm infants not affected by ROP and of term infants.

Case Report

From January 1987 to September 1992, 1385 prematures visited the Pediatry Institute of Catania University and the Pediatric Department of S. Bambino Hospital of Catania. 333 prematures were affected by ROP, with an incidence of 23.89%, which, according to the evolutive staging of the disease, were subdivided as follows:

Stage I: 183
Stage II: 87
Stage III: 53
Stage IV: 2
Stage V: 8

Echographical Staging

The echographic pattern relating to stages I and II is negative, both in the demarcation line and in the intraretinal ridge. The lesions are localized in the retina and they cannot be distinguished by means of ultrasound.

Instead, echography is particularly useful in the presence of retinal ridge with fibrovascular proliferation (stage III). In this stage, we can notice an alteration of the retinal profile in extreme perifery. This aspect can be observed easily by means of last generation B-scan, and evaluated by means of computerized processing, performable by these equipments. The contour enhancement is one of the most useful procedures for the study of this stage.

In fact, we can emphasize by means of a particular shade of grey, or pseudo-colour, the inner content of the ridge and subsequently, by other grey levels the interface between vitreous and retina, which makes a small lump at the ridge level.

We can observe, after the stage III, an anterior vitreous opacity which can be enhanced by means of particular image processing methods.

Stage IV is characterized by a partial retinal detachment, which may involve the macula. Naturally the echopattern will be like the retinal detachment echopattern, represented by a high reflectivity vitreal membrane.

Stage V is characterized by a total tractional retinal detachment, shape like an open or funnel anteriorly closed by medium-high reflectivity membranes. Also in this case, thanks to computerized programs and last generation equipment, we can observe the fibrovascular inner content in specific reflectivity, while the retinal profile can be distinguished at higher reflectivity. This aspect can be better analyzed by means of contour enhancement.

Post-Surgical Follow Up

According to the followed treatment (cyro, photocoagulation, encirclement, buckling, vitrectomy), the echographical aspects will be different: in the cases treated by cryo and or photocoagulation (stage III) we can monitor by echography the possible disappearance of the ridge, generally 10–15 days after treatment.

The echographical pattern of the cases treated by encirclement, shows both direct signs (evidence of encirclement), and indirect signs due to surgical treatment (ocular profile deformation, less pronounced than traditional detachments).

In the cases treated by vitrectomy the echographical pattern shows the lens absence and it can stress the retinal detachment persistence.

Experimental Study

A preliminary study to establish the thickness of the retina-choroid complex was carried out to investigate differences in choroidal thickness among preterm infants non affected by ROP, those affected by early stages of ROP and term infants.

In order to obtain accurate biometries on frozen B-scan images and exact measurement of the thickness, we used the 'Sonovision STT 100' equipment instead of standardized A-scan, because the frozen images could then by recorded on floppy disk, allowing further measurements, whereas A-scan following does require the patient's collaboration.

We set the equipment with the following parameters: Power 100%, low and variable gain values, persistence 0.

Thanks to the collaboration of the Paediatric Institute of Catania University, we performed B-scan examinations on 25 preterm infants (50 eyes), on

20 term infants (40 eyes) and on 5 preterm infants affected by early stages of ROP (10 eyes).

The study about preterm infants included 25 infants born between 28th and 37th week of pregnancy with an average pregnancy of 33 weeks.

The 25 preterm infants were in incubator and we performed the echography a week after birth, a successive echographical examination was carried out on 10 preterm infants after 10 days, without noticing any variation. The study on term infants included 20 infants non affected by disease and never put in the incubator.

We performed an echographical examination on 5 patients affected by ROP. Among these patients 3 had ROP stage II, 2 patients ROP stage III.

An echographical examination was performed in all the patients in 4 quadrants of the eye, to evidence differences in the choroidal thickness. In the same quadrant the measurement was performed three times and then we made the average.

According to statistical results the average thickness of retina-choroid complex in preterm infants is 1.11 mm.

For the average thickness of each sector we found:
superior sector: 1.09
inferior sector: 1.14
temporal sector: 1.11
nasal sector: 1.12
In term infants the retina-choroid average thickness was 1.23.

For the average thickness of each sector, we found:
superior sector: 1.24
inferior sector: 1.22
temporal sector: 1.21
nasal sector: 1.24
In preterm infants affected by ROP, the choroidal average thickness was 1.16.

For the average thickness of each sector, we found:
superior sector: 1.16
inferior sector: 1.15
temporal sector: 1.16
nasal sector: 1.16
We performed a statistical comparison between the differences of averages obtained in three groups, and calculating the t Student with these results:
1. Term infants vs. preterm infants:
    superior: 0.153 – t Student 7.65 (significant)
    inferior: 0.09 – t Student 3.69 (significant)
    temporal: 0.09 – t Student 4.33 (significant)
    nasal: 0.12 – t Student 5.41 (significant)
2. Term infants vs. ROP:
    superior: 0.08 – t Student 2.67 (significant)
    inferior: 0.07 – t Student 2.57 (significant)

temporal: 0.05 – t Student 1.85 (significant)
nasal: 0.08 – t Student 2.66 (significant)
3. ROP vs. preterm infants:
superior: 0.07 – t Student 2.26 (significant)
inferior: 0.02 – t Student 0.39 (non significant)
temporal: 0.04 – t Student 1.11 (non significant)
nasal: 0.03 – t Student 0.94 (non significant)

Conclusions

In our opinion, the indirect ophthalmoscopy is always the most important examination to obtain clinical data, plus signs, small haemorrhages, relation between retinal vessels and ridge, in particular to assess if they are behind the ridge or overtopping it. These aspects inform the ophthalmologist if and when it is necessary to perform a cryotherapy.

Echography was of fundamental importance when there are opaque media, in the study and monitoring of this disease, especially in its most serious stages, to give to the surgeon all the useful anatomical information whether surgery is necessary and for the post-surgical follow-up. Echography is essential when the examination must be carried out on non-cooperative patients, as in the case of children.

References

Berteny, A., Veli, M. and Fodor, M. A-mode ultrasonography and oculometry in retrolental fibroplasia. Ultrasound in Med. and Biol. 1980;6:19–24.

Brown, O. and Biglan, A. Retinography of prematurity: the relationship with intraventricular haemorrhage and bronchopulmonar dysplasia. J. Paediatric Ophthalmol. Strabismus 1990;27,5:268–299.

Committee for the classification of retinopathy of prematurity. The international classification of retinopathy of prematurity. Ach. Ophthalmol. 1984;102:1130-4.

De Juan, E., Shields, S. and Machemer, R. The role of ultrasound in ophthalmology. Ophthalmology 1988;95:884-8.

De Molfetta, V., Arpa, V. and De Casa, N.: Il trattamento chirurgico della retinopatia dei prematuri di grado elevato. Atti LXIV Congr. S.O.I. 1984;213-217.

Fledelius, H.C. Prematurity and the eye. Ophthalmic follow-up of children of low and normal birth weight. Acta Ophth. 1976;Suppl. 128.

Fledelius, H. Ultrasound imaging in retinopathy of prematurity. S.I.D.U.O. XII Program and abstracts, Iguazu, Argentina, September 1988.

Frazier, Byrne S., Hughes, J., Gendron, E.K., Welsey, C. and Clarkson, J. Echography protocol for eyes with severe retinopathy of prematurity (ROP). S.I.D.U.O. XII Program and abstracts, Iguazu, Argentina, September 1988.

Gitter, K.A., Meyer, D., White, R., Ortolan, G. and Sarin, L.K. Ultrasonic aid in the evaluation of leukokoria. Am. J. Ophthalmol. 1969;65:190-5.

Goes, F. Ultrasonographic aid in the diagnosis of retinoblastoma – suspected cases. Docum. Ophthalmol. Proc. Series 1984;38:81-91.

Gruppo di studio per la retinopatia del pretermine: La retinopatia del pretermine. Fogliazza editor, 1988.

136

Jabbour, N.M., Eller, A.E., Hirose, T., Schepens, C.L. and Liberfarb, R.: Stage 5 retinopathy of prematurity-prognostic value and morphologic findings. Ophthalmology 1987;94:1640–6.

International Committee for the Classification of the last stage of retinopathy of prematurity: Classification of retinal detachment. Arch. Ophthalmol. 1987;105:906–912.

Machemer, R. Fibroplasia retrolenticolare: terapia chirurgica. Basic and advanced vitreous surgery course, Rome, Italy, 7 September 1984.

Mazzeo, V., Ravalli, L., Faco, L. and Scorrano, R. B-scan in retinopathy of prematurity (ROP). Doc. Ophth. Proc. Series 1984;48:431–435.

Mazzeo, V. and Perri, P. Ecographic findings in infants with ROP. Doc. Ophth. 1990;74:235–244.

McPherson, A.R. and Hittner, H.M. Retinopathy of prematurity. Current concepts and controversies. B.C. Decker Inc., Toronto, 1987.

Pats, A. Retrolental fibroplasia. Surv. Ophthalmol. 1969;14:1–29.

Phelps, D.L. Vision loss due to retinopathy of prematurity. Lancet 1981;8:220,606.

Phelps, D.L. Retinopathy of prematurity: an estimate of vision loss in the United States – 1979. Paediatrics 1981;67:924.

Reese, A.B., King, M.J. and Owens, W.C.: A classification of retrolental fibroplasia. Am. J. Ophthalmol. 1952;35:1333–5.

Reibaldi, A., Santocono, M., Scuderi, A. and Pizzo, G. ROP-optimal timing of clinical evaluation and standard procedures. Doc. Ophthalmol. 1990;74:229–234.

Reibaldi, A., Avitabile, T., Cascone, G., Franco, L., Marino, C. and Scuderi, A. Ecografia e prematurita. Relaz. al VI Congr. Naz. S.I.E.O., Genova 23–24 November 1990.

Reibaldi, A., Avitabile, T., Cascone, G., Franco, L., Marino, C., Scuderi, A. and Pappalardo, A. Ecografia e prematurità. Lettura magistrale V Congr. Naz. S.I.E.O., Genova 23–24 November 1990.

Scuderi, A., Gagliano, C., Marano, F. and Reibaldi, A. La patogenesi della retinopatia del prematuro: up-date. Clin. Ocul. e Patol. Ocul. 1990.

Scuderi, A., Avitabile, T., Cascone, G., Franco, L. and Marino, C. La stadiazione ecografica nella ROP. Commun. XVI Congr. S.O.Si., Taormina 22–24 Febbraio 1991.

Shammas, J. Atlas of ophthalmic ultrasonography and biometry. The C.V. Mosby Co. St. Louis, 1983.

Steindler, P. Relievi ecografici ed elettroretinografici nella fibroplasia retrolenale. In M. Maione and J.C. Orsoni, eds. Simp. Inter. Oftalm. Ped.: CEM 1974;96–101.

Takao, Y., Hayashi, H., Oshima, K. and Kitagawa, Y. B-scan ultrasonographic findings in eyes with the rush-type of active. Doc. Ophth. Proc. Series 1987;48:437–441.

Terry, T.L. Extreme prematurity and fibroplastic of persistent vascular sheath behind each cristalline lens. Am. J. Ophthalmol. 1942;25:203–204.

Treese, M.T. Visual results and prognostic factors for vision following surgery for stage V retinopathy of prematurity. Ophthalmology 1986;93:574–579.

Catania University
Institute of Ophthalmology
Catania, Italy

3.6. The Analysis of Radiofrequency Ultrasonic Echosignals for Intraocular Tumors

E. MOTOLESE, A. BARTOLOMEI, G. ADDABBO,
R. FREZZOTTI S. ROCCHI,* A. FORT* and L. MASOTTI*

(Siena and Florence, Italy)*

Abstract. An algorithm has been developed for spectral analysis of backscattered radiofrequency signals. It has been tested on a tissue model, a gel suspension of calibrated latex spheres (between 20 and 100 μm in diameter), and on malignant intraocular tumours. The results so far appear promising regarding tissue differential diagnosis.

Key words: Radiofrequency ultrasonic signal, spectral map, intraocular tumor.

Introduction

Since its introduction into ophthalmology, ultrasonography has been used to differentiate various intraocular tumors and related lesions and to calculate tumor thickness to monitor the growth pattern.

In the past it was helpful for diagnosis mainly in eyes with opaque media. But now, with the wide use of conservative treatments, ultrasonography plays a primary role in the management of intraocular tumors because the most effective treatment of an intraocular mass can considerably vary according to the type of tumor, tumor dimension, and its position inside the eye. In particular, the modern use of ultrasonography regards the evaluation of tumor size by a 3-D reconstruction, the characterization of tumor tissue, and the estimate of regression patterns and quiescence after conservative treatment.

Conventional ultrasonography, whose principal characteristics for intraocular tumors are well known, is not able to provide sufficient data regarding histological characterization and tissue structure because of the filtering and averaging processes of the backscattered signal, with ensuing loss of information; these processes are however necessary to visualize and analyse the signal by the ophthalmologists as it is done in A&B-mode.

To overcome this problem we have the possibility of analysing the features conveyed by the radiofrequency backscattered signal. Some of these features, depending on the mean size, shape, elastic properties, and concentration of

J.M. Thijssen, H.C. Fledelius and S. Tane (eds.), Ultrasonography in Ophthalmology 14, 137–142.

the scattering particles in the tumor mass, can be extracted from the estimate of the power spectrum density (PSD). The spectral PSD estimator we propose is based on the autoregressive (AR) modelling technique. This technique is intrinsically insensitive to the windowing side-lobe effects. As a consequence, the centroid frequency estimate is meaningful also when the number of samples of the radiofrequency signal is drastically reduced allowing a local characterization of inhomogeneous media.

The above mentioned aspects make the AR technique particularly suitable for the online production of pathological maps based on spectral parameters.

The use of "Spectral Maps" in the management of intraocular tumors will be of great importance not only to obtain a correct differential diagnosis among rather similar pathologies but also to evaluate the regression patterns of conservatively treated tumors.

Theoretical Framework

Usually, for tissue characterization the estimate of the power spectral density (PSD) of the backscattered ultrasonic echosignal is obtained via the periodogram technique. This is based on the FFT (fast Fourier transformation) performed on the sampled measured signal windows. Depite the wide range of applications, this approach bears two main limitations:
- an increase in the PSD estimation quality decreases the frequency resolution;
- the implicit windowing of the data causes "leakage effects" in the spectral domain that may obscure and distort weak signal spectral responses.

The above limitations are particularly troublesome when analysing short data records, as it is the case for a local tissue characterization. Therefore we have used an alternative spectral estimation procedure, based on the fitting of the measured data to an assumed model. The PSD estimation, in the context of modelling, becomes a three step procedure:

(1) Selection of a time series model describing the process (measured data);
(2) Estimation of the parameters of the assumed model;
(3) Substitution of the estimated parameters into the theoretical PSD implied by the model.

By this approach, more realistic assumptions are made on the measured process outside the considered interval, and data windowing is intrinsically eliminated. Thus the improvement over the conventional periodogram approach can be quite noticeable especially for short data records.

In the present paper an AutoRegressive (AR) model with unknown and noisy input was selected to describe the backscattered ultrasonic echosignal. This choice is particularly indicated since the estimate of the AR parameters results in solving a set of linear equations. Here the backscattered echo is described by an AR model of order p:

$$x(n) = \sum_{k=1}^{p} a_k x(n - k) + u(n)$$

where $x(n)$ represents the measured data and $u(n)$ is the unknown imput sequence. Hence, the power spectral density is:

$$P_{\mathrm{AR}}(f) = \frac{T\sigma_u^2}{|1 + \Sigma_{k=1}^p a_k e^{-j2\pi fkT}|^2}$$

where T is the signal sampling period and σ_u^2 is the variance of $u(n)$, assumed to be a zero mean, white noise process.

The filter order p is not a-priori known, and is selected in relation to the particular application. Here a small value of p is chosen, namely $p = 2$ or 3, the main interest being emphasizing the signal high energy frequency, regardless of the spectrum details. To evaluate the AR parameters the modified covariance method (MCM) has been used, which, independently of the selected AR order, exploits the information of the whole data sequence.

This method leads to a linear system of order $p = 1$ whose coefficient matrix has entries which are combinations of all the available data. By expressing it as sums and products of Toeplitz and Hankel matrices, a fast computational solution of the MCM exists, only requiring Np + 6p2 operations and N + 4p data storage, N being the number of data samples.

This aspect makes the algorithm particularly suitable for real time application in the biomedical field.

The spectral maps based on the processing technique presented above are produced considering a set of RF backscattered signals obtained by linear or sectorial scan. Each echo line is divided into windows corresponding to tissue segments.

Second and third order AR models are used to estimate the PSD centroid. Finally a bidimensional spectral image is produced by associating the centroid value to a gray level or to a color coded scale.

Experimental Results

For ophthalmological clinical practice, differentiation is required between tissues characterized by particles with mean dimensions ranging from about 20 μm to 100 μm.

Commonly these tissues are investigated by conventional ultrasonography using ultrasonic transducers characterized by a central frequency of 10 MHz which implies a wavelength of 150 μm, which is well above the mean particle diameters. This choice is determined as a compromise between good resolution and low attenuation of ultrasonic waves in tissue.

For an experimental validation of the proposed technique a laboratory set-up was carried out using test-objects consisting of gel suspension of calibrated latex spheres (with diameters of 20–50–80–100 μm).

A linear scanning was performed on the test objects to gather the radio-

Fig. 1

MAPS A

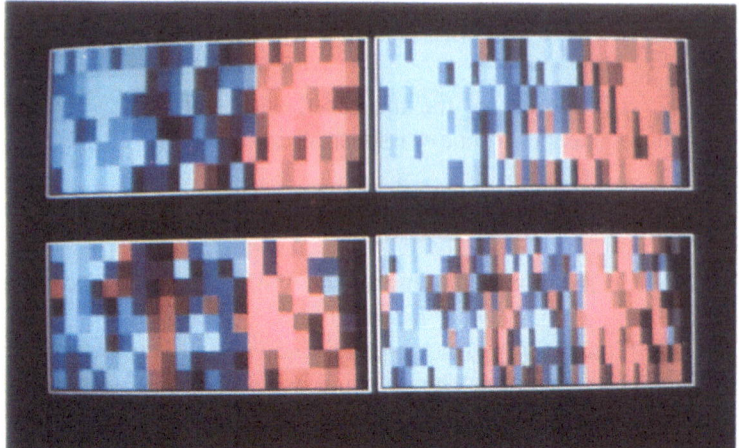

MAPS B

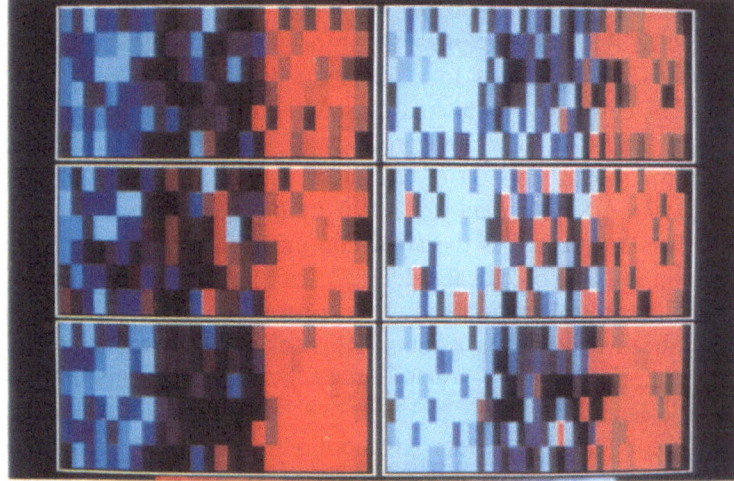

Fig. 2

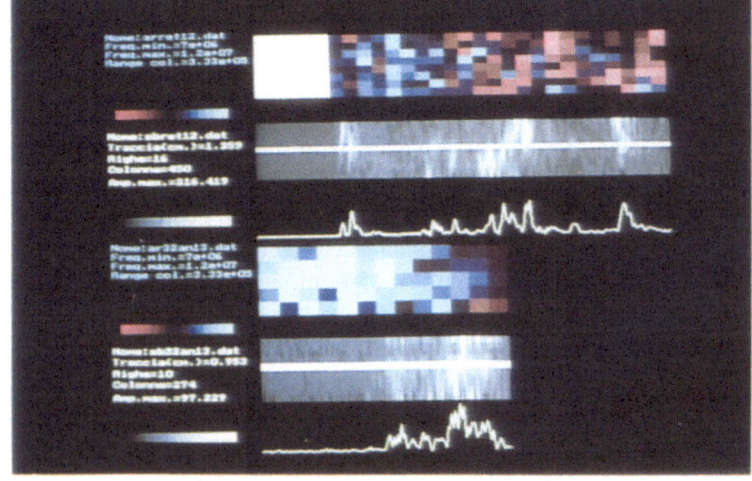

frequency signals that were digitized and stored in a computer memory for subsequent processing.

A wide band focused transducer (PANAMETRICS V311) was used; the technical characteristics were: −6 dB bandwidth of 7 MHz, central frequency equal to 9.9 MHz, −12 dB focal spot of 0.8 mm at the distance of 35 mm.

Finally, we have performed acquisitions with the same experimental set-up on eyes enucleated for intraocular tumors (malignant choroidal melanoma and retinoblastoma) using a linear scanning with a 4 mm step.

The B-mode image generated from the set of RF signals was useful to detect the signal's pattern regarding the pathological region from which the echosignals were extracted.

The spectral maps were simultaneously displayed with the B-mode images, preserving the topological references. Examples are shown in Fig. 1 (phantoms) and Fig. 2 (tumors).

A complete diagnostic tool has thus been obtained since the B-mode images exploit the information related to the echo amplitude, while the spectral maps outline the frequency dependence of the backscattered echoes.

This enables the differentiation between various pathological zones which with the conventional imaging technique are not resolved.

Conclusions

Usually the extraction of an ultrasonic spectral signature for the characterization of pathologic tissue is troublesome due to the complex nature of the biological media.

Hence, a spectral imaging technique is developed. Probably it will lead to the extraction of pathological features when the displayed information is filtered and interpreted by the physicians' experience.

The spectral images are based on the estimate of the power spectrum density (PSD) centroid frequency, which is related to the average scatterer

---

Figure 1 Spectral maps based on frequency centroid evaluation by AR estimators The maps are related to a fictitious tissue, made up of three zones containing scatterers with diameters of 20 μm, 50 μm, 80 μm, respectively Maps (A) are obtained analyzing simulated signals, Maps (B) are obtained by assembling spectral maps coming from 3 different test objects, consisting of a gel suspension of latex spheres of respectively 20 μm, 50 μm, 80 μm In the maps at the left a pixel corresponds to a 500 μm tissue segment (sequence of 64 data samples), in those at the right it corresponds to 250 μm (32 data samples)

Figure 2 Spectral maps based on frequency centroid evaluation by AR estimators related to two different intraocular tumors The upper one derived from a retinoblastoma, the lower one derived from a choroidal malignant melanoma The spectral maps clearly differentiate the two different pathologies

size. Spectral autoregressive estimators are propoosed for the PSD centroid evaluation.

The AR estimators, being intrinsically insensitive to the windowing side-lobe effects are suitable for local characterization of the investigated inhomogeneous media as well as for real time implementation.

The spectral maps emphasize both the average value of the scatterers size and degree of local inhomogeneity of the investigated pathology, thus providing an easy and effective diagnostic tool.

References

Cheung, A.T., Buchen, P.W., Macaskill, C. and Robinson, D.E. Backscattered spectrum of a randomly perturbed regular array of discrete scatterers. J. Acoust. Soc. Am. 1989;86(1):40.

Fort, A., Manfredi, C., Masotti, L. and Rocchi, S. Spectral maps by AR models as a support to conventional ultrasonic imaging. Proc. EUSIPCO 1992. Bruxells 24–27 August, 1992 in press.

Insana, M.F., Wagner, R.F., Brown, D.G. and Hall, T.J. Describing small-scale structure in random media using pulse echo ultrasound. J. Acoust. Soc. Am. 1990;87(1):179.

Kay, S.M. and Marple, S.L. Spectrum analysis – A modern perspective. IEEE Proc. 1981;69(1):1380.

Lizzi, F.L., Greenbaum, M., Feleppa, E.J. and Elbaum, M. Theoretical framework for the spectrum analysis in ultrasound tissue characterization. J. Acoust. Soc. Am. 1983;73(4):1366.

Lizzi, F.L., Ostromogilsky, M., Feleppa, E.J., Rorke, M. and Yaremko, M.M. Relationship of the ultrasound spectral parameters to features of tissue microstructure. IEEE Trans. on UFFC 1986;33(1):319.

Marple, S.L. Digital spectral analysis with applications. Prentice Hall. Englewood Cliffs, N.J. 1987.

Ueda, M. and Ichikawa, H. Analysis of an echosignal reflected from a weakly scattering volume by a discrete model of the medium. J. Acoust. Soc. Am. 1981;70(6):1768.

Wang, T., Saniie, J. and Jin, X. Analysis of low order autoregressive-models for ultrasound grain signal characterization. IEEE Trans. on UFFC 1991;38(2):116.

Dr. E. Motolese
Institute of Ophthalmology and Neurosurgical Sciences
University of Siena
Italy

3.7. Atypical Retinoblastomas

V. MAZZEO, P. PERRI, P. MONARI, L. RAVALLI and
M. CHIARELLI

(Ferrara, Italy)

Abstract. More cases of atypical retinoblastomas are documented, primarily characterized by the lack of calcifications. We presented our first case in 1984, a diffusely infiltrating form of retinoblastoma with dense vitreous opacities. Recently two other forms came to our attention. The first one looked like a complete retinal detachment. The other appeared as a cauliflower solid mass with a pedunculate distal part that oscillated around its stalk with eye movements. All these cases were detected in children older than 5 years.

Key words: Retinoblastoma, atypical, retinoblastoma without calcification

Introduction

In 1987 one of us (V.M.) reviewed the echographic literature concerning the presence of calcifications in Retinoblastomas (RB). The percentages reported ranged from 81 to 100%. A table containing the acoustic characteristics of non-calcified RB was published (Table 1). In the same year we reported our first case of noncalcified RB [8].

At SIDUO XI Abraham et al. (1990) reported that califications were evident only in 18 eyes among the 42 with RB [1]. In the same paper they described the case of a large necrotic tumour strictly resembling a vitreous hemorrhage, as did Lombardi et al. (1990) at the same meeting [5].

A masquerading syndrome was described in a 9-year-old girl who finally underwent enucleation. Both cases dealt with diffuse infiltrating RB.

Recently Nemeth et al. (1992) reported an unusual echographic form of diffuse RB that gave origin to a funnel shaped retinal detachment where the retina was enormously thickened while the vitreous and subretinal space appeared acoustically empty [7].

In our review of 16 RB seen during the past 17 years we have encountered three cases of non-calcified RB. The fourth case deals with a 5 month old girl who harboured a de hovo complex chromosome translocation and was

J.M. Thijssen, H.C. Fledelius and S. Tane (eds.), Ultrasonography in Ophthalmology 14. 143–147.
© 1995 *Kluwer Academic Publishers, Dordrecht.*

Table 1. Echographic characteristics of retinoblastoma without calcifications (A- and B-scan)

Diffused necrotic form	Mobile echoes in the vitreous Low to medium reflectivity Irregular coat at the site of the retina
Other diffused forms	Total or partial retinal detachment in which the retina "disappears" in the tumour, with acoustically clear vitreous and subretinal space Single or multiple masses, even pedunculated Irregular internal reflectivity

lost to follow-up after enucleation [2]. The patient returned after 4 years with a new tumour which looked like a diffuse infiltrating form.

Material

Case 1 was fully desribed in SIDUO X proceedings [3].

Case 2 deals with a 7-year-old boy who had complained of blurred vision for 6 months. A diagnosis of phacomatosis had been suggested elsewhere. Visual acuity was hand movements. Slit-lamp of the anterior segment was normal. Fundoscopy revealed a large dilated vessel going from the disk toward the inferior temporal quadrant where a solid whitish mass was present along with a satellite serous detachment.

On echography the solid mass showed a medium reflectivity. The detached retina was thickened and showed only very little after-movements. The subretinal space was acoustically empty.

An aqueous puncture was then performed to evaluate both LDH level and cellularity. The enzyme titer was only slightly elevated in comparison to serum and no cells were found.

The patient was sent home for close follow-up, but he was lost for two controls. When he returned, ultrasonically the detached retina had increased its thickness, its surface towards the choroid was highly irregular, and the subretinal space was still empty. The solid mass had increased in volume and its internal reflectivity decreased (Fig. 1). The eye was enucleated and an undifferentiated RB with necrotic areas was found.

Case 3. Male, 6-year-old. For two months the mother had seen a kind of 'peek-a-boo' white mass through the pupil. At initial examination, a diagnosis of vitreous cyst had been made. Visual acuity was 1.0. On slit lamp examination the anterior segment was normal; through the dilated pupil vitreous seeding was clearly visible and a solid white roundish mass moving with eye movements could be seen.

On echography the lesion had a pedunculated appearance, being composed of two parts: one was arising from the retina; it had a cauliflower

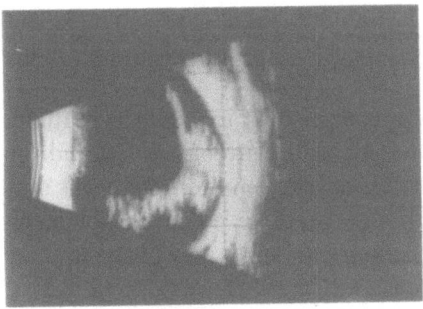 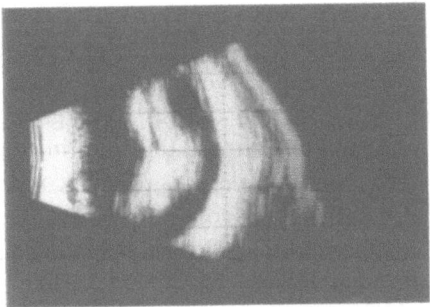

Figure 1. RB of the diffuse form causing an almost complete retinal detachment. The retina is enormously thickened but still shows aftermovements. Vitreous and subretinal spaces are acoustically empty.

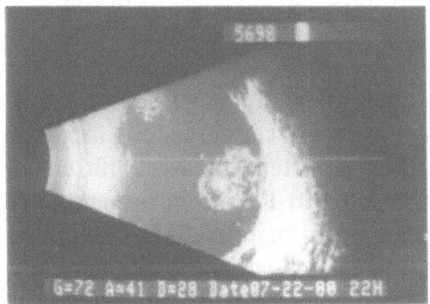 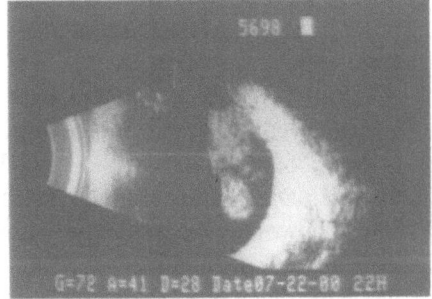

Figure 2. RB in a 6-year-old boy. On the left: cauliflower-like solid lesion. Vitreous seeding is present near the lesion. On the right: longitudinal section of the same lesion showing a very irregular "sausage-like" lesion. A solid oval lesion is connected through a thin stalk to the lesion attached to the eye wall. The distal part of the lesion oscillated on its stalk.

shape. The other was connected to the first through a short collar. It was oval and moving on its axis. Tumour debris was found surrounding the mass (Fig. 2).

Discussion

In 1987 after describing our case of the diffuse type of RB, we stated that "this atypical echographic behaviour of RB should be considered one of the possible echographic types of this tumour".

Our case was very similar to the ones described by Abraham *et al.* [1] and Lombardi *et al.* [5] while quite different from the one described by Nemeth *et al.* [7].

Their case is more similar to our case number two. In both cases the tumoral retina was thickened and detached; the main difference between the two cases was the presence of small aftermovements of the retina in our case, even at a very advanced stage before enucleation. No aftermovements were present in Nemeth *et al.*'s case.

While in the diffuse type, giving origin to a masquerading syndrome, moving particles are the rule, in the other type the vitreous cavity and the subretinal space can be found acoustically clear. These peculiar patterns may depend on the amount of necrosis that produces seeding and/or haemorrhage. Inflammatory exudation, haemorrhage and tumour debris may have the same echopattern.

Case three seems to have more peculiar clinical features. It deals with a solid lesion with aftermovements. Two mushroom-like RB were already described by Kerman and Fishman in 1984 [4]. To the best of our knowledge our case is the first one described with this sausage-like appearance.

Apart from the complete absence of calcifications these cases have another peculiar clinical pattern: they all deal with children older than 5 years. Carol Shields *et al.* (1991) reported that the average patient's age at diagnosis of retinoblastoma is 24 months in unilateral cases and 13 months in bilateral cases [9].

Almost 90% of all patients with retinoblastoma are diagnosed before the age of 5 years. Shields and coworkers pointed out certain unique aspects in a group of older patients with RB. They reported 26 cases with clinical histories and features similar to the non-calcified RB we have mentioned. They, however, did not report any echographic features. Accordingly, we may infer that either they had not undergone echographic examination, or the acoustic characteristics were not pathognomonic for RB (otherwise they would have been correctly diagnosed.

References

[1] M Abraham, M Sriram, S M Oke, Ch Abraham and S S Bradinath Ultrasonography in intraocular tumours Ultransonography in Ophthalmology 12 R Sampaolesi (ed), Kluwer Academic Publishers, 1990,269–279

[2] E Calzolari, P Palazzi, V Aiello, V Mazzeo, P Perri, A Minelli, L Del Senno, P Patracchini and F Bernardi De novo complex autosomal translocation involving chromosomes 8, 13 and 15 in a girl with a sporadic retinoblastoma Human Genetics 1987,77 51–54

[3] G Galli, P Perri and V Mazzeo Retinoblastoma of the diffused type on the A and B-scan K C Ossoinig (ed), Ophthalmic Echography Martinus Nijhoff - Dr W Junk Publishers, Dordrecht, 1987,419–423

[4] B M Kerman and M L Fishman Non melanomatous collar-button tumors, K C Ossoinig (ed), Ophthalmic Echography Martinus Nijhoff – Dr W Junk Publishers, Dordrecht, 1987,413–416

[5] A Lombardi, L A Irarrazaval, J O Croxatto, R Hulsbus, R Fernandez Meijide and E S Malbran Ultrasonographic findings in selected cases of masquerading syndrome Ultrasonography in Ophthalmology 12 R Sampaolesi (ed), Kluwer Academic Publishers, 1990,313–319

[6] V Mazzeo Ecografia dell'apparato oculare Testo Atlanta Fogliazza (ed), Milano, 1987 264–269

[7] J Nemeth, A Szabo and M Vegh Unusual echographic form of retinoblastoma Acta Ophthalmologica Suppl 204, Vol 70 Ophthalmic Ultrasound 1992 107–109

[8] P Perri, F Marozzi, P Monari and V Mazzeo Su due casi di retinoblastoma non calcifico Atti IV Congresso Nazionale Otalmologia Pediatrica O I C Medical Press, 1987,201–206

[9] C L Shields, J A Shields, P Shah Retinoblastoma in older children Ophthalmology 1991,98/3 395–399

University Eye Clinic of Ferrara
Ferrara
Italy

3.8. Ultrasonic Diagnosis in Breast Carcinoma Metastatic to the Choroid
Clinical Experience from 20 Cases

B. ANHALT, CH. JACKISCH, B. AWE, S. CLEMENS, and
H. BUSSE

(Munster, Germany)

Abstract. The present report summarizes the experience with ultrasonic examination of the eye in 20 cases of ocular metastases from our clinic 1977–91. Ultrasonography appears as the most useful, non-invasive test in early diagnosis of disease dissemination and an efficient means of following palliative treatment, and therefore helpful also for the oncologist in establishing an adequate therapy regimen in treatment of breast carcinoma. In 11 of the 20 the uveal metastasis represented the first clinical evidence of hematogeneous generalization.

Key words: Uveal metastasis, breast cancer dissemination, ultrasonography.

Introduction

Though metastatic cancer is generally recognized as the most common form of intraocular malignant tumor in adults, in many clinics the role of ocular examination is ignored.

Ocular metastases have been known for more than a century. In 1872 Perls reported a metastatic lung carcinoma in the eye, and in 1884 the first known metastatic breast cancer to the eye was reported [8].

We reviewed our clinical experience in 20 patients from 1977–1991 with breast cancer metastatic to the uvea in order to study the role of ultrasonic examination in the early diagnosis of hematogenous generalisation and to evaluate the optimal management of palliative oncologic treatment

Materials and Methods

From December 1977 until March 1991, 20 female patients were examined at our Department of Ophthalmology, University Münster, because of suspicion of choroidal metastasis. All patients had ophthalmological symtoms, in 19 of the 20 cases with relation to known breast carcinoma.

The patients underwent complete ophthalmic evaluation including clinical history, slit-lamp and fundus examination, A- and B-scan ultrasonography, and fluorescein angiography (Figs. 1–3). In more than 90% the diagnosis

J M Thijssen, H C Fledelius and S Tane (eds), Ultrasonography in Ophthalmology 14, 148–152

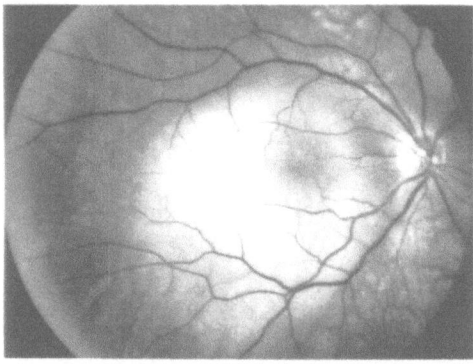

Figure 1 Fundus photograph of a posterior choroidal tumor in the right eye of a 37 year-old woman with breast carcinoma diagnosis one year before

was found by non-invasive means: history, ophthalmoscopy, and ultrasonography.

In our ultrasonic examinations we looked for the known differential diagnosis criteria for metastatic, choroidal tumors. In A-scan for the medium to high reflectivity and climbing posterior spike, in B-scan for the missing excavation and the quiet zone or orbital shadow.

Results

For our 20 patients with choroidal metastases the average age at cancer diagnosis was 47 years. At ocular diagnosis it was 49 years. The median interval from primary to choroidal metastasis was 2.8 years (range from 5 months to 7 years) and the median survival after ocular diagnosis 15.6 months (range from 2 months to 4.8 years). These figures are in accord with literature [2, 6].

Only one case dealt with an unknown breast cancer at the time of ocular diagnosis of metastasis. In more than 50% (11 cases) the ocular symptoms were the first representation of hematogenous generalisation.

The most common presenting symptom of our 20 patients was defective vision, followed by reduced visual field, detached retina and pain. With 15 left to 12 right cases, in this study the left eye was not significantly more often involved. The incidence of bilateral metastasis was 35% (17 cases).

As known from literature, the posterior pole has a predisposition of neoplastic metastasis [6]. In 13 patients we found the lesion in the posterior fundus. Further, the temporal retina between the vascular arcades was over-represented. The average tumor height was 2.7 mm, range from 0.05 to 8 mm.

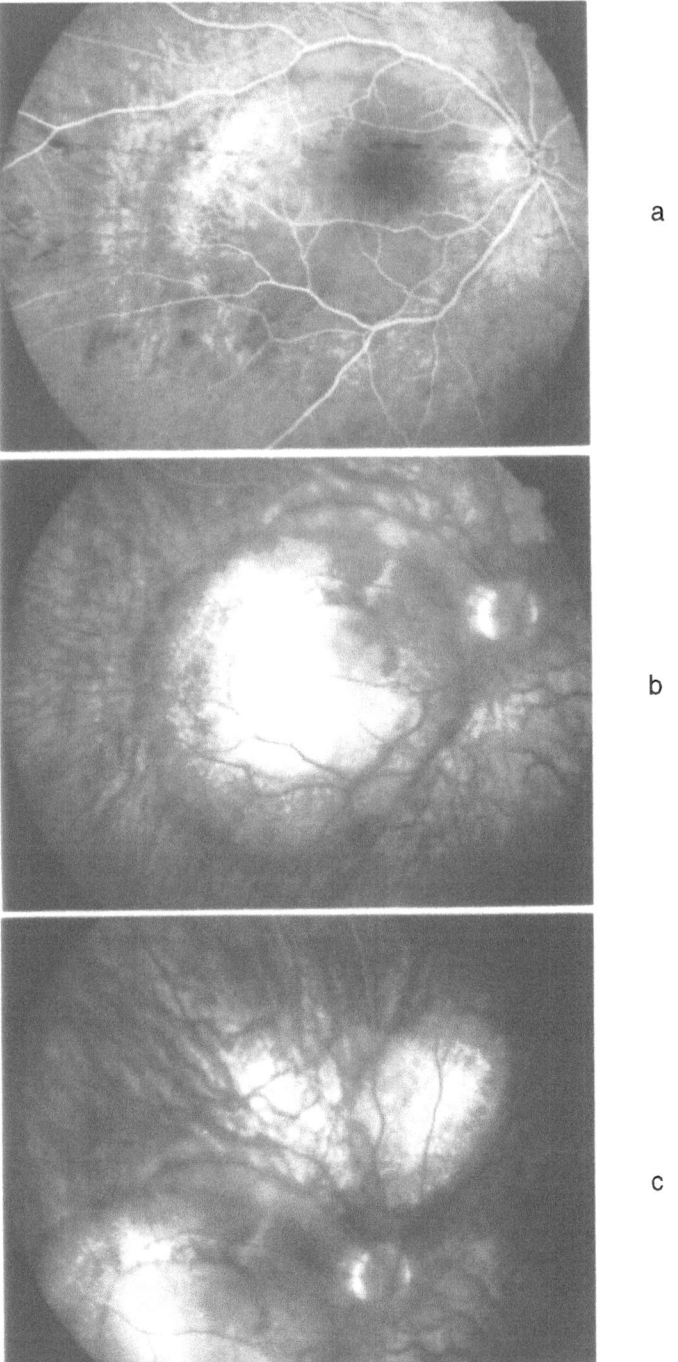

a

b

c

Figure 2. Fluorescein photograph of the central metastatic lesion of the right fundus; top, in arterial phase; two pictures at bottom, in late phase (same tumours as in Figs. 1 and 3).

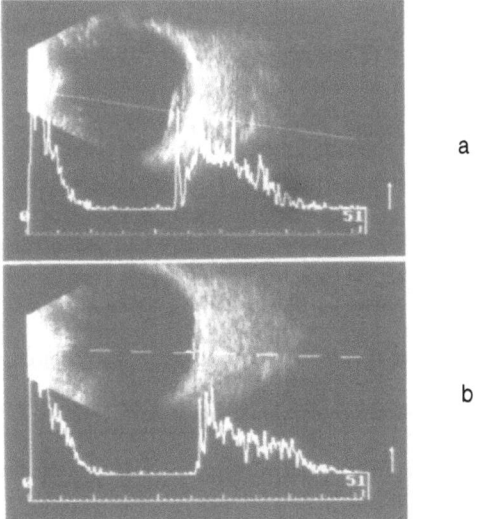

Figure 3 A- and B-scan ultrasonogram of the metastatic tumor of the choroid, before and 3 weeks after irradiation and chemotherapy

Discussion

In females, 85% of the metastatic tumors of the uvea were primarily situated in the breast, while in men, 47% originated from the lung, as reported in a literature study in our clinic of 745 cases [9]. The incidence of such lesions in patients with known malignancies elsewhere have ranged from 0.07% to 12% in clinical or postmortem studies [1].

All patients with ultrasound examination showed most of the typical diagnostic criteria for choroidal metastasis: the variation of the reflectivity and the climbing posterior spike (A-scan) on the one hand, on the other hand the missing choroidal excavation (as differentiation towards malignant melanoma) and finally the orbital shadow [3, 4, 7].

With these characteristics respected, the reliability of ultrasonography in choroidal tumor diagnosis is near 90% [5]. Together with other methods, including the newer techniques of ultrasound, in about 90% differentiation can be made between choroidal metastasis and malignant melanoma.

Even today the prognosis at the time of ocular metastasis is poor. So we should find the best palliative way of therapy for, as indicated by our study, the remaining average 15 months of life. In our follow-up of 11 patients/15 eyes, it was possible with irradiation and/or chemotherapy in 10 of 15 eyes to improve or stabilize the visual acuity for the short average life expectancy.

To save our patients from painful diagnostic procedures and useless treatments, we need an early and exact staging of the choroidal lesions. Therefore, ocular examination including atraumatic methods like ultrasonography is our recommendation to the oncology teams in patients where metastases are suspected.

References

[1] R S Bloch and S Gartner The incidence of ocular metastatic carcinoma Arch Ophthalmol 1971,85 673–675

[2] J D Bullock, M D Facs and B Yanes Ophthalmic manifestations of metastatic breast cancer Ophthalmology 1980,87 961–973

[3] S Chang and D J Coleman Ultrasonography of vitreoretinal disease Company, NY, 1988, pp 404–428

[4] D J Coleman, D H Abramson, R L Jack and L A Franzen Ultrasonic diagnosis of tumors of the choroid Arch Ophthalmol 1974,91 344–354

[5] D J Coleman Reliability of ocular tumor diagnosis with ultrasound Tr Am Acad Ophth Otol 1986,77 677–683

[6] A P Ferry and R L Font Carcinoma metastatic to the eye and orbit Arch Ophthalmol 1974,92 276–286

[7] R Guthoff Ultraschall in der ophthalmologischen diagnostik Enke, Stuttgart, 1988

[8] J Hirschberg and A Birnbacher Ueber metastatischen aderhautkrebs Albrecht v Graefe's Arch Ophthal 1884,30 113–122

[9] H P Schiffer, H Busse and J Weihmann Karzinommetastasen in der Aderhaut Klin Mbl Augenheilk 1978,173 195–207

Dr B Anhalt
Department of Ophthalmology
University of Munster
Munster, Germany

3.9. Analysis of Ocular Circulatory Kinetics in Glaucoma by the Ultrasonic Doppler Method

AKEMI TOMATSU, MASAYA HIRATA and SADANAO TANE

(Kawasaki, Japan)

Abstract. Sixty patients with varying degrees of glaucomatous visual field damage had their vascularity in a fundus artery and in a branch of the ophthalmic artery evaluated by an ultrasound Doppler method. They were compared to 17 cases of simple optic atrophy and to 30 normal controls. Decreased vascularity dynamics appeared to occur with increasing glaucoma damage.

Key words: Ocular haemodynamics, Doppler ultrasound method, glaucoma, visual field damage, excavation of optic disc, optic atrophy.

Introduction

The present study was performed to elucidate some aspects of ophthalmic hemodynamics related to progress in the pathological course of primary open angle glaucoma (POAG), using an ultrasonic Doppler method. The correlation was evaluated between blood flow velocity obtained from flow velocity pulses of a fundus artery (FA), primarily the central retinal artery, as well as the peripheral frontal medial artery, of a branch of the ophthalmic artery, and visual field disorder, pulse rise time and the degree of optic cupping.

Material and Methods

The study was performed on 60 cases (100 eyes of 28 male and 32 female subjects aged 20–70 years, the G group) with primary open angle glaucoma, 17 cases of simple optic atrophy (19 eyes of 11 male and 6 female subjects, the A group). As control, 30 normal subjects of matching age (60 eyes, the N group) were included. The G group was further subdivided into G1, G2, G3 classification of stages I–IIa, IIb–IIIa, IIIb–IV, and V–VI, respectively, according to the extent of glaucomatous visual field disorder (Kosaki classification).

J.M. Thijssen, H.C. Fledelius and S. Tane (eds.), Ultrasonography in Ophthalmology 14, 153–155.
© *1995 Kluwer Academic Publishers, Dordrecht.*

Acccording to the vertical cup/disc ratio (D/C ratio) showing the degree of glaucomatous atrophy of the optic disc, the group was further divided into g1 and g2 groups, for C/D ratio of 30–60% and 60–90% respectively.

The ultrasonic Doppler diagnostic device used for the study was Vasoflo-3; the frequency of the transducer was 4.0 MHz.

The pulses of ophthalmic blood flow velocity were measured in the fundus artery (FA) on the disc surface and ophthalmic artery (OA) in the peripheral ophthalmic artery. To measure flow velocity pulses of OA, the probe was applied to the skin surface of the superior medial wall of the orbit. For the measurement in the FA, a hollow cylindrical eye cap was used and the measurement was made via the corneal surface. The parameters used for analysis were: mean frequency (Mean F) from the average of two heart beats in FA and OA, and pulse rise time (PRT), i.e. the time from end-diastole to systole. To minimize fluctuation between individuals, the ratio of FA to OA was taken, and the blood flow velocity was calculated from Mean F. The ratio of Mean F between FA and OA was used as fundus blood flow index [V(FA/OA)], and the ratio by PRT was used as pulse rise time index [T(FA/OA)].

The study was performed to evaluate the correlation between V(FA/OA) and staging by visual field (Kosaki classification) and the stage according to T(FA/OA) and C/D ratio.

Results

We found a significant inverse correlation between V(FA/OA) and the degree of visual field disorder (Kosaki classification). In A group and G group, the values in FA were lower than those of OA compared with N group. Significant difference from the N group was noted in A group and G group ($p < 0.01$). Among the cases of the G group, many cases with severe visual field disorder due to late or terminal glaucoma showed remarkable decrease in FA compared with the N group. T(FA/OA) revealed a significant inverse correlation with the C/D ratio. PRT in FA was shorter in the G group than in N group or A group; a significant difference ($P < 0.01$) from the G group was found in the N group and the A group.

Discussion

In order to identify the results of our analysis of ophthalmic hemodynamics in the cases of glaucoma in terms of pathological stages, we used the ultrasonic Doppler method. The sites of measurement were fundus artery (FA) and ophthalmic artery (OA).

It is considered that FA plays an important role in supplying blood flow into the eye in the vascular system of the optic nerve, and our OA value is interpreted as showing blood flow in the ophthalmic artery. It is assumed that fundus blood flow velocity index V(FA/OA) and pulse rise time T(FA/OA) provide important indices to elucidate hemodynamics in the cases of glaucoma.

Compared with normal controls (N), V(FA/OA) decreased in the A group (simple optic atrophy) and in the G group (glaucoma) as well. This means that blood flow velocity in the fundus artery had a trend to decrease and was related to a filling defect of capillaries on the optic disc, suggesting circulatory disorder of the optic nerve.

The decrease of V(FA/OA) was linearly correlated to the degree of visual field disorder. Obviously, the circulatory disorder, i.e. one of the causes of glaucoma, tended to progress in parallel to the development of a pathological course. Compared with the N group, T(FA/OA) decreased in the G group; this trend became more conspicuous with the increase of C/D ratio. Again, this may reflect the blood flow condition of blood vessels relatively stenosed and bent by the progress of disease at the site of the optic cup. In the A group, no decrease of T(FA/OA) was found, and there was an apparent difference in blood flow pulse near the optic disc comparing simple optic atrophy and glaucomatous optic atrophy associated with optic disc cupping.

It appears that optic disc cupping, one of the causes of glaucoma, may mechanically influence the blood flow in the central retinal artery and this shortens the PRT.

It is interesting that, the more advanced the stage of glaucoma is, the stronger this trend appears to be.

There have been very few reports on glaucoma using the ultrasonic Doppler method. Our results suggest that this technique may represent a useful diagnostic approach for physiopathological studies of glaucoma in the near future.

Department of Ophthalmology
St. Marianna University School of Medicine
2-16-1, Sugao Miyamae-ku
Kawasaki-city, 216 Japan

3.10. High Resolution B-Mode Evaluation of Macular Holes

O. BERGES, C. BOSCHER, A. LEMOINE, J.Y. PERICHON,
Ph. GIRARD, O. LE QUOY, J.F. KOROBELNIK, D. BARON
and G. BRASSEUR

(Paris, France)

Abstract. High resolution ultrasound B-mode was performed in 62 patients who had manifest or impending macular holes. Changes in retinal contour or condensed posterior hyaloid were the main findings. Assessing the minute changes, ultrasound appeared superior to biomicroscopy, even when in the hands of experienced retinal surgeons.

Key words: Ultrasound, high resolution, retinal macular hole

Introduction

Recently, macular holes have become a challenge for the retinal surgeon. Indications of surgery are based on fundoscopy, fluorescein angiography and biomicroscopic evaluation of the vitreoretinal relationships [2, 3, 4, 5, 6].

In this multicentric study, the authors present the echographic findings of the macula and of the vitreo retinal relationships of macular holes (MH). They also want to stress the usefulness of echography in the planning of surgical treatment.

All the cases were seen in 4 centers (2 centers in Paris, Nantes and Rouen), but all the echograms were performed by O. Berges and C. Boscher.

Material and Methods

Our material includes 62 patients: 64 eyes with true macular holes and 27 eyes with impending macular holes, as listed in Table 1.

Clinical criteria of true macular holes included (1) a loss of visual acuity of 20/200 to 20/100, (2) in biomicroscopy, a macular hole surrounded by a rim of serous detachment of the neuro-epithelium, and (3) in fluorescein angiography, a window defect. The echograms evaluated the appearence of the macula plus the existence and extension of a posterior vitreous detachment, if present.

The technique utilized 2 orthogonal sections perpendicular to the macula and 2 orthogonal sections parallel to the macula (Fig. 1) as previously de-

J.M. Thijssen, H.C. Fledelius and S. Tane (eds.), Ultrasonography in Ophthalmology 14, 156–160.
© 1995 *Kluwer Academic Publishers, Dordrecht.*

Table 1. True and/or impending MH in the two eyes were evaluated

Bilateral True M.H.	**2**
True MH / Impending M.H.	**17**
True M.H. / Normal *	**43**
Impending M.H. / Normal *	**10**

*Normal appearance of the macula sometimes included subtle changes of the region.

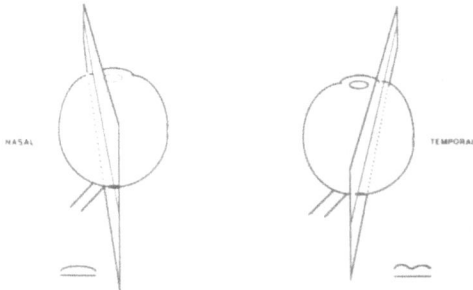

Figure 1. Drawing showing the usefulness of perpendicular and oblique ultrasonic beams to evaluate the macular region.

scribed [1]. The probe was placed directly on the conjunctiva to prevent any absorption of the ultrasound beam energy by the eye lid and to increase the signal-to-noise ratio. All the examinations were performed with an OPHTA-SCAN S machine by ALCON/BIOPHYSIC MEDICAL with a 10 MHz probe focused at 22 mm. Sections were performed at high sensitivity setting (usually 90 dB) and at tissue sensitivity settings (usually 76 dB) in all cases.

Results

US Appearence of True Macular Holes (64 eyes)
The US appearence of true MH is summarized in Fig. 2. There was a convex elevation of the macula, in all cases, corresponding to the serous detachment of the neuro-epithelium (Fig. 3). In 22 eyes, there was an excavation, central, or sometimes slightly excentric corresponding to the macular hole. In 24 eyes, the excavation was replaced by a slight diminution of density at the dome of the convexity. This is explained by the lack of spatial resolution of the probe in regards to the size of the hole itself. In 18 eyes, it was possible

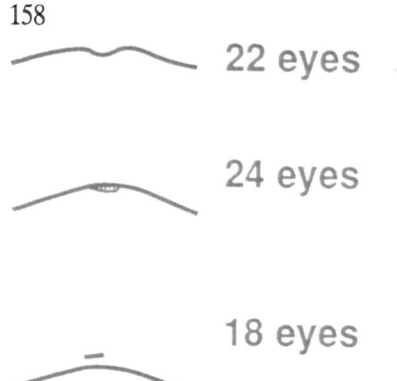

22 eyes

24 eyes

18 eyes

Figure 2. Echographic appearance of true macular holes.
9

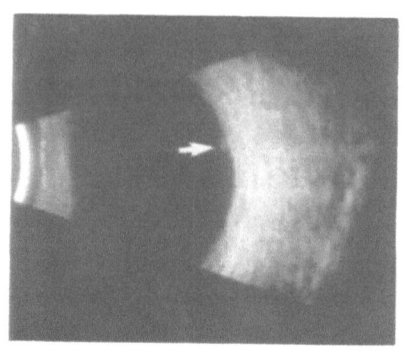

Figure 3. True macular hole. Slight elevation of the macula with a small central depression corresponding to the hole (→).

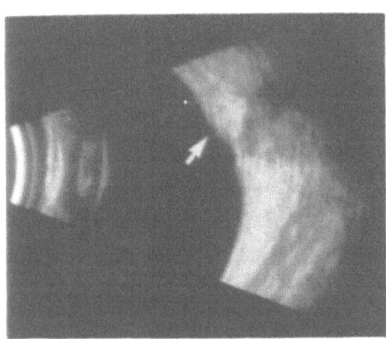

Figure 4. Operculum facing a macular hole (→).

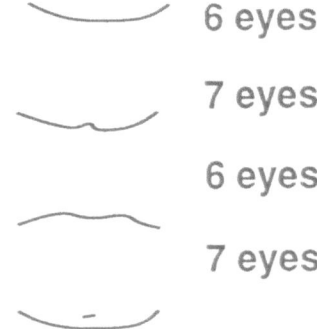

6 eyes

7 eyes

6 eyes

7 eyes

Figure 5. Echographic appearance of impending macular holes (27 years).

to detect some echogenic material facing the dome of the convexity. It was mainly a strongly reflecting retinal material (operculum), but in some cases (Fig. 4), it was considered only as a small part of the condensed hyaloid membrane, usually less reflective than the above retinal material.

US Appearance of Impending Macular Holes (27 eyes)
The US appearance of impending MH is summarized in Fig 5. The appearance of the macula was considered as smooth and normal in 6 eyes, slightly irregular in 7 eyes. In 6 eyes, an irregular elevation of the macula was demonstrated. In 7 eyes, it was possible to detect a reflective membrane in front of the macula, possibly of retinal or hyaloidal origin.

Table 2. Relation between posterior vitreous detachment and true macular holes, subdivided by echographer

	CB	OB	Total
• Total P.V.D	20	8	28
• Peripheric Partial P.V.D.	5	3	8
• Central Partial P.V.D.	5	3	8
• No P.V.D	13	7	20

Note the similarity of the results of the series evaluated by Boscher (C.B.) and Berges (C.B.).

Discussion

Differential Diagnosis

Differential diagnosis of macular holes has to include pseudo macular pseudo-hole, cystoid macular oedema, age related macular degeneration, and other macular lesions such as tumors, serous pigmented epithelium detachment, or localized retinal detachment.

The diagnosis of pseudo-hole due to epiretinal membranes is usually easy since it has not the convex appearance typical for detachment of the neuro-epithelium. It usually appears as a small linear membrane at the level of the macula.

Age-related macular degeneration is an easy diagnosis when the lesion is disciform since it usually appears more elevated, hypereflective and heterogenous, with an irregular surface without any central excavation. However, the atrophic form of age-related macular degeneration is sometimes difficult to separate from impending macular holes.

Cystoid macular oedema is usually very difficult to differentiate from macular holes since there is an elevation of the macula with sometimes the visualization of a central excavation.

The other macular lesions are usually not a difficult diagnosis.

Evaluation of Posterior Vitreous Detachment in Case of True Macular Holes and Impending Macular Holes

The results are summarized in Tables 2 and 3.

First of all, it is interesting to compare the results of the 2 echographists (C.B. and O.B.) and to realize that they are very similar. Secondly, it is interesting to note that total posterior vitreous detachement is much more frequent in case of true macular holes than in impending macular holes. Finally, echography proved to be superior to biomicroscopic evaluation in 3 of 6 of the 11 cases with peripheric partial posterior vitreous detachment, in the 14 cases with central partial PVD, and in 1 case of total posterior vitreous detachment. The biomicroscopic evaluations of the vitreous were all

Table 3. Relation between posterior vitreous detachment and impending macular holes. PVD is less frequently encountered in impending holes than in true macular holes

	CB	OB	Total
• Total P.V.D	2*	3	5
• Peripheric Partial P.V.D.	2	1	3
• Central Partial P.V.D.	3	4	6
• No P.V.D	10	3	13

performed by experienced retinal surgeons (CB, PhG, OLQ, JFK, GB). The technical problem is to ascertain the central partial posterior vitreous detachment really being central, since the angle with the surrounding wall usually cannot be shown. This is mainly due to the low reflectivity of the membrane and to the angle of incidence of the ultrasound beam.

In conclusion, high resolution B-mode of the macula proved to be efficient in evaluating and grading macular holes as well as to analyze the vitreo-retinal relationships. The superiority of ultrasound to biomicroscopic evaluation of total and central posterior vitreous detachment leads the authors to propose performing ultrasound examination as support for the planning of surgical treatment of macular holes.

References

[1] O. Berges and E. Nau. High resolution B Mode echography and colour Doppler (CDFI) of the macula. Acta Ophthalmologica. 1992(Suppl. 204);70:745.
[2] Sy. Cohen, G. Soubrane and G. Coscas. Les trous maculaires. J. Fr. Ophthalmol. 1989;12:477–488.
[3] J.D.M. Gass. Idiopathic senile macular holes. Its early stages and pathogenis. Arch. Ophthalmol. 1988;106:629–39.
[4] B.M. Glaser and coll. Transforming growth factor-B2 for the treatment of full thickness macular holes. Ophthalmology. 1992;99:1162–1172.
[5] D.R. Guyer and coll. Histopathologic features of idiopathic macular holes and cysts. Ophthalmology. 1990;97:1045–1051.
[6] W.E. Smiddy and coll. Vitrectomy for impending idiopathic macular holes. Retina. 1991;11:192–197.

Fondation A. de Rothschild
Paris
France

3.11. Contact B-Scan Ultrasound Evaluation of the Vitreoretinal Interface in Emmetropic and Normal Eyes

J.Y. PERICHON, J. UZZAN, M. DUCHAMP, S. AOUIDIDI,
O. BERGES* and G. BRASSEUR

(*Rouen and Paris*, France)

Abstract. Ultrasound characteristics of the posterior and peripheral vitreous structure was evaluated in a prospective study comprising 220 healthy emmetropic eyes from subjects aged 20–80 years. Normative data are given for vitreous detachments, partial and complete, and for giant vitreous lacunas.

Key words: Ultrasonography, posterior vitreous detachment, giant lacuna, emmetropia

Introduction

The evaluation of the vitreoretinal relationship can be achieved by biomicroscopic examination (90 D and the El Bayadi Kajiura lenses) and by ultrasound. Anyhow, the position of the posterior hyaloid membrane is sometimes difficult to assess whatever the lenses used.

We performed a contact B-scan ultrasonography on 220 emmetropic eyes without any ophthalmic diseases to study the vitreoretinal relationships in a population ranging from 20 to 80 years.

The *aim* of our prospective study was
– to establish a reliable examination method
– to define the ultrasonic characteristics and position and morphology of the vitreous body according to the age
– to define the criteria of differential diagnosis between posterior vitreous detachment (P.V.D.) and giant lacuna.

Material and Methods

Selection of the Patients

All patients were from neurology and E.N.T. departments. We excluded all those who had an eye disease (diabetic retinopathy, exudative age related macular degeneration, vitreous haemorrage, hyalitis, retinal detachment.) Then, we performed a biometry or a refraction. Included were only those

J M Thijssen, H C Fledelius and S Tane (eds), Ultrasonography in Ophthalmology 14, 161–168
© 1995 *Kluwer Academic Publishers, Dordrecht*

162

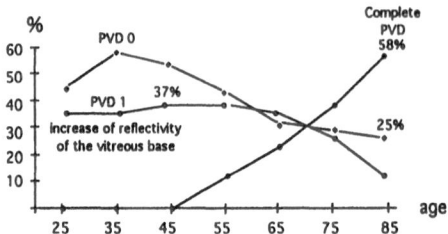

Figure 1. Graph showing the frequency of various types of posterior vitreous detachment with age, cf. text. PVD 0 = absence of PVD. PVD 1 = in one quadrant only.

with ocular axial lengths between 22.2 and 23.8 mm or with refraction between −2 and +2 diopters.

Technique

For this study we used the *mini B* machine by *Alcon Biophysic Medical*.
We performed all examinations in the same way:
– *maximum* gain,
– probe put directly on the *conjunctiva* and not through the lids, to get optimum reflectivity from the vitreous body,
– in supine position.
We performed for each eye
– *4 coronal* probe examining positions (one per quadrant),
– *4 meridian* probe examining positions,
– 1 horizontal and *para-axial* section, to avoid the lens artifacts for the study of the posterior pole,
– a *kinetic* examination when the diagnosis was difficult.

Results

The results are condensed in four graphs (Figs 1, 4, 5 and 9) and in five B-scan photos (Figs. 2, 3, 6, 7 and 8), to be discussed in the following.

Discussion

Partial and peripheral P.V.D. – high reflectivity of the vitreous base.
Coronal probe examining positions provide a very good *general* approach of the vitreous body position because they allow a very wide sectorial scan of the quadrant. They can detect a very partial and very peripheral P.V.D. The results are given in Fig. 1.
We found that 71 of the 220 examined eyes (32%) had such a very partial and very peripheral P.V.D. localized only at one quadrant, and with an incidence for the nasal sector, 51 of the 71 eyes (70%).

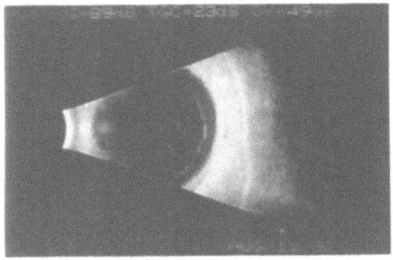
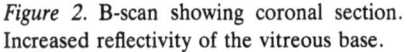
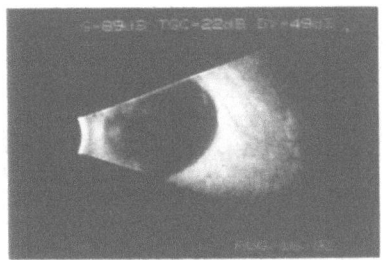

Figure 2. B-scan showing coronal section. Increased reflectivity of the vitreous base.

Figure 3. B-scan, meridian section. Vitreous base as in Fig. 2, increased reflectivity.

The percentage of this kind of P.V.D. is very high, 37 % for young subjects, then decreasing for older subjects because the frequency of the larger P.V.D. is increasing with age.

This kind of P.V.D. has always the same appearance:
- on a coronal section, the posterior hyaloid membrane always follows the curvature of the eye ball. The distance between this membrane and the retinal surface is always very short (Fig. 2).
- The posterior hyaloid membrane often has a high reflectivity compared with a usual P.V.D. with collapse for example. Moreover, it has often a relatively continuous appearance (Fig. 2).
- On a meridian section, its visualization at the level of the vitreous base is always very short and very localized (Fig. 3).

In fact, we suggest that these very partial and peripheral P.V.D.s are corresponding to a simple *increase of the reflectivity* of the vitreous base and not to a real P.V.D. because:
- In most cases (51/71 eyes – 70%), we detected them in the nasal quadrant. The frequency of real P.V.D. would certainly be higher in the superior quadrant.
- However, the reason we detected them predominantly in the nasal sector may be due to the fact that the examination of the other quadrants is more difficult because of the orbital walls and the nose.

Moreover, we performed a biomicroscopic examination in 20 of the 71 eyes with such a P.V.D. We detected a partial P.V.D. in 2 eyes only, whatever the lenses used. So this is probably a *normal variant* of the appearance of the vitreous base and not a real peripheral P.V.D.

Absence of P.V.D. – Partial P.V.D. – Complete P.V.D.
- The frequency of the absence of P.V.D. is progressively decreasing to reach 25% for patients over age 80 (Fig. 1). This percentage is higher than the one reported by most of the large biomicroscopic studies.
- The frequency of the complete P.V.D. is increasing very much for patients

164

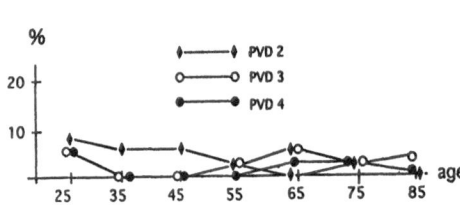

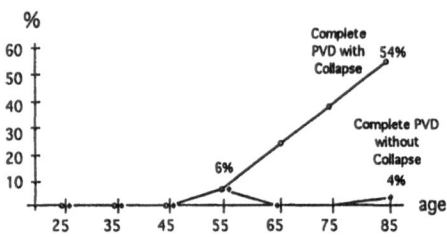

Figure 4. Posterior vitreous detachment, in 2, 3 or 4 quadrants (PVD 2, 3 or 4). The graph shows frequency and age.

Figure 5. PVD, with and without vitreous collapse, and the association with age.

over age 55 to reach 58% for patients over age 80 (Fig. 1). This percentage is clearly lower than the one reported by most of the large biomicroscopic studies.

– The frequency of the partial P.V.D. localized at 2, 3 and 4 quadrants, except the posterior pole, is staying very low whatever the age (Fig. 4). So, partial P.V.D. appear transitory.

Indirectly, therefore, Figs. 1 and 4 show us that the P.V.D extension into a complete P.V.D. is probably very quick.

Moreover, we found only one papillary attachment for a 65 year old man out of our 220 examinations. So like in other large biomicroscopic studies, ours seems to prove that the P.V.D. extension happens around age 60–65.

Complete P.V.D. with/without Collapse

With reference to the graph in Fig. 5, in most cases of complete P.V.D. (35/38 eyes – 92%), this extension ends up in a complete P.V.D. *with* collapse:

– The percentage of the complete P.V.D. *without* collapse is low whatever the age: 6% for patients 65 years old, 4% for patients over age 80.

– The percentage of the complete P.V.D. *with* collapse is increasing throughout to reach 54% for patients over age 80.

A prepapillary ring has been detected in 32 of the 38 cases (84%) of complete P.V.D. with or without collapse. Its appearance changed from a simple high reflective point along the posterior hyaloid membrane to a real ring. But in most of the cases, this prepapillary ring was not localized in front of the optic nerve. We never saw a prepapillary ring when there was not a complete P.V.D. So we believe that this is a specific sign of complete P.V.D. with or without collapse. But its absence does not imply that there is no P.V.D.

All our examinations were performed in the supine position, never in upright position. But when the vitreous body position was difficult to define, we always used a kinetic examination. So, in case of complete P.V.D., especially for the inferior sector, even when the vitreous body is directly applied on the retinal surface because of its weight, the posterior hyaloid

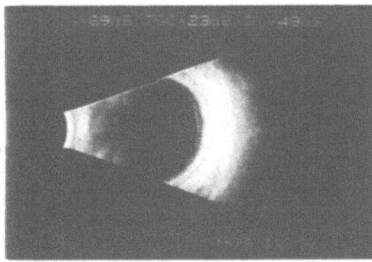

Figure 6. B-scan showing coronal section, common type of posterior detachment.

membrane becomes visible with the kinetic examination. Acoustically we can see an empty space between the retinal surface and the posterior hyaloid membrane. Therefore, we do believe that we have described the real frequency of complete P.V.D. for emmetropic and normal eyes in our study.

This frequency (58% for patients over age 80) is however clearly smaller than the one reported in most of the large biomicroscopic studies giving percentages ranging from 55 to 80%.

A few reasons to explain this:
- First, our study includes normal and emmetropic eyes only. The other studies always included myopic and pathologic eyes. This will markedly increase the frequency of P.V.D.
- Secondly, we believe that this over-estimation is partly due to the difficulty between P.V.D. and giant lacuna during a biomicroscopic examination. We did not have this problem because the visualization of the vitreous body of the emmetropic eye is easier than that of myopic eyes. So with the probe put directly on the conjunctiva, and not through the lids, we have clearly seen the echoes of the vitreous body except for 4 eyes. The ultrasonic differential diagnosis between P.V.D. and giant lacuna appeared relatively easy in the great majority of cases.

Ultrasonic Differential-Diagnosis between P.V.D. and Giant Lacuna
- In favour of a P.V.D. is the visualization on a coronal section of the posterior hyaloid membrane with an acoustically empty space behind it (B-scan, Fig. 6). This sign must always be confirmed by a meridian section where you *must* see the peripheral connection of the posterior hyaloid membrane to the retinal surface (B-scan, Fig. 7). This is the *only formal* sign of P.V.D.
- In favour of a giant lacuna is the absence of a peripheral connection of its posterior limit to the retinal surface and the presence of echoes behind it (Fig. 8). This last sign is not absolute because we have got a few cases of real P.V.D. with some echoes behind the posterior hyaloid membrane. But these cases are rare.

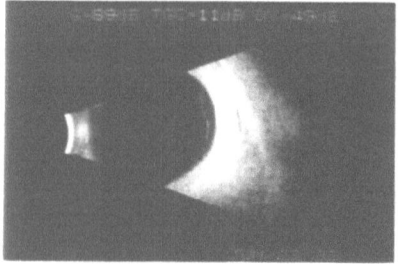

Figure 7. B-scan, meridan section. Connection between posterior hyaloid membrane and retinal surface.

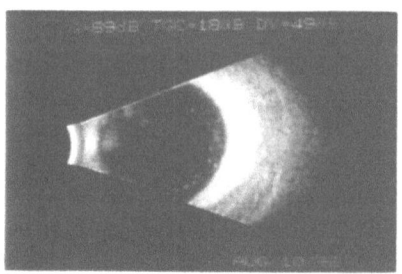

Figure 8. B-scan showing typical giant vitreous lacuna in a young male. There is a thick and relatively discontinuous posterior limit.

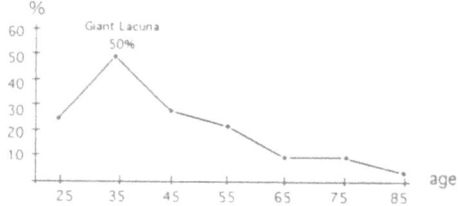

Figure 9. Graph on the occurrence of giant vitreous lacuna in emmetropic eyes, peak value in the early thirties, a marked decrease with age.

– Another criterion in favour of a giant lacuna is the appearance of its posterior limit. In most cases it is relatively less membrane-like and thicker than a posterior hyaloid membrane (Fig. 8).

Of course, all these signs are not absolute, and the examination for a giant lacuna is more difficult than the one of a real P.V.D. because a giant lacuna has not its own limit. This is contrary to a real P.V.D. where the posterior hyaloid membrane can easily be seen in emmetropic eyes.

Frequency of Giant Lacunas

The frequency of the giant lacunas is at its highest level (16/32 eyes – 50%) for young people between 30 and 40 years old. It is then decreasing when the P.V.D. becomes complete (Fig. 9).

Reflectivity of Vitreous Body

It is usually stated that the reflectivity of the vitreous is higher for old people. In the present study, however, the average level of the reflectivity of the vitreous body changed only little. It was highest for patients between 70 and 80 years old, when the P.V.D. becomes complete. But the variation of reflectivity was small only.

Conclusion

We performed a contact B-scan examination of the vitreous in 118 patients.

Because of poor cooperation, it was impossible to put the probe directly on the conjunctiva in 3 cases. So the examination could not be performed in ideal conditions, and these 3 patients have been excluded.

In five other cases, the vitreous body morphology was too difficult to define even by kinetic examination. In most of these cases there was a line with some echoes in front of and behind it, with all the characteristics of a posterior hyaloid membrane: appearance, connection, and movements. In these cases, we performed a biomicroscopic examination and there was always a complete P.V.D. So we suggest that the echoes behind the posterior hyaloid membrane are due to vitreous material which has escaped behind this membrane through a hole.

In conclusion, 5 among 115 patients is a very small percentage and for this reason we believe that contact B-scan ultrasonography makes the position and morphology of the vitreous body easier to define than by biomicroscopic examination of emmetropic eyes.

Summary

The evaluation of the vitreoretinal relationships can be achieved by biomicroscopic examination and by ultrasound. Several studies demonstrated a good agreement between ultrasound and biomicroscopy,

We analyzed 220 normal and emmetropic eyes in a population ranging from 20 to 80 years to evaluate the position of the posterior vitreous face (prospective study).

We found that:

- Most of the partial and peripheral P.V.D (71/220 eyes – 32%), especially those localized in the nasal quadrant, are rather corresponding to a simple increase of the reflectivity of the vitreous base and not to a real P.V.D.
- The frequency of the absence of P.V.D. is progressively decreasing with age. Only 25% of subjects over age 80 escape P.V.D.
- The frequency of the partial P.V.D. localized at 2, 3 and 4 quadrants, except the posterior pole, is staying low whatever the age. These partial P.V.D.s are transitory.
- The frequency of complete P.V.D. is increasing markedly for patients over age 55 to reach 58% for patients over age 80. This percentage is clearly lower than reported in most biomicroscopic studies. Like these, ours seems to prove that the P.V.D. extension happens around age 60–65. In most cases of complete P.V.D. (35/38 eyes – 92%), this extension ends up in a complete P.V.D. *with* collapse.
- A prepapillary ring is a specific sign of complete P.V.D. with or without collapse, but its absence (5/38 eyes) does not mean that there is no P.V.D.
- The frequency of the giant lacunas is at its highest level (16/32 eyes –

50%) for young people between 30 and 40 years old, then decreasing when the P.V.D. becomes complete.
- The average level of the reflectivity of the vitreous body is highest for patients between 70 and 80 years old. But variation is small.

References

[1] O. Berges. Echographie de l'oeil et de l'orbite. Ed. Vigot, Paris, 1986.

[2] C. Boscher. Echographie et décollement postérieur du vitré. Oral communication presented at the Ophthalmology society of Paris, September 1991.

[3] Y.L. Fisher, J.S. Slakter, R.A. Friedman and L.A. Yannuzzi. Kinetic ultrasound evaluation of the posterior vitreoretinal interface. Ophthalmology 1991;98:1135–1138.

[4] M. Favre and H. Goldman. Zur genese der hinteren Glaskörperabhebung. Ophthalmologica 1956;132:87–97.

[5] R.Y. Foos. Posterior vitreous detachment. Tr. Am. Acad. Ophth. & Otol. 1972;76:480–497.

[6] R. Guthoff. Ultrasound in ophthalmologic diagnosis. Ed. Thieme, 1991.

[7] J. Poujol. Echographie en ophtalmologie. Ed. Masson, 1984.

[8] J.Y. Perichon, M. Mehech and G. Brasseur. Approche échographique du vitré. Film presented at the Ophthalmologic Society of France, Paris, May, 1992.

[9] J.Y. Perichon. Diagnostic échographique d'un D.P.V. Visions Internationales n° 30 – November 30th, 1992; Ed. Girold, Mutzig.

[10] M. Roldàn and M. A. Hernàez, Rapports vitreorétiniens chez le sujet normal. Ophtamologie 1988;2:321–325.

Dr. J.Y. Perichon
Hospital Charles Nicolle
Rouen
France

3.12. Dynamic Interaction of Vitreoretinal Adhesions

U.K. FRIES and R. MAKABE
(Frankfurt/Main, Germany)

Abstract. Experience is presented from a series of ophthalmic patients presented with vitreoretinal adhesions. Imaging is difficult by previous generations of ultrasound machines, but with high-resolution real-time echography (B-model) of today it is possible. In particular, the movements and after-movements are stressed, as clues to early diagnosis of traction detachment of the retina. The results are discussed.

Key words: Vitreoretinal surgery, vitreoretinal adhesion, ultrasonography, high-resolution B-scan, kinetic dynamics of vitreous structure.

Introduction

Echographical examinations are mostly done in the non-moved eye. The aim is the tissue-characterisation which has reached a high level in the combination of A- and B-mode [1–3, 5, 8, 11, 13].

The examinations evaluate pathological findings in the globe, especially in uvea and sclera, as well as in the orbit. As electronics have developed with better techniques regarding gain and noise-reduction, structures of the vitreous can be examined in more detail. These structures are important in our understanding of the dynamic pathology behind PVR and PDVR [6]. In inflammation (posterior uveitis), for instance, the vitreous is more concerned than clinically expected [7].

Material and Methods

The tissue-examination is done in a combination of A- and B-mode combined with dynamic echography of the moved eye.

By high-resolution B-mode real-time echography with good noise-reduction and a quality amplifier (logarithm, 10 MHz, vector-scanner) the pathological findings in the vitreous can be evaluated during eye-movement. In the last two years it was possible to study in more detail the dynamic of the vitreous, due to a better amplifier.

J.M. Thijssen, H.C. Fledelius and S. Tane (eds.), Ultrasonography in Ophthalmology 14, 169–172.
© 1995 *Kluwer Academic Publishers, Dordrecht.*

After the usual tissue-characterisation the patients were asked to move the eyes rapidly during the echographical examination of the lesion. The amplifier's settings were elected to guarantee a best-possible picture with the lowest level of noise.

The documentation was done by on-line video and by freeze-frame giving a frozen picture of the kinetic process.

The examination was done with the patient lying, with a contact-agent (methylcellulose) and through the closed lids in order to avoid corneal damage.

In about 200 out of some 2500 eyes a vitreoretinal adhesion was found either in the posterior pole and/or periphery.

Most patients with adhesions had diabetes mellitus (about 2/3) of which 55% had a known vitreous haemorrhage before the traction appeared. Other cases of vitreoretinal traction had a vitreal haemorrhage associated to trauma, thrombosis or partial posterior vitreous-detachment and subhyaloidal-preretinal haemorrhage.

Results

Documentation of the dynamics of the vitreous body during movement of the globe gives further information in addition to the usual tissue-characterization. The change in the posterior vitreous-membrane's motility gives the proportion of morphological changes such as fibrosis and consecutive sails and/or tractions. One can see the foot-point and the traction's rigidity, its size, and direction during movement.

Most eyes with a vitreoretinal adhesion had it in the posterior pole (80%). About 1/3 had vitreoretinal tractions with two or more foot-points. The behavior of the attached vitreous showed strong differences as compared to the age-related normal group.

With the vitreous attached only at the posterior pole, a rather free floating was found following eye-movements. Globes with two or more vitreoretinal-adhesions showed less dynamics of the posterior vitreal membrane. The forces caused by acceleration during the change of the movement's direction at the saccade's final point were transformed to the retina as forces of traction and gravitation.

Regarding physics there are, when the saccade stops, point accelerations to change the movement's direction. The eye's movement is no steady process; it is a series of quick movements in different directions. There are rotation moments, accelerations, centrifugal and centripetal forces. The axis is in the vitreous body.

During the movements the behaviour of the vitreous and the traction can be specified (Fig. 1). Very important is the examination of the foot-points when the movements stop, in order to detect short-term retinal tractions. As the first step of severe PVR/PDVR causing retinal ablation, it gives information of importance for deciding the surgical approach

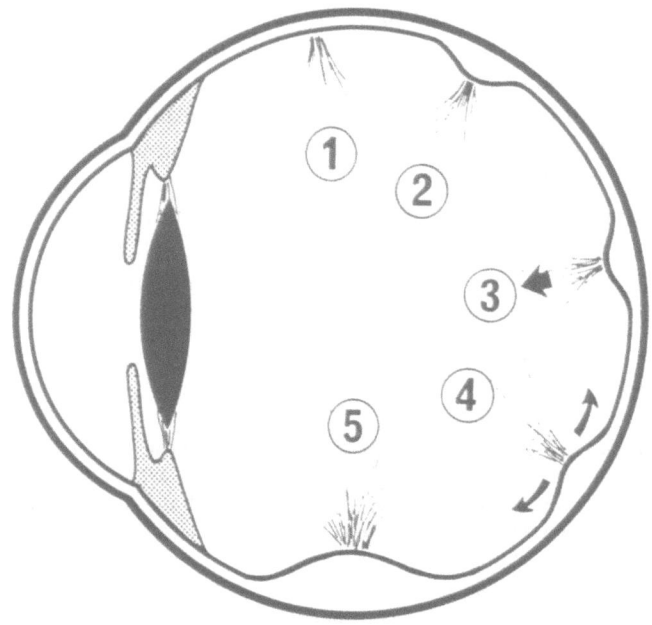

Figure 1. (1) Vitreoretinal adhesion; (2) vitreal traction onto the retina; (3) traction in steady state (arrow: centripetal force); (4) traction in movement (arrows: actions of highest energy); (5) beginning retinal detachment.

Repeated kinetic examination of a traction will show the change of dynamics with increasing fibrosis and tension.

Discussion

The examination of the three-dimensional globe is done mainly by standardized A-mode echography [12], B-mode echography [1, 5] or by a combination of both.

Examining the globe in various directions in addition to the tissue-characterisation information may be obtained about the vitreous-structures' quality and mobility [2]. The pioneers of ophthalmic ultrasound described the vitreous body as acoustically homogenous [11], but a further technical development made pathological findings as well as age-related degenerations detectable [10].

With improved amplifiers and resolution, fluctuations of the vitreous structures could be imaged in the second half of the 1980s [3]. With high resolution, real-time presentation, sufficient gain, and good noise-reduction the interactions at the vitreoretinal interface can be seen and documented.

Further, dynamic ophthalmological video-echography allows additional information about the vitreo-retinal lesions and their dynamics [3], through

172

analysis of the forces in the moment of their highest energy. This is very important as the eye does complex rotations during the saccades.

The vitreous body has an inert relative counter-movement, which is braked by vitreoretinal adhesions. These adhesions transmit vectors of forces onto the retina. If there is short-term lifting of the retina while the highest energy is on, a traction and PVR-ablation on its way can be detected early, and possibly prevented by pars plana vitrectomy. The echographical diagnoses of a retinal ablation by traction is admitted [1, 2, 5, 8, 9, 14].

The higher developed diagnostics make a safer early diagnosis as well as prevention possible.

References

[1] N.R. Bronson, Y.L. Fisher, N.C. Pickering and E.M. Trayner. Ophthalmic contact B-scan ultrasonography for the clinician. Intercontinental Publ., Westport, 1976.

[2] W. Buschmann and H.G. Trier. Ophthalmologische ultraschalldiagnoastik mit atlas, standardisierung und einordnung in den augenärztlichen untersuchungsgang. Springer, Berlin – Heidelberg – New York – Tokyo, 1989.

[3] S.F. Byrne and R.L. Green. Ultrasound of the eye and orbit. Mosby, St. Louis, 1992.

[4] S. Chang and D.J. Coleman. Beurteilung des vitrektomie-patienten. In W. Buschmann and H.G. Trier (Hrsg) Ophthalmologische ultraschalldiagnostik mit atlas, standardisierung und einordnung in den augenärztlichen untersuchungsgang. Springer, Berlin – Heidelberg – New York – Tokyo, 1989, pp. 111–118.

[5] D.J. Coleman, F.L. Lizzi and R.L. Jack. Ultrasonography of the eye and orbit. Lea & Febiger, Philadelphia, 1977.

[6]. U. Fries, O.-E. Schnaudigel and R. Makabe. Echographische darstellung von dynamischen glaskörpertraktionen. Spektrum Augenheilkd. 1992;6(4):161–163.

[7] U. Fries, H. Gümbel, M. Rodenbach and R. Makabe. Frühveränderungen des glaskörpers bei patienten mit CMV-retinitis nach gancyclovir-therapie in der echographischen darstellung (hochauflösende B-bild-echography). Ophthalmolog (in print).

[8] R. Guthoff. Ultraschall in der ophthalmologischen diagnostik. Ein leitfadebn für die Praxis. Encke, Stuttgart, 1988.

[9] R. Guthoff. Ultrasound in ophthalmologic diagnosis. A practical guide. Thieme, Stuttgart – New York, 1991.

[10] A. Oksala. Ultrasonic findings in the vitreous at various ages. Arch. Clin. Exp. Ophthalmol. 1978;197:83–87.

[11] A. Oksala and A. Lehtinen. Investigations on the structure of the vitreous body at various ages. Am. J. Ophthalmol. 1958;46:361–366.

[12] K.C. Ossoinig. Echography of the eye, orbit and periorbital region. In P.H. Arger (ed.), Orbit roentgenology. Wiley, New York, 1977, pp. 224–269.

[13] K.C. Ossoinig. Standardized echography: basic principles, clinical applications and results. Int. Ophthalmol. Clin. 1979;19(4):127.

[14] R. Rochels. Ultraschalldiagnostik in der Augenheilkunde – Lehrbuch und Atlas. Ecomed, Landsberg, 1986.

Universitäts-Augenklinik Frankfurt/Main
Theodor Stern Kai 7, H8b
D-W-6000 Frankfurt/Main 70
Germany

3.13. Echographic Characteristics of Perfluorodecalin: A Case Report

JÁNOS NÉMETH, MIHÁLY VÉGH* and ILDIKÓ SÜVEGES

(*Budapest and Szeged*; Hungary)

Abstract. The echographic findings are described which occured after surgical removal of a dislocated eye lens by using perfluorodecalin

Key words: Lens dislocation, surgery, perfluorodecalin

Introduction

Echography is a very useful tool in the examination of patients with vitreoretinal diseases. It may provide valuable help in the planning of vitreoretinal surgery and in the postoperative control of the patients, even in the most difficult cases. In the case of opaque optical media, it is the only chance for the surgeon to orientate before and after operation.

In case of artificial endotamponade materials, echographists meet with various difficulties. Gas tamponade materials, such as air, perfluorocarbon gases (perfluoroethane, perfluoropropane) or sulphur hexafluoride, give a very high reflection of ultrasound beam at their anterior surface, which results in an extended empty area in the echographic picture behind the bubble. If the intraocular gas bubble is large, ultrasound examination of the eyeball is impossible. In case of silicone oil, there are many well known artefacts which cause trouble during ultrasonography. The high surface spike of the silicone oil at its posterior surface hampers detection of the retinal position behind the material. Silicon oil often greatly distorts the echographic picture of the eyeball.

Perfluorocarbon liquids, new surgical materials, are indicated during vitreoretinal surgery [2, 6, 10, 14]. In our present case report, the startling echographic characteristics of perfluorodecalin are described.

Case Report

A case of a 61-year-old woman with dislocation of the lens because of a head contusion is presented.

The lens was located in front of the macula in the lying position and could

J.M. Thijssen, H.C. Fledelius and S. Tane (eds.), Ultrasonography in Ophthalmology 14, 173–176.

174

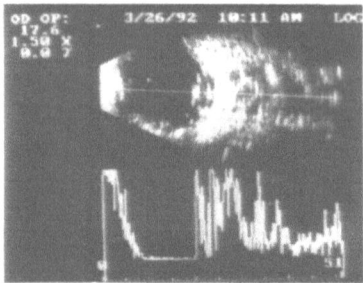 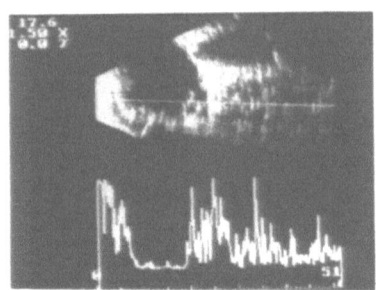

Figure 1. A/B-scan ultrasonogram of an eye with perfluorodecalin residue after vitrectomy and lens removal (vertical plane).

Figure 2. The same eye as in Fig. 1 in an oblique section displaying the optic nerve and perfluorodecalin at the same time.

move to the equator after the patient sat up. During surgery, the dislocated lens was lifted up and removed using perfluorodecalin, which was injected behind the lens, through the vitreous. The surgical technique was similar to the method described by Shapiro and colleagues [15–16]. The removal of perfluorodecalin was not complete and after surgery a little quantity of perfluorodecalin could be found in the eye.

Echography was performed with Ultrascan Digital B equipment with 10 MHz A/B-scan probe. Ultrasonographic examinations displayed a startling picture. The surface spike of the perfluorodecalin was very high and the inside echo pattern was inhomogenous (echo-free spaces and echogenic lines) (Fig. 1). The backward displacement of the ocular wall behind the material indicated that the ultrasound velocity was lower in perfluorodecalin than in the vitreous. The sectoral chain of echogenic artefacts behind the perfluorodecalin were very similar to the artefacts behind spherical metal foreign bodies (Figs. 1–2). The perfluorodecalin did not display any movement during or after eye movements and it always occupied the lowest possible area in the eyebal.

Some days after surgery, perfluorodecalin bubbles appeared in the anterior chamber after down-gaze of the patient. The perfluorodecalin bubbles were well visible in the anterior chamber. On B-scan pictures, the echogenic sectoral artefacts of perfluorodecalin now started from the anterior chamber (Fig. 3). The bubbles were easily removable in a second minor operation.

Discussion

Perfluorodecalin is a clear colourless fluid with a high specific gravity. It does not mix with gas, blood, water, or any other fluid used in vitrectomy. Its low viscosity permits easy injection and removal with microsurgical equipment [8]. The advantages of perfluorocarbon liquids are [2–3, 6, 8–10]: easy flattening of the retina; it eliminates the subretinal fluid, provides excellent

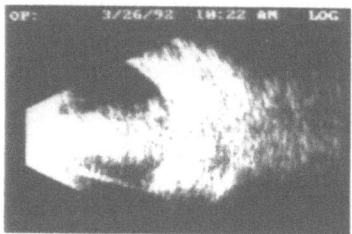

Figure 3. Echographic picture of the eye after the perfluorodecalin has moved into the anterior chamber. The echogenic chain of the artefacts caused by the material starts at the anterior segment of the eye.

reapposition of the tear, and allows effective endophotocoagulation under optimal visual conditions. Posterior retinotomies can be avoided. It facilitates retinal reattachment without manipulation of the posterior retinal flap and edge of the giant retinal tear, thus decreasing the risk of iatrogenic retinal breaks, hemorrhage, and retinal trauma [8]. In the management of a dislocated lens, perfluorodecalin allows removal of the lens with minimal manipulation, even in case of poor medium clarity [5, 13–16].

Since perfluorodecalin and perfluorocarbon liquids are new surgical materials, only few articles have been published about their usage [2–6, 8–10, 15–16]. To date, only few reports have appeared about the echographic signs of such materials. We described it in the XVI Alpe-Adria Congress in September, 1992 [11–12]. Hasenfratz [7] explained the acoustic criteria of perfluorocarbon liquids in the German Ophthalmological Congress, also in September. He found similar signs. Avitabile and colleagues published their experimental results [1], not only with echography but also by CT and MRI [14]. Noske and colleagues described the detection of perfluorodecalin with 19F-MRI [13].

To summarize our experience, perfluorodecalin can be displayed by ultrasonography during and after surgery knowing its special echographic characteristics. It is important to have this knowledge because perfluorocarbon liquids are toxic agents [4] and the chain of the artefacts behind them can give the false impression of a metal foreign body. There are marked differences in the appearance of the echographic signs and artefacts of perfluorodecalin depending on the place, amount, number and size of the bubbles of the material and also on the direction of the ultrasound probe.

Summing up, the typical echographic characteristics of perfluorodecalin are as follows:
– very high surface spike
– inhomogenous inside echo pattern (echo-free spaces + echogenic lines)
– apparent ocular wall displacement behind the material (low sound velocity)

- sectoral chain of echogenic artefacts behind the material
- no movement during or after eye movements
- it occupies the lowest possible space in the eyeball.

References

[1] T. Avitabile, L. Franco, V. Russo and A. Reibaldi. Aspetti ecografici del perfluorocarbone liquido: studio sperimentale. Clin. Ocul. 1992;13:203–206.

[2] S. Chang, H. Lincoff, N.J. Zimmerman and Fuchs. Giant retinal tears. Surgical technique and results using perfluorocarbon liquids. Arch. Ophthalmol. 1989;107:761–766.

[3] S. Clemens. Giant tear retinal detachment reproliferation with and without temporary perfluorocarbon endotamponade. German J. Ophthalmol. 1992;1:266.

[4] C. Eckardt and U. Nicolai. Clinical and histological findings after long-term vitreous replacement with perfluorodecalin. German J. Ophthalmol. 1992;1:268.

[5] E. Frau, J.F. Korobelnik and L. Nabet *et al.* Perfluorocarbon liquids in the management of dislocated lens. German J. Ophthalmol. 1992;1:267.

[6] H. Greber. Perfluorodecalin als raumtaktische Substanz bei komplizierten netzhautablösungen. Fortschr. Ophthalmol. 1991;88:350–353.

[7] G. Hasenfratz and M. De La Torre. Echography of eyes harbouring perfluorocarbonliquid. German J. Ophthalmol. 1992;1:267.

[8] A.E. Krieger and H. Lewis. Management of giant retinal tears without scleral buckling. Ophthalmology 1992;99:491–497.

[9] Y. Le Mer, D. Kuhn, J. Siegert and J. Chofflet. Vitrectomy, PFCL, diode laser endophotocoagulation and gas injection in the management of complicated retinal detachment. German J. Ophthalmol. 1992;1:267.

[10] A. Mathis, V. Pagot and J.L. David. The use of perfluorodecalin in diabetic vitrectomy. Fortschr. Ophthalmol. 1991;88:148–150.

[11] J. Németh, M. Végh and I. Süveges. Echographic detection of perfluorodecalin. 16th Alpe-Adria International Ophthalmological Meeting, Györ, 1992.

[12] J. Németh and I. Süveges: A perfluorodecalin echográfiai jelei. Szemészet, 1993.

[13] W. Noske, B. Gewiese and D. Schilling *et al.* Perfluorodecalin revealed by 19F-MRI. German J. Ophthalmol. 1992;1:267.

[14] A. Reibaldi, T. Avitabile, L. Franco, G. Fabbri, L. Manfré and G. Pero. Echography and N.M.R. in vitrectomized eyes with internal tamponade. XIV SIDUO Congress. Tokyo, 1992.

[15] M.J. Shapiro, K.I. Resnick, S.H. Kim and A. Weinberg. Management of the dislocated crystalline lens with a perfluorocarbon liquid. Am. J. Ophthalmol. 1991;112:401–405.

[16] I. Süveges, Á. Szabó and A. Facskó. Removal of lens dislocated into the vitreous. IXth Congress of SOE, Brussels, 1992.

1st Department of Ophthalmology
Semmelweis Medical University
Tömö u. 25–29
H-1083 Budapest
Hungary

3.14. The Diagnosis and Management of Intraocular Inflammation with Standardized Echography, with Emphasis on Macular Thickness

G. CENNAMO, N. ROSA and G. IACCARINO

(Naples, Italy)

Abstract. The clinical evaluation of an ocular disease in a patient with uveitis is often difficult due to opacities of the dioptric media. Hence standardized echography can be very important in the study of uveitis. The most common macular lesion associated with uveitis being the macular edema. Our results are presented from 42 eyes with uveitis. Our study points out a relation between visual acuity and retino-choroidal thickness in the macular area. In particular, our results show that a thickening of the macula may appear before a decrease in visual acuity.

Key words: Uveitis, standardized echography, macular thickness, cystoid macular edema.

Introduction

Cystoid macular edema is by far the most common lesion of the posterior pole associated with uveitis.

The mechanism of the development of macular edema during ocular inflammatory relapses is not clear. Inflammatory cell products in uveitis may very well induce an extracellular fluid accumulation and/or widespread swelling and necrosis of the Müller cells, along with vascular abnormalities.

In most cases, the presence of macular edema can be evaluated by usual clinical examination, although we have some patients in whom further evaluations were needed to fully confirm its presence.

It should be stressed that the presence of edema does not necessarily indicate poor vision. Further, a major clinical question is: which one is a 'reversible' disease, and therefore, how aggressive should a therapeutic approach be?

The goal in the evaluation of patients with uveitis and macular involvement is to determine the decrease in vision and the timing of treatment. Obviously, important parameters in this evaluation include the examination of the best visual acuity. Visual acuity is the main criterium concerning the decision to start, continue or stop therapy.

J.M. Thijssen, H.C. Fledelius and S. Tane (eds.), Ultrasonography in Ophthalmology 14, 177–180.
© 1995 Kluwer Academic Publishers, Dordrecht.

178

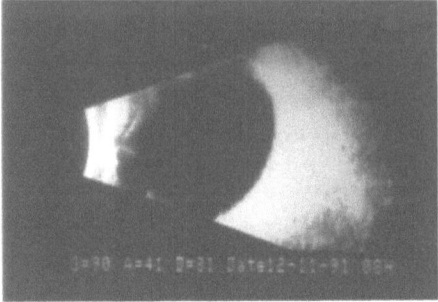 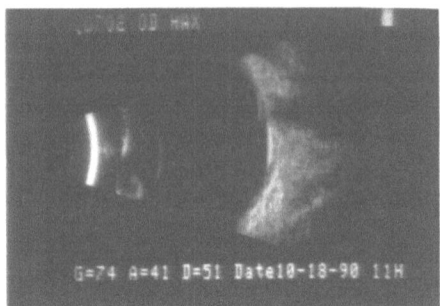

Figure 1. Contact B Scan in a patient with uveitis and normal macular thickness.

Figure 2. Contact B Scan in a patient with uveitis and macular thickening.

Fluorescein angiography gives us a typical image: fluorescein leakage and accumulation is still the widely accepted criterion of cystoid macular edema. However, we have not found this approach helpful, either in predicting the actual visual acuity in many patients, nor the ultimate visual outcome after therapy. Probably the macular thickening rather than diffuse fluorescein leakage could be significant in predicting visual loss [6].

Standardized A-scan was introduced as a method for the echographic screening of the posterior eye segment in the mid-1960's by Ossoinig [7]. Since then it has been regularly used for the evaluation and measurement of the retino-choroidal layers throughout the entire fundus [2, 4, 8].

Over the years the normal thickness range of these layers and the critical measuring values that help distinguish between normal and abnormally thick layers were established for different portions of the eye.

Sometimes a thickening of the macular area can be detected by B Scan echography, but cannot be measured (Figs. 1–2). With standardized A scan echography alone, it is possible to distinguish pseudomembranes from a melanomatous lesion when the thickness of the retino-choroidal layer is 0.75 mm above the normal values. In the macular region a retino-choroidal thickness more than 1.5 mm should be considered abnormal and compatible with a disease (Figs. 3–4).

Materials and Methods

We have compared the thickness of the macular area and the visual acuity in 31 eyes with intermediate uveitis. The patients showed a visual acuity ranging from 20/240 to 20/20, clinically with no significant abnormalities in the optic media. All patients were examined with Mini-A and the Ophthascan 'S from Biophysic Medical.

The examination of the macular area was performed with the echographic beam through the lens at T minus sensitivity.

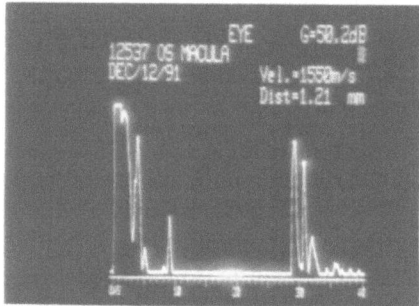 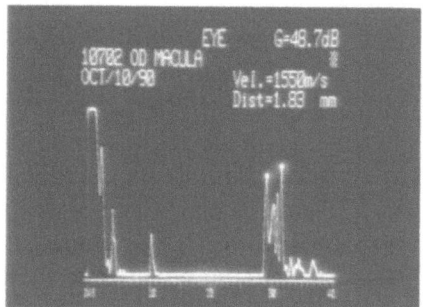

Figure 3. Standardized A Scan in a patient with uveitis and normal macular thickness.

Figure 4. Standardized A Scan in a patient with uveitis and macular thickening.

Table 1. The association between thickness and visual acuity (42 eyes)

Normal V.A. Macula ≥1.5 mm	–	Normal V.A. Macula >1.5 mm	–	Decreased V.A. Macula ≥1.5 mm	–	Decreased V.A. Macula >1.5 mm
17	–	14	–	2	–	9

Results

Out of 42 eyes, 17 eyes had a normal macular thickness with a good visual acuity.

Two eyes had a normal macular thickness with a decrease in visual acuity.

Out of 23 eyes with a macular thickness >1.5 mm, 14 had a normal visual acuity, 9 had a decrease in visual acuity (Table 1).

Discussion

Our results in eyes with intermediate uveitis show that a thickening of the macula may appear before a decrease in visual acuity.

Firstly, our results point out a definite correlation between macular thickness and visual acuity (e.g. increased thickness = decreased vision, cf. Table 1). But secondly, the cases with a thickening of the macula and a good visual acuity show that the macular edema may precede the visual acuity decrease.

Why then is macular edema present in a great number of patients with intermediate uveitis after a variable period of time from the appearance of the disease?

Probably the vitreous alteration found in this disease plays an important role. Sometimes (more frequently than described in literature) it is possible to detect a vitreoschisis.

According to Favre and Goldmann [1] and Rossi and Gallenga [9] senile vitreal degeneration begins with fiber degeneration and cavity formation in the central and superior vitreous body. This liquifying process, or syneresis, could be caused by loss of water-containing capacity, due to gravity. The fluid-filled cavities can separate the vitreous gel [5]. When part of the normal vitreous is attached to the retina, a vitreoschisis will occur that can become so large that it simulates a posterior vitreous detachment (PVD, Figs. 3, 4).

However, this disease is easily differentiated from a PVD using standardized echography, that shows the posterior hyaloid and part of the vitreal cortex still close to the retina. In the case of vitreoschisis a low reflective spike close to the retina with no after movements will be found by A scan, and a thin low reflective area close to the retina by B scan [3].

This particular condition can allow the migration and the "capture" in the macular area of toxic substances and cells coming from the anterior part of the eye and/or from the pigment epithelium. In these cases, the evolution will be a cystoid macular edema, or a macular pucker if only a thickening of the posterior hyaloid is present.

References

[1] M. Favre and H. Goldman. Zur Genese Der Hinteren Glaskorperabhebung. Ophthalmologica 1956;132:87–97.
[2] P.E. Gallenga, L'ecografia nelle malattie uveali. Atti XXIV Congegno S.O.M. – Scalea, 1–3 Guigno 1990.
[3] P.E. Gallenga, G. Cennamo, M. Rosa and G. de Crecchio, Echographic study of the vitreoretinal interface. Advances in vitreoretinal surgery. Acta III Intercontinental Congress on Vitreoretinal Surgery. M. Stirpe (ed.), A. Brucker Publ. 107–112, 1992.
[4] G. Iaccarino, A. Pezone, D. Ciatto, G. Marotta and A. Del Prete. Uveiti ed ecografia. Clin. Ocul. 1992;4:213–215.
[5] A. Nettens and C.L. Schepens. The vitreous and vietreoretinal interface. Bull. Soc. Belge Ophthalmol. 1987;223-1:85–102.
[6] R.B. Nussenblat. Macular alterations secondary to intraocular inflammatory disease. Ophthalmology, Vol. 93, 7–July, 1986.
[7] K.C. Ossoinig. Standaridized echography: basic principles, clinical applications and results. Int. Ophth. Clin. 1979;19:4.
[8] A. Pezone, G. Iaccarino, A. Mele, A. Del Prete, T. Foá and A. La Rana. Studio ecografico delle uveiti. Clin. Ocul. 1991;4:261–265.
[9] A. Rossi and P.E. Gallenga. Ultrasonographic features of the senile vitreous body. Ultrasonographia Medica 1969;2:247–253.

Dr. G. Cennamo
Eye Department
University Federico II
Naples, Italy

3.15. Posterior Scleritis Monitoring of Systemic Steroid Treatment with Standardized Echography: A Case Report

JAN SCHUTTERMAN

(Stockholm, Sweden)

Abstract. The usefulness of standardized echography for the diagnosis of posterior scleritis is illustrated by the findings in a 30-year-old female. Clinically and ultrasonographically there was a good response to systemic corticosteroid therapy.

Key words: Posterior scleritis, ultrasound diagnosis, standardized echography.

Case report

A 30-year-old woman presented with increasing pain in her left eye. On clinical examination she had 20/20 V.A. Posteriorly and temporally there was a slight injection of the globe. There was no impairment of muscle function.

Local steroid treatment with eye-drops gave a slight improvement in globe appearance, but did not relieve her pain.

Standardized echography was performed and revealed an area about 5 mm in diameter posteriorly temporally, behind the equator, where scleral reflectivity was reduced to about 50% of display height (medium reflectivity) with standardized A-scan (Fig. 1). Also with B-scan the area could be clearly shown (Fig. 2).

Systemic steroid treatment (oral prednisolone starting with 60 mg daily) resulted in almost instant pain relief. However reflectivity remained reduced for a few weeks and oral prednisolone was tapered according to echography results.

There have been a few recurrences which were promptly diagnosed with standardized echography and treated without delay. No increased injection was seen on the sclera on these occasions.

J M Thijssen, H C Fledelius and S Tane (eds), Ultrasonography in Ophthalmology 14, 181–182
© 1995 *Kluwer Academic Publishers, Dordrecht*

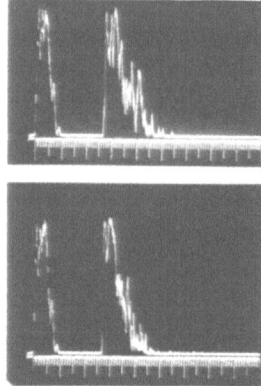

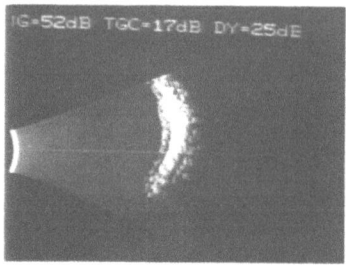

Figure 1. Standardized A-scan (Kretztechnik 7200MA) shows widened sclera with medium high reflectivity (top), with fellow eye as control (bottom).

Figure 2. The area affected, on B-scan (Ophthascan mini-B), at a low sensitivity setting.

Conclusion

Standardized echography is an excellent tool to diagnose posterior scleritis, to monitor treatment, and also to manage recurrencies.

Standardized echography can be performed again and again, without reservation, in contrast to e.g. CT-scan which has the well-known risks of radiation side effects.

Dept. of Ophthalmology
Sodersjukhuset Hospital
S-118 83 Stockholm
Sweden

3.16. Ultrasonographic Analysis of Glaucomatous Eyes

SADANAO TANE and YOHTARO KIMURA
(Kawasaki, Japan)

Abstract. A review is given of various glaucoma types, mainly based on the authors' own ultrasonographic investigations. Ultrasound is extremely useful regarding measuring eye dimensions as well as by rendering imaging for differential diagnosis.

Key words: Glaucoma, open angle (POAG), glaucoma, angle closure (PACG), congenital glaucoma, secondary glaucoma.

Introduction

Useful analytical information has been obtained by applying ultrasonic methods to the examination for glaucoma. The following items will be discussed:
(1) Axial length measurement of various glaucomatous eyes.
(2) Axial length measurement of the buphthalmic eyes.
(3) Comparison of the values obtained by microbiometry of ocular wall thickness between normal eyes and glaucomatous eyes
(4) Ultrasonic diagnosis of the eyes with secondary glaucomas.

1. Axial Length Measurement in Various Types of Glaucoma

As reference, Table 1 shows the results of measuring axial length in normal eyes of Japanese subjects. The mean axial distances for 244 eyes (110 eyes of adult men and 134 eyes of adult women) are 3.24 mm for anterior chamber depth, 4.10 mm for lens thickness, 16.30 mm for axial vitreous length, and 23.65 mm for the total axial length of the eyeball. The axial measurement value of each refractive compartment was significantly higher in men than in women.

Axial length was measured in 62 eyes with primary angle closure glaucoma and 48 eyes with primary open angle glaucoma. The results demonstrated that the anterior chamber depth and total axial length of the eyeball were significantly lower in eyes with angle closure glaucoma when compared to normal eyes, and to those with open angle glaucoma as well, whereas the

J.M. Thijssen, H.C. Fledelius and S. Tane (eds.), Ultrasonography in Ophthalmology 14, 183–187.
© 1995 *Kluwer Academic Publishers, Dordrecht.*

Table 1. The results of measuring axial length in normal eyes of Japanese subjects.

sex & number of eyes	M & σ	anterior chamber depth	lens thickness	vitreous thickness	total axial length
♂ (110 eyes)	M	3.36	4.15	16.39	23.90
	σ	0.47	0.54	1.02	1.00
♀ (134 eyes)	M	3.14	4.06	16.23	23.45
	σ	0.49	0.50	1.04	1.07
♂♀ (244 eyes)	M	3.24	4.10	16.30	23.65
	σ	0.49	0.52	1.04	1.06

M Means   σ Standard Deviation

Table 2. Comparative study of axial dimension in primary angle-closure glaucoma and primary open-angle glaucoma.

Comparative Study of Axial Dimension in PACG and POAG

Toe of Glaucoma	Age (YR)	No of Eyes	Range of Refraction (D)	Average Depth of Anterior Chamber (Range, mm)	Average Lens Thickness (Range, mm)	Average Total Axial Length (Range, mm)	Relative lens Position (Ronge)
PACG	32~82	62	+2.75~ −2.50	2.29±0.35 (1.1~3.2)	4.85±0.16 (3.3~6.1)	22.17±0.86 (19.4~25.6)	0.213±0.014 (0.1431~ 0.2348)
POAG	24~78	48	+1.75~ −2.2	2.91±0.32 (1.8~4.1)	4.59±0.22 (3.7~5.6)	23.33±0.94 (19.8~25.5)	0.223±0.031 (0.1981~ 0.2636)
T·Test Between				Highly Significant	Highly Significant	Highly Significant	Significant

lens was thicker in the 62 eyes with PACG than in the other two groups of eyes (Table 2). In the eyes with angle closure glaucoma the mean anterior chamber depth was as shallow as 2.29 mm, the lens was slightly thickened, up to 4.85 mm, and the mean total axial length of the eyeball was was only 22.17 mm. As Lowe had stated, "the eye with closed angle glaucoma is a hypoplastic eye".

2. Axial Length Measurement of Buphthalmic Eyes

The echometric findings in congenital glaucoma are classified into the following three groups, as based on 58 eyes examined:
(1) A-group: with complete healing and normal vision.
(2) B-group: at the end the appearance is like in open angle glaucoma, with normal axial length.
(3) C-group: with a very enlarged eye. They have retinal changes in the posterior pole due to ocular elongation.

(Block diagram of the data acquisition system)

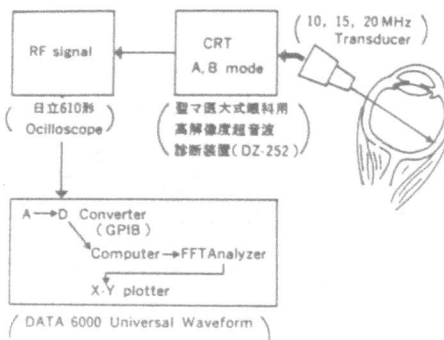

Figure 1 The block-diagram of the microbiometry of ocular wall thickness

Table 3 The thickness of the retina, choroid and sclera in living normal human eyes by means of ultrasonic radio-frequency signal analysis

age groups (cases)	Sclera		Retina		Retina + Choroid	Choroid		
	t₁	µm	t₂	µm	t₃	t₃ t₂	µm	
30y ≥	848.6	700 1	175 4	135 5	670 8	500 0	392 5	
(6 cases, 9 eyes)	±11 53	±95 23	±34 26	±26 56	±118.09	±97 82	±76 80	
31 − 50y	854 3	+704 9	194 2	149 9	714 0	460 5	361 5	
(14 cases 23 eyes)	±14 19	±11 70	±34 68	±26.94	±202 11	±16 56	±13 01	
51 − 70y	850 3	701 5	201 2	155 0	708 1	469 3	368 5	
(21 cases. 39 eyes)	±13 53	±11 16	±40 06	±30 98	±14 12	±97 56	±76 57	
71y ≤	904 0	745 8	201 8	155 4	677 1	478.9	376 0	
(5 cases 10 eyes)	±16 05	±13 25	±22 98	±17 93	±78.67	±84 16	±65 91	
Average	858 1	708.0	196 1	151 2	702 8	471 3	370 0	
(46 cases 81 eyes)	±13 75	±11 34	±36 23	±28.03	±15 49	±11 73	±92 08	

3. Comparison of the Values Obtained by Microbiometry of Ocular Wall Thickness in Normal Eyes and in Glaucomatous Eyes

The block-diagram of the microbiometry is shown in Fig. 1. In order to carry out automatic processing of radio-frequency (RF) signals of ultrasonic waves by computer, and to determine precisely the thickness of an ocular wall even when thinner than 1 mm, we used a DATA 6000 universal wave-form analyzer containing a computer linked with St. Marianna's high resolution ultrasonic diagnostic equipment.

The mean values for the measurements in 81 eyes of 46 healthy subjects in all age groups was 151 ± 28 µm for the retina, 370 ± 92 µm for the choroid and 708 ± 11 µm for the sclera. These values indicate the thickness of the ocular wall of a normal eye *in vivo*, at a site slightly posterior to the pole of the equator (Table 3).

As shown in Table 4, the choroid of the eye with open angle glaucoma was significantly thicker than that of the normal eye.

Table 4. The thickness of the retina, choroid and sclera of the eyeball with non-operated primary open angle glaucoma.

Case No.	Name	age sex	Retina (μm) R	Retina (μm) L	Choroid (μm) R	Choroid (μm) L	Sclera (μm) R	Sclera (μm) L
1	T. Y.	69 ♀	123.2	134.8	471.0	302.2	792	660
2	F. M.	73 ♀	160.9	207.5	338.3	511.0	726	759
3	M. M.	68 ♀	98.6	123.2	527.5	471.0	759	990
4	M. T.	47 ♀	164.2	185.5	303.8	282.6	858	825
5	T. A.	62 ♀	123.2	123.2	471.0	471.0	660	660
6	Y. M.	68 ♀	123.2	123.2	408.2	282.6	825	858
7	T. H.	42 ♂	123.2		596.6		891	858
8	K. K.	38 ♂	164.2	123.2	492.2	282.6	693	660
9	K. M.	51 ♀	159.3	164.2	339.9	303.8	693	660
10	T. T.	38 ♀	164.2	197.1	680.6	489.8	792	759
11	M. S.	40 ♂	123.2	123.2	361.1	314.0	693	544
	mean		144.4		414.3		755.3	
	+SD		±29.32		±114.94		±102.34	

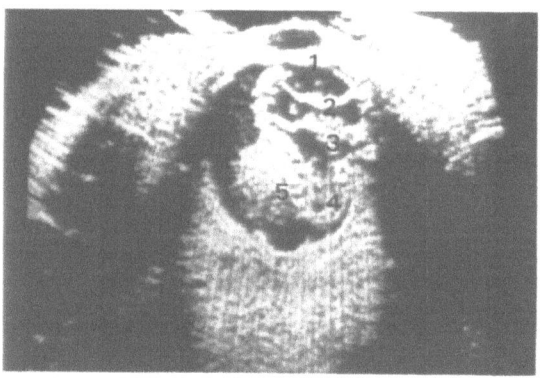

1 iris
2 luxated lens
3 ratinal detachment
4 vitreous hemorrhage
5 choroidal melanoma

Figure 2. B-scan ultrasonogram of a globe with a solid choroidal melanoma, vitreous hemorrhage and retinal detachment, showing acute secondary glaucoma attack.

4. Ultrasonic Diagnosis of Eyes with Secondary Glaucomas

Intraocular lesions of eyes with secondary glaucoma are discussed with reference to imaging diagnosis ($n = 18$ eyes). Figure 2 shows the B-scan right eye finding of a 62-year-old female who presented with an acute attack of angle-closure glaucoma.

A choroidal tumor was detected in her right eye by ultrasonography. The

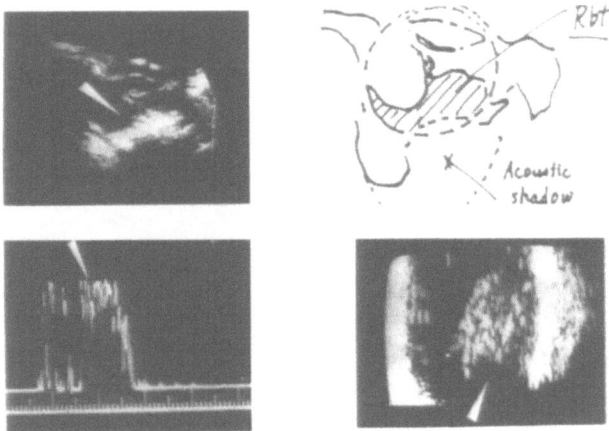

Figure 3. B-scan ultrasonogram of a globe with retinoblastoma showing a solid mass at the posterior pole, with intraocular tension elevation.

iris was pushed from behind by the tumour and a dislocated lens. The posterior lesion was a malignant choroidal melanoma.

Figure 3 shows the ultrasonograms and eyeball findings in a 7-month-old girl with monolateral leucocoria associated with elevated intraocular tension. We were obliged to carry out enucleation of the eyeball because the tumor had grown markedly. B-scan and A-scan immersion findings are shown to the left and a B-scan contact finding is shown at bottom, right. A solid tissue pattern with acoustic shadowing is demonstrated.

Summing up, ultrasonography is very useful clinically for performing measurements in glaucomatous eyes and for diagnosing by imaging.

References

Coleman, D.J. and Lizzi, F.L. In vivo choroidal thickness measurement. Am. J. Ophthalmol. 1979;88:369–376.

Sampaolesi, R. Echometry in congenital glaucoma: Long-term results after 10 to 17 years of surgery. In R. Sampaolesi (ed.), Ultrasonography in Ophthalmology 12, Kluwer, Dordrecht, 1990, pp. 181–191.

Tane, S., Kohno, J. and Horikoshi, J. The study on the microscopic biometry of the thickness of the human retina, choroid and sclera by ultrasound. Acta. Societatis Ophthalmologicae Japonicae 1984;1412–1417.

Tane, S. *et al*. In vivo measurement of the thickness of the retino-choroidal layers by RF-signal analysis. In J.M. Thijssen, J.S. Hillman, P.E. Gallenga and G. Cennamo (eds.), Ultrasonography in Ophthalmology 1988;11:91–94.

Dept. of Ophthalmology
St. Marianna University, School of Medicine
2-16-1 Sugao Miyamae-ku
Kawasaki-city, 216 Japan

4.1. Standardized Optic Nerve Echography in Patients with Empty Sella

D. DORO, M. SALA, E. MANTOVANI and M. VACCARO

(Padua, Italy)

Abstract. A complete neuro-ophthalmological evaluation was performed in 12 female symptomatic patients with MRI evidence of empty sella; mild intracranial hypertension was monitored in 3 patients with increased subarachnoid fluid (1) and sheathing sign (2) on standardized A-scan examination of retrobulbar optic nerve. All patients showed moderate to severe visual field defects. 17 out of 24 eyes retained full visual acuity but 20 out of 24 had reduced contrast sensitivity. Retrobulbar thickened optic nerve sheaths were echographically noted mostly in eyes with pale disc, severe field constriction and reduced VEPs amplitude. Seven eyes showed a normal standardized A-scan display of the optic nerve. Our findings indicate that axoplasmic flow impairment due to stretching of the optic nerve at the level of the empty sella may explain the absence of increased subarachnoid fluid in eyes with swollen disc eventually turning pale.

Key words: Empty sella syndrome, standardized echography, visual evoked potentials, automated perimetry, optic disc, intracranial hypertension.

Introduction

The so called empty sella is a normal sized or enlarged sella, partly or totally filled with cerebrospinal fluid. Empty sella may be primary or secondary to surgery or irradiation. Increased intracranial pressure with deficient sellar diaphragm and pituitary adenoma necrosis are believed to be involved in the pathogenesis of primary empty sella. However, empty sella is also regarded as a simple anatomical variant [1].

It is known that empty sella syndrome (ESS) is revealed by a combination of headache, obesity, visual disturbances, benign intracranial hypertension and pituitary insufficiency or hypersecretion [1]. The opthalmoscopical finding of a swollen optic disc in patients with ESS may indicate intracranial hypertension, a condition that can be detected and differentiated with standardized echography [2, 4].

The aims of our study were (1) the correlation between the results of

J.M. Thijssen, H.C. Fledelius and S. Tane (eds.), Ultrasonography in Ophthalmology 14, 189–194.

standardized echography of optic nerve, ophthalmoscopy, automated perimetry, contrast sensitivity, visual evoked potentials (VEPs) and visual acuity in patients with ESS, and (2) the comparison between the findings of echography and intracranial pressure (ICP) monitoring in selected patients with ESS.

Patients and Methods

12 symptomatic female patients with MRI evidence of empty sella, aged between 32 and 62 years (average 47 years), were evaluated at least twice with binocular ophthalmoscopy, standardized echography of the optic nerve (Coopervision Ultrascan Digital IV B^{TM}; Biophysic Medical Ophthascan Mini A), automated perimetry (Octopus 2000 R, program 24), pattern reversal evoked potentials (amplitude and latency of P100 at full field; T.F. 2Hz; S.F. 10', 33'; contrast 10%, 20%, 30% and 100%; active electrode Oz, O1, O2), contrast sensitivity (Vistech 6500 charts) and Snellen visual acuity recording.

Pituitary hormones were assayed in all patients; ICP was continuously (24 hours) monitored in three patients only.

Results

Table 1 summarizes all the clinical results in the 24 examined eyes, as far as standardized echography of the optic nerve, optic disc appearance, automated perimetry, VEPs, contrast sensitivity and visual acuity are concerned.

Eight out of the 12 patients with ESS (nos. 1, 2, 4, 5, 6, 7, 9, 11) (67%) suffered from headache, 6 patients (nos. 2, 3, 5, 7, 8) (50%) were obese, 2 patients (nos. 3, 4) (17%) had hyperprolactinemia.

A-scan standardized echography of the retrobulbar optic nerve displayed increased subarachnoid fluid (ISAF) of the retrobulbar optic nerve in two eyes (mean arachnoidal diameter 6.70 ± 0.44 mm), some separation between pia and arachnoid, called "sheathing sign" [5], in 5 eyes (mean arachnoidal diameter 4.47 ± 0.73 mm), thickened perineural sheaths in 10 eyes (mean arachnoidal diameter 4.21 ± 0.47 mm) and normal appearance in 7 patients (mean arachnoidal diameter 3.51 ± 0.17 mm) (Figs. 1 and 2).

Ophthalmoscopically swollen disc was noted in 14 eyes (6 of them also with retinal venous congestion), pale disc in 6 eyes and normal disc in 4 eyes.

Mild intracranial hypertension (20–25 mmHg during 24 hour monitoring) was found in the only three monitored patients (nos. 2, 4, 11). All three patients had swollen disc and patient no. 4 had also retinal venous congestion.

Twenty out of 24 eyes (83%) (including three amblyopic eyes – patients nos. 2, 6. 11) showed impaired contrast sensitivity on Vistech charts. On the other hand, 19 eyes (79%) retained full visual acuity. In 4 out of 6 eyes with pale disc visual acuity was reduced to 0.5 or less; among these the right

Table 1. Clinical results in the 24 examined eyes of patients with empty sella syndrome

Pat.	Eye	Optic nerve echography	Optic disc appearance	Automated perimetry*	VEPs A. / L.		Contrast sensitivity	Visual acuity
1	R	Sheathing	Swollen**	++				1.0
	L	Thick sheaths	Swollen**	++				1.0
2	R	Sheathing	Swollen	+			<<	0.3***
	L	Sheathing	Swollen	+			<	1.0
3	R	Thick sheaths	Normal	+++			<	1.0
	L	Thick sheaths	Normal	+++			<	1.0
4	R	I.S.A.F.	Swollen**	+++	<	>	<	1.0
	L	I.S.A.F.	Swollen**	+++	<	>	<	1.0
5	R	Sheathing	Swollen**	+	<		<	1.0
	L	Normal	Swollen**	+	<			1.0
6	R	Thick sheaths	Swollen	+			<	1.0
	L	Sheathing	Swollen	+	<		<	0.7***
7	R	Thick sheaths	Pale	+++			<	0.5
	L	Thick sheaths	Pale	+++			<	0.3
8	R	Normal	Swollen	+				1.0
	L	Normal	Swollen	+	<		<	1.0
9	R	Normal	Normal	+			<	1.0
	L	Normal	Normal	+			<	1.0
10	R	Thick sheaths	Pale	+++	<		<	1.0
	L	Thick sheaths	Pale	+++	<	>	<	1.0
11	R	Sheathing	Pale	+++	<<	>	<<	CF***
	L	Thick sheaths	Pale	+++	<		<	0.4
12	R	Normal	Swollen	+++	<		<	1.0
	L	Normal	Swollen	+++	<	>	<	0.9

*+ = slight peripheral defects; ++ = nasal defects; +++ = severe constriction.
**Swollen optic disc plus venous congestion.
***Amblyopia.

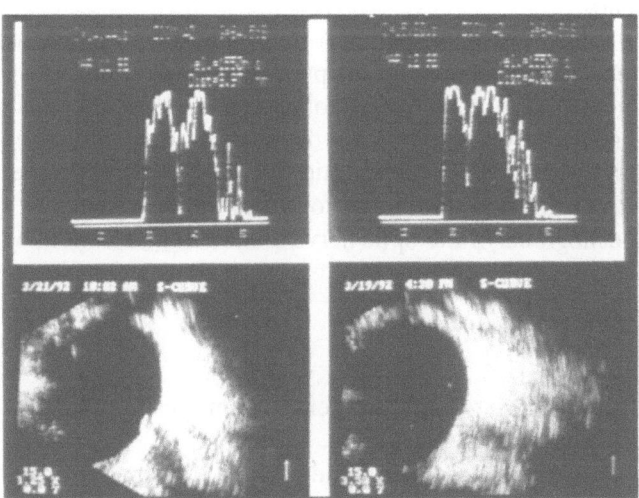

Figure 1. Left: A-scan showing nasal sheathing of optic nerve. B-scan evidence of elevated optic disc and optic nerve void (patient no. 1; RE). Right: A-scan evidence of thickened optic nerve sheaths with non elevated optic nerve head on B-scan imaging (patient no. 7; RE).

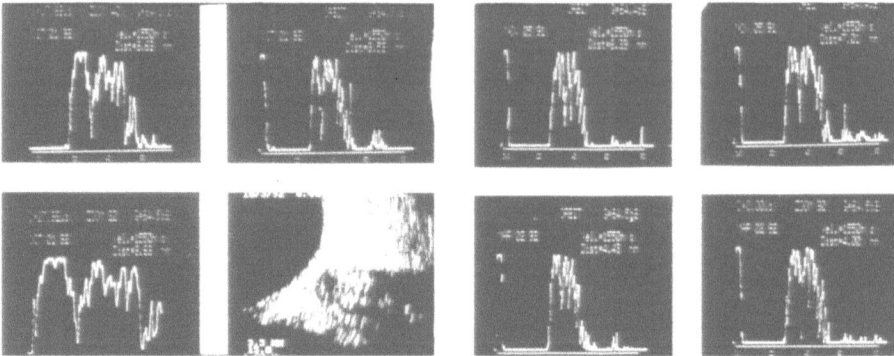

Figure 2. Patient no. 5. On A-scan sheathing sign (top left), better evidenced when zoomed (bottom left) and visible also with B-scan (bottom right). Normal A-scan optic nerve display in the controlateral eye (top right).

Figure 3. Patient no. 4. (Top) November 1991: standardized A-scan showing increased left and right subarachnoid fluid of retrobulbar optic nerve. (Bottom) March 1992: subarachnoid fluid is clearly decreased.

amblyopic eye of patient no. 11 showed a reduction of visual acuity to counting finger.

Automated perimetry bilaterally revealed nasal defect in patient no. 1, moderate peripheral sensitivity loss in 5 patients (42%) and severe generalized field constriction in the remaining 6 patients (50%).

VEP recording showed reduced P100 amplitude in 50% of eyes and increased P100 latency in 5 out of 24 eyes (21%); these 5 eyes including an amblyopic eye (patient no. 11) had both VEP reduced amplitude and increased latency.

During a follow up ranging from 6 to 24 months no noteworthy change was observed in ophthalmoscopical, perimetric and VEP findings. In both eyes of patient no. 4 there was retrobulbar increased subarachnoid fluid, with 30 degree positive test, which reduced at the four month examination (Figs. 3 and 4), and the swollen optic disc turned pale. The echographic findings were unchanged during the follow up in the remaining 11 patients and A-scan echograms of the optic nerve looked similar both in anterior and posterior sections.

Discussion

We judged the following four considerations interesting, which were made on the basis of our data.

1. Only one of our 12 female patients with ESS (patient no. 4) showed bilateral standardized A-scan evidence of ISAF with positive 30 degree test. Mild intracranial hypertension was monitored in this patient and in other two patients (nos. 2, 11) with swollen or pale optic disc and sheathing signs

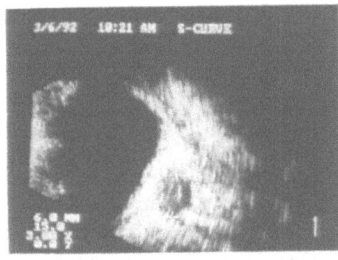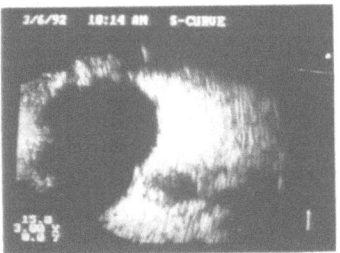

Figure 4. Patient no. 4. (Left) March 1992: cross section of left optic nerve showing subarachnoid fluid nasally ("doughnut sign"). (Right) Same optic nerve in longitudinal section with accentuation of optic nerve sheaths.

on echographic examination. So echographic evidence of subarachnoid fluid was found in all patients with mild intracranial hypertension, but, on the other hand, sheathing sign is also reported as a physiological finding [5].

2. Thickened optic nerve sheaths were noted in 5 out of 6 eyes with pale disc and in 7 out of 10 eyes with severe visual field constriction. This finding indicates that long standing optic nerve damage is associated with echographically thickened optic nerve sheaths. We can speculate that thickened retrobulbar sheaths may result as a reaction to persistent axoplasmic flow impairment at the level of the empty sella where the optic nerve is stretched. The axoplasmic flow blockage can also explain the swollen optic disc eventually turning pale in patients with EES without intracranial hypertension.

3. A normal standardized A-scan display of retrobulbar optic nerve with a mean 3.5 mm arachnoid diameter was found in 7 eyes with normal or swollen disc. Thus, standardized echography seems important to rule out intracranial hypertension which is reported in 10% of patients with ESS [1]. However, we have no information on ICP monitoring of our patients with swollen disc and normal A-scan display of the optic nerve.

4. It is important to remind that all our 12 patients with ESS showed visual field defects on automated perimetry. Interestingly, VEPs amplitude was reduced especially in eyes with severe field constriction (6 out of 12 patients) and retaining normal visual acuity. VEPs latency was bilaterally increased only in the patients with ISAF, thus indicating damaged conduction in optic pathways as in 30% of reported cases of pseudotumor cerebri [6]. Reduced contrast sensitivity found in 20 out of 24 eyes of our symptomatic patients seems to be a good but aspecific indicator of impaired visual function in ESS.

In conclusion, according to our experience different patterns of A-scan display of the retrobulbar optic nerve may be found in patients with EES; the interpretation of the echograms is not always easy, and the echographic finding of really increased subarachnoid fluid is rare [3]. ICP monitoring seems advisable in these cases in order to decide for a surgical procedure to lower ICP.

References

[1] P Bjerre The empty sella A reappraisal of etiology and pathogenesis Acta Neurol Scand 1990,130 1–25

[2] S F Byrne The echographic measurement and differential diagnosis of optic nerve lesions In K C Ossoing (ed) "Ophthalmic Echography", Doc Opthalmol Proceed Series vol 48, Martinuus Nijhoff/Dr W Junk Publishers, Dordrecht, NL, 1987,571–585

[3] G Cennamo, N Rosa and L De Palma Echographic and ophthalmodynamometric study in the Empty Sella syndrome Doc Ophthalmol Proceed Series (SIDUO XIII), in press

[4] K C Ossoing, G Cennamo and S Frazier-Byrne Echographic differential diagnosis of optic nerve lesions In "Ultrasonography in Ophthalmology", Doc Ophthalmol Proceed Series Vol 29, Dr W Junk Publishers, Dordrecht, NL, 1981,327–335

[5] K C Ossoing Oral communication Advanced Course on Standardized Echography of the Optic Nerve (Naples, Italy, Sept 3, 1989)

[6] P S Sorensen, W Trojaborg, F Gjerris and B Krogsaa Visual evoked potentials in pseudotumor cerebri Arch Neurol 1985,42 150–153

Clinica Oculitica
Università di Padova
Via Giustiniani 2
I35128 Padova
Italy

4.2. Ultrasonographic Follow-up of Orbital Rhabdomyosarcoma in a Child

YOSHIE USUKI, KAZUIKO TOYOTA, HARUMI NOSE,
SACHIKO HOMMURA and MICHIO KANEKO*

(Tsukuba, Japan)

Abstract. Ultrasound examination was performed in addition to MRI for the primary diagnosis of rhabdomyosarcoma in a young child. The echographic findings are described during a follow-up on chemotherapy and proton beam irradiation treatment.

Key words: Ultrasonography, rhabdomyosarcoma, follow-up, chemotherapy, proton beam irradiation.

Introduction

Recent advances in diagnostic imaging have had great impact in ophthalmology [1]. However, computed tomographic scanning (CT-scan) and magnetic resonance imaging (MRI) sometimes can not be performed in children, because they cannot keep still even for a moment. The use of hypnotic drugs for sedation of children during imaging is common, especially for those under 6 years old. In such cases, ultrasonography can easily provide information concerning the evolution of ocular disease, and facilitate diagnosis.

We report on a child with rhabdomyosarcoma, evaluated by ultrasonography. Rhabdomyosarcoma is the most common primary malignant tumor of the orbit [2]. Over 90% of orbital rhabdomyosarcomas occur in children under the age of 16 years [3]. It is necessary to diagnose such tumors accurately and ultrasonography is an effective technique for examining children without anesthesia.

Case Report

A 3-year-old boy was hospitalized on December 18, 1989, because of progressive swelling of the left eye lid, sudden painful proptosis and severe vomiting. The swelling of left eye lid was associated with subcutaneous hemorrhage, proptosis (right eye 8 mm, left eye 16 mm by Hertel), and dislocation of the eyeball toward the upper lateral portion (Fig. 1). The left bulbar conjunctiva was slightly infected, diffuse superficial keratitis was seen in the center of

J.M. Thijssen, H.C. Fledelius and S. Tane (eds.), Ultrasonography in Ophthalmology 14, 195–199.
© 1995 *Kluwer Academic Publishers, Dordrecht.*

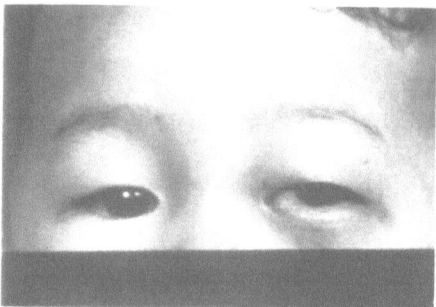

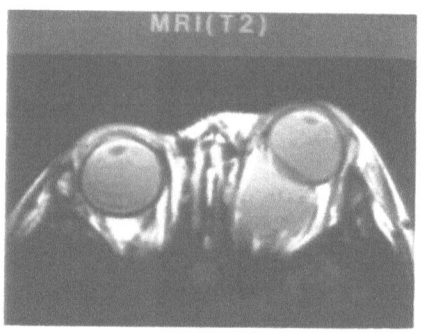

Figure 1 Left proptosis with subcutaneous hemorrhage

Figure 2 MRI (T2) showing involvement of the tumor filling most of retrobulbar, infero-nasal space

the left cornea. Hyperemic and unclear margin of the optic disc and dilatation and tortousity of the retinal vessels were noted in the left eye. MRI revealed that most of the retrobulbar, infero-nasal space was filled by tumor which had not extended beyond the orbit (Fig. 2). From the sudden onset of proptosis, CT and MRI findings and the result of biopsy, this tumor was diagnosed a rhabdomyosarcoma.

Chemotherapy was initiated using a combination of drugs. This was a combination of adriamycin, vincristine, and cyclophosphamide administered until October 1991. During this period, we continued ophthalmic examinations. Proptosis continued until March, but optic disc edema decreased and abnormal findings of retinal vessels improved. Visual acuity was 20/600 in the left eye against 20/20 in the right eye. Ultrasonographic examination could not start until February in 1991. Because of the number of examinations during therapy, frequent injections terrified the child, and he would not permit us to touch his eye. Using the DESITAL B-scan, we performed the examination. The image of the tumor was relatively good, and had clear margins (Fig. 3). The tumor appeared to be solid. Almost simultaneously, MRI showed that the tumor size had gradually decreased. At the inner part of tumor, fluid-fluid niveau formation was seen on MRI, T2 weighted image, indicating that chemotherapy was effective (Fig. 4).

After chemotherapy, he was discharged and followed through the out-patient clinic. Figure 5 shows the ultrasonogram 2 years after onset. His left visual acuity decreased to 20/600, because the optic nerve was lifted and the eye ball was pressed by tumor. We covered the right eye, and 4 months later, his left visual acuity improved to 20/20. In March 1992, his mother noticed a slight swelling of the left eye lid. Ultrasonographic examination showed that the tumor was characterized by good outline, acoustic solidity, high transmission and by compression of the nasal inferior wall of the eyeball (Fig. 6). Fundus examination was performed.

The inferior optic disc margin was blurred, and venous dilatation was seen.

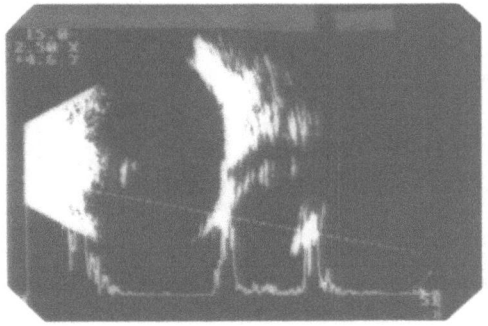

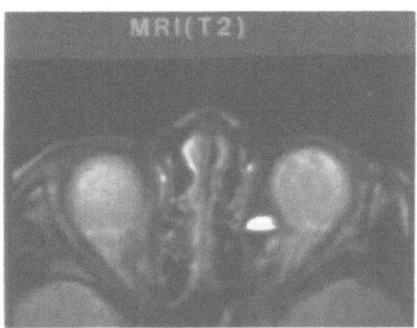

Figure 3. Ultrasonographically, the image of this tumor was relatively low reflective and had a clear margin. The tumor appeared to be solid.

Figure 4. MRI (T1, T2) showing fluid-fluid niveau formation in the inner part of tumor.

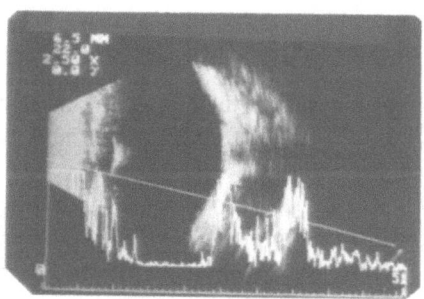

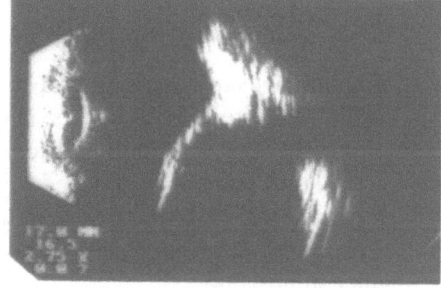

Figure 5. Ultrasonographically, acoustic shadow was slightly decreased compared to that 9 months earlier.

Figure 6. Tumor was characterized by good outline, acoustic solidity, low attenuation and by compression of the nasal inferior wall of the eye ball.

On enhanced CT, the recurrence was observed. The tumor was enlarged and compressed the infero-nasal portion of the eye ball. After admission, a one month course of chemotherapy was initiated and proton beam irradiation was performed. From 14 May to 12 June, the total dose was 45 gray with irradiation being performed every other day.

During proton beam irradiation, ultrasonographic examination was performed almost every week. In response to irradiation, the tumor size gradually reduced. The changes in the tumor are shown in Figs. 7 and 8; it was clearly outlined and contained more calcification. The sound transmission improved after proton irradiation. By July, the tumor did not show further reduction. There were no improvements on other examinations.

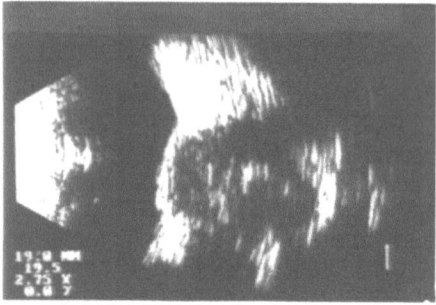 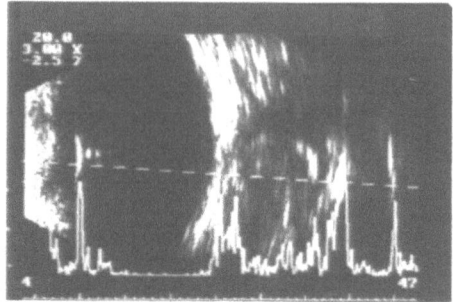

Figure 7. The changes in the tumor during proton beam irradiation.

Figure 8. The tumor size did not show further change.

Enucleation was performed on July third, and the tumor was totally removed.

Discussion

Rhabdomyosarcoma is the most common primary malignant tumor of the orbit, and frequently occurs in childhood. Treatment is performed with chemotherapy, radiation and resection [4, 5].

Therapy can be prolonged. For example, combined chemotherapy requires at least 2 years to complete and many complications can arise during treatment, i.e. bone hypoplasia, cataract, keratoconjunctivitis or lacrimal duct stenosis [4].

Proton beam irradiation is a new therapeutic method [6]. In our case, after proton beam irradiation, there was a slight redness similar to sunburn, but without pain or disorder in the affected area. The redness disappeared in a few weeks [7]. Usually, CT and MRI examinations are performed under hypnotic drugs to check therapeutic efficacy. Regarding CT examination, we must avoid excessive radiation effects on children, so it's use was reduced to the minimum. In contrast, ultrasonography is performed quickly and easily [8]. This was the first case in our clinic where the therapeutic efficacy of proton beam irradiation was evaluated by ultrasonography without sedation. Every week, we evaluated the features of this tumor. We observed the rapid decrease in size and the progressive inner calcification. In measuring the tumor size, we were restricted in direction by the transducer, so we measured in a slightly oblique direction.

Now, we are using ultrasonography to follow 4 children with rhabdomyosarcoma treated by proton irradiation and chemotherapy. All of the children can endure this examination easily. We conclude that proton beam irradiation may be an effective new treatment for orbital rhabdomyosarcoma and it is further suggested that ultrasonography is very useful for evaluating therapeutic efficacy in children with orbital tumor.

References

[1] R M Quencer In Computed tomography in the diagnosis of orbital tumors in children pediatric ocular tumors, Masson Pub , New York, 1981, pp 187–206

[2] D H Nicholson In Rhabdomyosarcoma pediatric ocular tumors Masson Pub , New York, 1981, pp 247–254

[3] D M Knowles II *et al* Ophthalmic striated muscle neoplasma Surv Ophthalmol 1976–77,21 219

[4] J Brazier In Rhabdomyosarcoma pediatric ophthalmology, Blackwell Scientific, Inc , Massachusetts, 1980, pp 261–265

[5] Y A Salahudin *et al* Orbital rhabdomyosarcoma improved survival with combined pulse chemotherapy and irradiation Bri J Ophthalmol 1985,69 557–561

[6] M Kiribuchi Radiation therapy for orbital tumor orbital disease Ganka Mook No 13, Kanehara, Tokyo, 1980, pp 213–221 (in Japanese)

[7] K Toyota *et al* Orbital rhabdomyosarcoma treatment course and ultrasonographic evaluation Jap J Clin Ophthalmol 1993, in press (in Japanese)

[8] R Guthoff Ultrasound diagnosis of orbital diseases ultrasound in ophthalmologic diagnosis, Georg Thieme Verlag, Stuttgart, 1991, pp 116–149

Department of Ophthalmology and *Pediatric Surgery
Institute of Clinical Medicine
University of Tsukuba
Tennodai 1-1-1, Tsukuba-shi
Ibaraki 305, Japan

4.3. Findings in Standardized Echography for Orbital Hemangioperycytoma

TOMOMI CHUMAN, HIDEKI CHUMAN, JO FUKIYAMA,
NOBUHISA NAO-I and ATSUSHI SAWADA

(Mɩyazakɩ, Japan)

Abstract. A case of orbital hemangiopericytoma in a 59-year-old woman is reported. Echography showed encapsulation and low internal reflectivity. Echography was useful in differentiating round-shaped, well-circumscribed orbital tumors. Histology of the resected tumor showed a characteristic feature of staghorn appearance.

Key words: Echography, MRI, hemangiopericytoma, orbital tumor.

Introduction

Orbital hemangiopericytoma is a relatively rare tumor that arises from the pericytes of the vessels. We recently experienced a case of orbital hemangiopericytoma of a middle-aged woman. We present the echographic and radiologic findings, clinical course, and the result of the histopathologic findings of this unusal orbital tumor.

Case Report

A-59-year-old woman was referred to us with a complaint of left upper lid swelling and proptosis of one month duration. She denied orbital pain, diplopia, decreased vision, and other physical symptoms.

On examination, her best-corrected visual acuity of both eyes was 20/20. Her left upper lid was swollen and an elastic hard mass was palpable in the superonasal aspect of the anterior orbit and superior conjunctival vessels were injected. There was no relative afferent pupillary defect. There was 8 mm forward proptosis of the left eye. The supraduction of the left eye was slightly restricted. The slit-lamp examination of the cornea, anterior chamber and lens of her left eye revealed no abnormality. Her left fundus showed no abnormality. She had no systemic disease and her family history was non-contributory.

The urine, blood analysis and chest X-ray were normal.

On axial CT scan, a round-shaped, well-circumscribed, high density mass

J M Thɩjssen, H C Fledelɩus and S Tane (eds), Ultrasonography ɩn Ophthalmology 14, 200–205

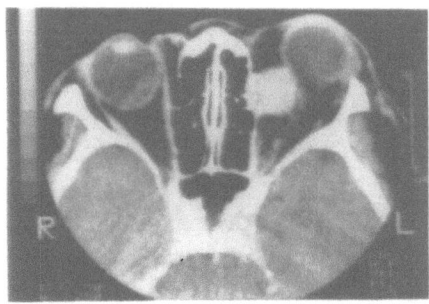

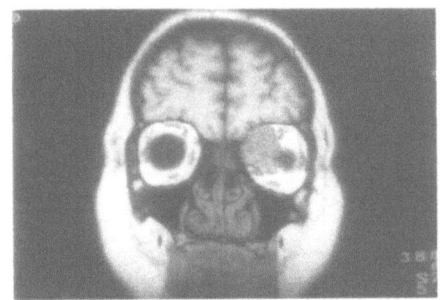

Figure 1. Axial CT scan shows a round-shaped, well-circumscribed, high density mass on the nasal side of the optic nerve in the retrobulbar space.

Figure 2. T$_1$-weighted coronal MRI reveals a low-intensity mass occupying the nasal aspect of the orbit. Note the mass involves the superior rectus muscle.

existed on the nasal side of the optic nerve in the retrobulbar space (Fig. 1). The nasal side of the mass lay on the medial orbital wall. A higher horizontal section revealed that the mass extended anteriorly toward the orbital septum and posteriorly toward the orbital apex. There was no bony erosion or destruction.

T$_1$-weighted coronal MRI (Fig. 2) revealed a low-intensity mass occupying the nasal aspect of the orbit, involving superior rectus and superior oblique muscles, and compressing the medial rectus muscle inferiorly. The mass was isointense to extraocular muscles and almost isointense to the white matter. After gadolinium administration, the tumor enhanced well. The tumor seemed to be highly vascularized.

A left internal and external carotid angiogram showed an arterial blood supply from the ophthalmic artery in early arterial phase and also a well-defined, long-lasting tumor stain in the capillary-venous phase.

The contact B-mode echogram of the orbital extension revealed a retrobulbar tumor having a high reflective posterior wall, suggestive of encapsulation (Fig. 3). The low internal reflectivity of the tumor was detected by standardized A-mode echogram. The contact A-mode echogram showed more reflective areas within the tumor at high gain setting but they diminished at tissue sensitivity (Fig. 4).

A tiny part of the mass displaying acoustic shadow suggested a calcification.

In February, 1991 the tumor was surgically removed by frontal craniotomy. It was a red-brown encapsulated vascular tumor. The tumor involved the superior oblique muscle and was impossible to remove without cutting a part of the superior oblique muscle's tendon.

Histopathological examination showed the capillary channels of various size (Fig. 5). According to its characteristic configuration of dividing vascular pattern, so-called 'staghorn appearance', the diagnosis was hemangiopericy-

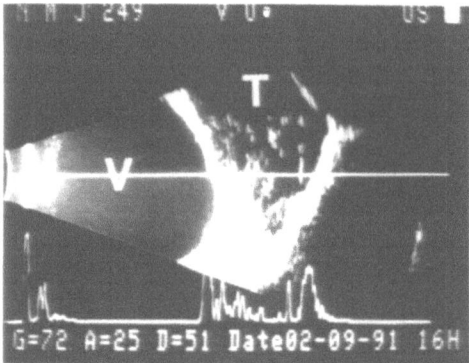

Figure 3. The contact B-mode echogram reveals the retrobulbar tumor having a high reflective posterior wall, suggestive of encapsulation.

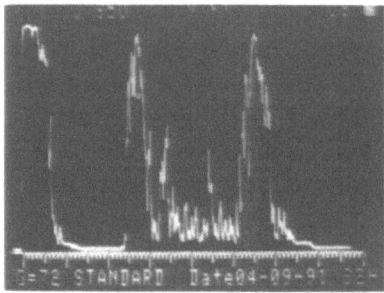

Figure 4. Standardized A-mode echogram shows the low internal reflectivity of the tumor.

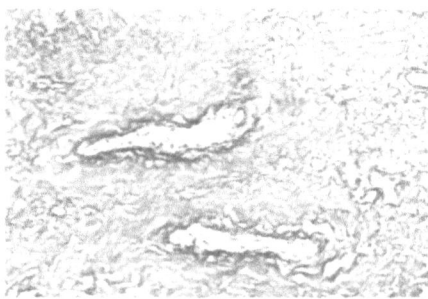

Figure 5. Histopathological examination shows the capillary channels of various sizes. Note the characteristic 'staghorn appearance'. (Hematoxylin and eosin stain ×40).

toma. At higher magnification, capillary channels lined by flattened endo-thelium and spindle-shaped tumor cells proliferating around them could be seen. Occasional mitotic appearance was noted. Reticulum stains showed the reticulum fibers outlining the basement membrane of the vascular spaces. With TPHA stains, a tumor origin from muscles was denied. After surgery, cobalt radiotherapy (total dosis 60 Gy) was administered. Postoperative vis-ual aquity was the same as preoperative and proptosis of both eyes was deviated 5 mm. Further, the left lid was 5 mm downward, and there was a paralysis of the left oblique muscle although the eye position was orthophoric.

Discussion

Orbital hemangioperycytoma was first described by Goodman and his col-leagues in 1955 [1]. The tumor may occur at any age, but mostly in middle-aged and rarely in infants [2]. The incidence is approximately 3% of primary orbital neoplasma and approximately 1.7% of orbital tumors [3]. The tumor has been rarely reported in the orbit, except for the retrobulbar space. For example 3 cases were reported in the choroid [4–6], 4 cases in the lacrimal sac [7–10] and 2 cases in the conjunctiva [11, 12].

The most common location is in the upper orbit [12]. In our case, however, it developed within the superior oblique muscle. There are no previous reports describing an orbital intramuscular hemangioperycytoma [2].

On CT scan, the tumor is well-demarcated and isointense or hyperintense to the brain with homogeneous enhancement [13–17].

On T_1-weighted magnetic resonance imaging (MAI), the tumor tend to be hyperintense to the vitreous and the cerebral white matter, whereas on T_2-weighted MRI, the tumor is hypointense compared to the vitreous and the cerebral white matter [13–15]. Since there are no characteristic findings in radiological features, it is difficult to distinguish the tumor from benign tumors like cavernous hemangioma and schwannoma which are well-circum-scribed and encapsulated.

Generally echography in hemangioperycytoma shows low to medium in-ternal reflectivity on the A-mode echogram. Contact B-mode echogram shows a well-circumscribed, round shaped mass having partially cystic spaces [2, 18, 19]. In the presented case, similar findings were imaged. Calcification, seen in our case, is characteristic in this tumor [13]. The differential diagnosis of orbital calcification includes varix, hemangioma, lymphangioma and or-bital vessels themselves [20]. The differential diagnosis of round-shaped, well-circumscribed orbital tumors includes cavernous hemangioma, fibrous histiocytoma, meningioma and schwannoma. The echographic findings are useful to distinguish orbital hemangioperycytoma from these tumors. First, cavernous hemangioma show a well-encapsulated and round-shaped mass on the B scan, however on the standardized A-scan it shows more solid, high amplitude internal echoes. So, it could be distinguished by A-scan [21, 22]. Second, fibrous histiocytoma shows low to medium internal reflectivity on the standardized A-scan [23], but is less encapsulated [24, 25]. Third, meningioma produces irregular internal structure, and the reflectivity is high to low on the standardized A-scan [26]. Fourth, schwannoma shows low to medium reflectivity with long spikes produced by the smooth cavity walls by standardzed A-scan and often shows partially cystic spaces on the B-scan [27]. Hemangiopericytoma could metastasize regardless of its histopathological findings; either benign, borderline or malignant. Setzkorn and his fellows reported distant metastasis of 7% even in presumed benign tumors [28]. This tumor is also characteristic in slow progress, Rice and his fellows reported a case recurring after 33 years [14]. Therefore, a long-standing follow-up is necessary. Echograms are also useful in monitoring recurrence.

References

[1] S A Goodman Hemangiopericytoma of the orbit Am J Ophthalmol 1995,40 237–243

[2] F A Jakobiec and G M Howard Hemangiopericytoma of the orbit Am J Ophthalmol 1974,78 816–834

[3] J W Henderson and G M Farrow Primary orbital hemangiopericytoma An aggresive and potentially malignant neoplasma Arch ophthalmol 1987,96 666–673

[4] J J Papale and A R Frederich et al Intraocular hemangiopericytoma Arch Ophthalmol 1983,101 1409–11

[5] S C GiGier and T J Hufnagel et al Hemangiopericytoma of the ciliary body Arch Ophthalmol 1988,106 1269–72

[6] H H Brown and M C Brodsky et al Supraciliary hemangiopericytoma Ophthalmology 1991,98 378–382

[7] N Gurney and T Chalkley et al Lacrimal sac hemangiopericytoma Am J Ophthalmol 1971,71 757–9

[8] L Carnevali and F Trimarchi et al Hemangiopericytoma of the lacrimal sac a case report Br J Ophthalmol 1988,72 762–5

[9] C Ni and D J D'Amico et al Tumours of the lacrimal sac a clinicopathological analysis of 82 cases Int Ophthalmol Clin 1982,22 121–40

[10] S I Roth and C Z August et al Hemangiopericytoma of the lacrimal sac Ophthalmology 1991,98 925–927

[11] H E Grossniklaus and W R Green et al Hemangiopericytoma of the conjunctiva Ophthalmology 1986,93 265–267

[12] J O Croxatto and R L Font Hemangiopericytoma of the orbit, A clinicopathologic study of 30 cases Hum Pathol 1982,13 210–213

[13] M Kubo and F Yamamoto et al A case of orbital hemangiopericytoma Jpn Rev Clin Ophthalmol 1988,82 1068–1077

[14] C D Rice and R C Kersten et al An orbital hemangiopericytoma, Recurrent after 33 years Arch Ophthalmol 1989,107 552–556

[15] I S Jones and F A Jakobiec Disease of the orbit Philadelphia JB Lippinco 1988,tt 291–293

[16] D J Coden and A H Hornblass Orbital hemangiopericytoma JAMA 1990,264 1861

[17] I Morino and A Nakayama et al A case of orbital hemangiopericytoma Acta Soc Ophthalmol Jpn 1990,94 532–536

[18] E G Grant et al Sonographic findings in four cases of hemangiopericytoma Ultrasound 1982,142 447–451

[19] S F Byrne and R L Green Ultrasound of the eye and orbit St Louis Mosby 1992,339–342

[20] J A Garrity and Kennerdell Orbital calcification associated with hemangiopericytoma Am J Ophthalmol 1982,102 126

[21] J A Shields Diagnosis and management of orbital tumors Philadelphia W B Saunders Company, 1989,128–132

[22] S F Byrne and R L Green Ultrasound of the eye and orbit St Louis Mosby 1992,329–331

[23] S F Byrne and R L Green Ultrasound of the eye and orbit St Louis Mosby 1992,284, 291

[24] F A Jakobiec and I S Jones Clinical ophthalmology mesenchymal and fibroosseous tumors, Vol 2, Chap 44 Philadelphia JB Lippincott Company, 1991,3–10

[25] F A Jakobiec and I S Jones Clinical Ophthalmology Vascular tumors, malformation, and degenerationeous, Vol 2, Chap 37 Philadelphia JB Lippincott Company, 1991,23–25

[26] S F Byrne and R L Green Ultrasound of the eye and orbit St Louis Mosby 1992,403

[27] K C Ossoinig, ed Ophthalmic echography Proceedings of the 10th SIDUO Congress, 1987,483–492

[28] R K Setzkorn and D J Lee *et al* Hemangiopericytoma of the orbit treated with conservative surgery and radiotherapy Arch Ophthalmol 1987,105 1103–1105

Dr Tomomi Chuman
Department of Ophthalmology
Miyazaki Medical College
Miyazaki, Japan

4.4. Respective Roles of Echography, CT Scanner, and MR Imaging in the Diagnosis of Orbital Space Occupying Lesions

O. BERGES

(Paris, France)

Abstract. The respective roles of various medical imaging modalities, i.e. echography, X-ray computed tomography and magnetic resonance imaging, are outlined and decision schemes for the procedures to follow in various clinical conditions are presented.

Key words: Orbit, space occupying lesion, echography, CT, MRI.

1. Introduction

Echography (B and standardized A mode) and recently color Doppler flow imaging (CDFI), CT scanner and MR imaging are actually the three modern techniques for imaging orbital space occupying lesions (SOL). In some instances, plain radiographs, phlebography and selective carotid arteriography are also useful. For economic reasons, it is desirable not to perform all these modalities on every patient initially, but to choose the one or two which gives the most valuable results at the most reasonable cost and which are least invasive for the patient.

This study reviews a 13 years experience of orbital processes diagnostic evaluation using different generations of echographic, scannographic and magnetic resonance units. During this period (from September 1978 till September 1992) 1269 orbital SOL were seen, using one or several of the techniques. Echography should be performed immediately after the analysis of the clinical symptoms and should play a strategic role in order to follow logic diagnostic algorithms.

Plain radiographs are still useful in the evaluation of traumatisms and malformations. They also are useful to the neurosurgeon to evaluate the size of the frontal sinuses. Tomographies are still useful to explore the state of the lacrimal ducts.

J M Thijssen, H C Fledelius and S Tane (eds), Ultrasonography in Ophthalmology 14, 206–210
© 1995 *Kluwer Academic Publishers, Dordrecht*

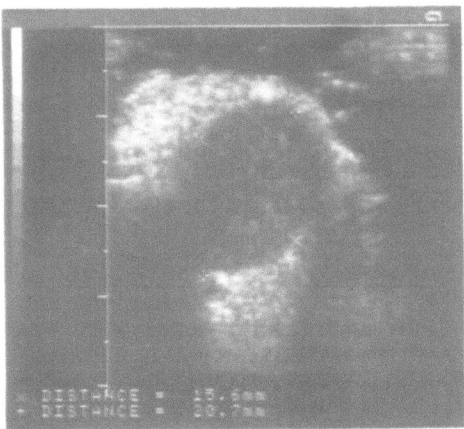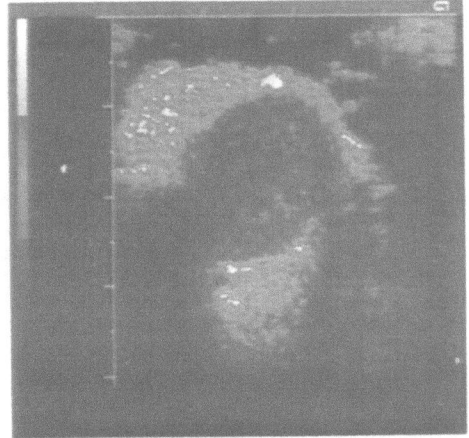

Figure 1. B mode echogram performed on a modern equipment of an anteriorly located orbital tumor. (a) Normal gray scale pictures with measurement of the lesion in two orthogonal directions. (b) Reflectivity coded picture. The lesion appears hyporeflective. This is confirmed by the reflectivity coded picture. The most reflective elements do not exceed the red level (which is less than 50% of the maximum reflectivity). The orbital fat appears green, blue and white ranging from moderate to high reflectivity levels. These informations are equivalent to what is given by standardized A mode.

2. Imaging Techniques

2.1. *Echography* is a simple, quick and cheap technique that gives wonderful information for the exploration of ocular, as well as orbital tumors and disorders. One of its main advantages is the possibility to obtain dynamic information in real-time. However, the quality of the obtained information is undoubtedly related to the experience of the echographist and to the quality of the machines. Training of the echographist is therefore very important. Recent technical improvements: gray scale up to 256 gray levels, high resolution, high energy beam, high image repetition rate, variable focusing of electronic probes and color coded reflectivity (Fig. 1) allow us to reduce this examiner dependency, to popularize the method and to broaden its indications (Berges and Torrent 1986). Color Doppler units that superimpose a color coded imaging of vascular flow on a conventional B mode picture appear to be very useful in the evaluation of orbital SOL (Fig. 2 and Table 1) (Berges 1992). These new techniques are a supplement to Standardized Echography that gives valuable topographic, quantitative and kinetic information (Table 2).

2.2. *CT Scanner* is an excellent technique to explore orbital SOL, but care must be taken with the techniques. Axial sections should follow the neuro-ocular plane. Direct coronal scans are always useful. Sections should be thin

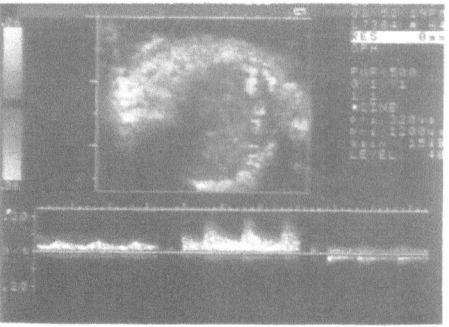

Figure 2. Color Doppler and pulsed Doppler of the same lesion. Vascular flows of different amplitude are detectable within the tumor.

Table 1.

INDICATIONS OF CDFI

* DIAGNOSIS (+ & ≠) OF OCULAR TUMORS
* FOLLOW UP OF MM POST CONSERVATIVE TREATMENT
* EVALUATION OF VASCULAR DISORDERS :
  Diabetes, Horton, Atheroma, Myopia, Glaucoma...
* ≠ DIAGNOSIS OF ORBITAL MASSES (vascularization)
* DIAGNOSIS AND FOLLOW UP OF CCF (post embolization)

Table 2.

		US	CT	IMRI
TOPOGRAPHY	LOCALISATION MORPHOLOGY LIMITS	+	++	++
QUANTIFICATION	ECHOSTRUCTURE REFLECTIVITY ATTENUATION	+++		
	DENSITY CONTRAST ENHANCEMENT		+	
	SIGNAL INTENSITY ρ, T1, T2,			++
KINETIC	COMPRESSIBILITY VASCULARIZATION	+	+/-	+/-

(1–2 mm), and reconstructed on a high resolution matrix. Recent computed programs allow to obtain coronal and sagittal reconstructed sections of good quality. Three dimensional reconstructions are particularly useful in cases of trauma, malformations and tumors with intra and extra-orbital compartments. Excluding the analysis of orbital fractures and Graves' disease where constrast medium injection is useless, it is advisable to realize sections before

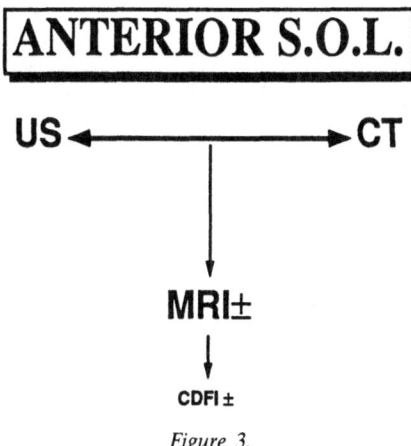

Figure 3.

and after contrast medium injection in order to demonstrate the vascularity of a lesion.

2.3. *Magnetic Resonance Imaging (MRI)* of the orbit, with its multiplanar capability, and its superior soft tissue discrimination is an excellent modality for demonstration of the complex orbital anatomy and for evaluation of orbital lesions. In fact, in some categories of orbital abnormalities, such as vascular, hemorrhagic, optic nerve complex, periorbital and apex lesions, MRI has a clear advantage on CT. It is necessary to perform T1 (spin echo dependant and gradient echo dependant) as well as T2 weighted sections in different planes. The use of surface coils permit acquisition of thin sections with improved signal to noise ratio and acquisition times of 1–2 minutes. Injection of contrast medium: Gadolinium DTPA, can be useful especially when associated to fat suppressed sequences. It is also advisable to perform cerebral sections in order to study the chiasm, the optic pathway, and the brain stem (Cabanis *et al.* 1992, Newton and Bilaniuk 1990).

Figures 3–7 are diagnostic algorithms that we recommend to follow in different clinico-echographic situations (Berges 1990).

3. Discussion

We want to stress that it is important to organize a multidisciplinary team, including ophthalmologists, radiologists, pathologists, radiation therapists, chemotherapists and orbital surgeons (ophthalmologist, neuro surgeon, ENT surgeon, maxillo facial surgeon). Such teams help to understand the complexity of orbital SOL's, which are rare, and help to find the most appropriate treatment for each patient.

210

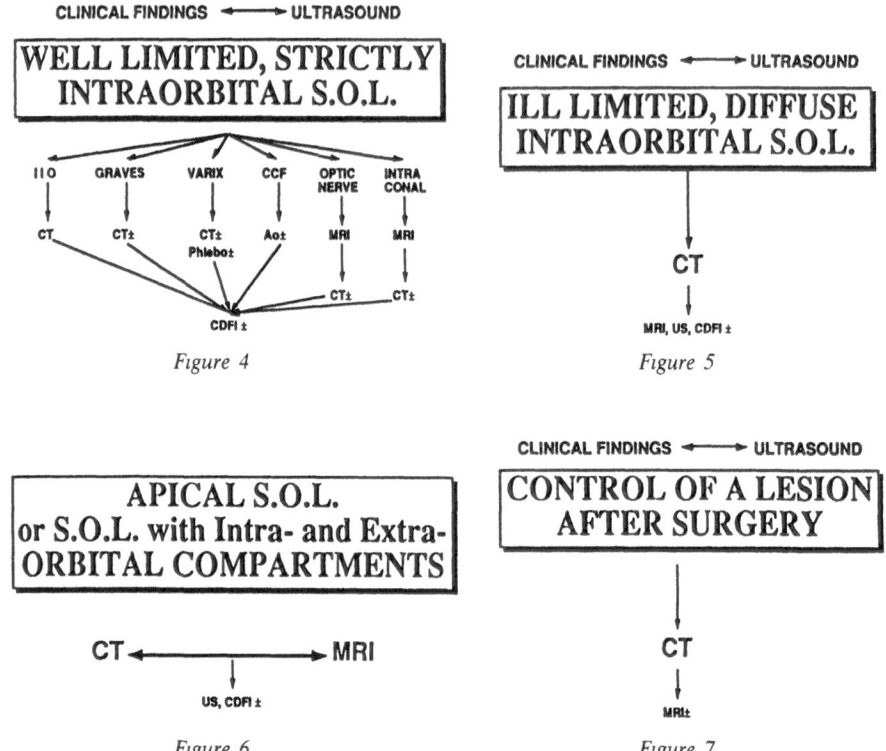

Figure 4

Figure 5

Figure 6

Figure 7

References

Berges, O and Torrent, M Echographie de l'oeil et de l'orbite Vigot, Paris, 1986

Berges, O Exploration de l'oeil et de l'orbite Scan/Echo/IRM Rev Prat 1990, 40 2631–2639

Berges, O Echo-Doppler couleur (EDC) en ophtalmologie Aspect des vaisseaux orbitaires normaux-Apport diagnostique de l'EDC a l'etude des tumeurs oculaires, de la pathologie vasculaire orbitaire et des tumeurs de l'orbite J Echogr Med Ultrasons 1992, 13 264–274

Cabanis, E A , Massinm, Iba-Zizen M T , Flament, J and Arnaud, D L'Imagerie par Resonance Magnetique (IRM) en ophtalmologie une introducation Bul Soc Ophtalmol France Rapport annuel, 1992 (920 references bibliographiques)

Newton, T H and Bilaniuk, L T (eds) Radiology of the eye and orbit 1990 A Clavadel Book Raven Press, New York

Fondation A de Rothschild
Paris
France

4.5. Diagnosis of Carotid-Cavernous Sinus Fistula Using Ultrasound, Color Doppler Imaging, CT-Scan and Digital Subtraction Angiography

JÁNOS NÉMETH, ENDRE NAGY,* ZITA MORVAY* and
ZOLTÁN HORÓCZI*

(*Budapest and Szeged*, Hungary)

Abstract. The results of diagnosis of 7 cases of carotid-cavernous sinus fistula are presented. The diagnosis was based on A- and B-mode and color Doppler echography, CT-scan and X-ray digital subtraction angiography. It is concluded that B-mode echography is the primary diagnostic modality for this disease.

Key words: Fistula, carotid-cavernous sinus, echography, color Doppler, CT-scan, digital subtraction angiography.

Introduction

The carotid-cavernous sinus fistula is a well-defined disease [11]. Its ophthalmological diagnostic signs are pulsating proptosis, chemosis, external muscle paresis, decrease of vision, headache and thrill. The clinical signs of the disease are sometimes very typical (mainly in the high-flow type or direct fistulas), but in many cases the diagnosis is difficult because of the incomplete clinical picture (mainly in the slow-flow type, indirect or dural fistulas). In such cases, echography (A/B-scan and color Doppler) and other imaging examinations (CT and digital subtraction angiography) of the orbit and brain may be of considerable help in the diagnosis. In the present paper, we summarize our experience concerning the clinical place and value of these diagnostic modalities in carotid-cavernous sinus fistulas.

Patients and Methods

A total of 7 cases with unilateral proptosis caused by carotid-cavernous sinus fistula (1 post-traumatic and 6 spontaneous) were examined. The age of the patients varied from 7 to 75 years. The sex distribution was 2 males and 5 females. Successful radiological intervention (closing the fistula with two detachable balloons) was performed in 1 patient After angiography, spontaneous occlusion was observed in 2 cases and a slow improvement in 1 case. In the other 3 cases, the further history is unknown.

Ophthalmic echography was performed with Ultrascan Digital B ultra-

J.M. Thijssen, H.C. Fledelius and S. Tane (eds.), Ultrasonography in Ophthalmology 14, 211–215.
© 1995 *Kluwer Academic Publishers, Dordrecht.*

Ophthalmic echography was performed with Ultrascan Digital B ultrasound equipment with 10 MHz A and B-scan probe. For color-coded Doppler imaging of the orbital circulation, an Acuson 128 with a 7 MHz linear probe and a Toshiba SSH-65A with a 5 MHz sector probe were used. Computerized tomography was carried out with a Siemens Somatom DRG (512*512 matrix). Digital subtraction angiography was performed with a Siemens Polytron instrument (1024*1024 matrix, 6 pictures/sec), and a Siemens Angiotron (512*512 matrix, continuous).

Results and Discussion

The *A-mode criteria* of carotid-cavernous fistulas were described by Ossoinig [15], and later by MacNeill [10]: steeply rising and falling surface spikes and low or very low spikes with fast-flickering vertical motion between them. Non-specific congestive signs may also be displayed, such as enlargement of the extraocular muscles and optic nerve.

The *B-mode signs* were detailed by Phelps and colleagues [16] and by Guthoff [6–7]. The picture is very typical: uniformly dilated ophthalmic vein(s) travelling from the nasal anterior part of the orbit to the temporal, and then to the posterior part. In our patients, dilated veins could also be detected contralaterally in 4 of the 7 cases.

In our experience, ophthalmic B-scan echography, as a quick screening method, is a suitable technique for establishment of the diagnosis of carotid-cavernous sinus fistula in all cases with high-flow (direct) fistulas and in most cases with slow-flow (indirect) fistulas.

Ossoinig [15] described the usefulness of continuous Doppler examination. Balazs and colleagues [1] examined the haemodynamic changes secondary to carotid-cavernous fistulas by using 2 MHz pulsed transcranial Doppler. The first publication on the use of *color-coded Doppler* in this disease was that of Erickson [4] in 1989. We likewise described our first patients four years ago [12–14]. Other authors too have published their experience [2, 5, 7–9]. The color Doppler signs of carotid-cavernous fistulas are as follows: reversal of the blood flow and arterialization of the blood flow. In our patients, we found relatively high velocities (15–35 cm/sec), see Fig. 1.

In our experience, the use of color-coded Doppler imaging permits the very easy demonstration of arterialized and reversed blood flow in ophthalmic veins. The spectra are typical of arterial or shunt circulation. Color Doppler has some advantages over conventional diagnostics and also over the other diagnostic imaging techniques: it is quick and non-invasive and can be repeated as frequently as needed; at the same time, it gives both topographic and haemodynamic information about arteries and veins.

On *CT-scans*, the pathological vessel dilatation in the orbit can be displayed, usually only through the use of contrast material. Although this makes the examination invasive, the results are poor, as frequently only part of the vessel can be visualized, and only in one scan plane. Enlargement of

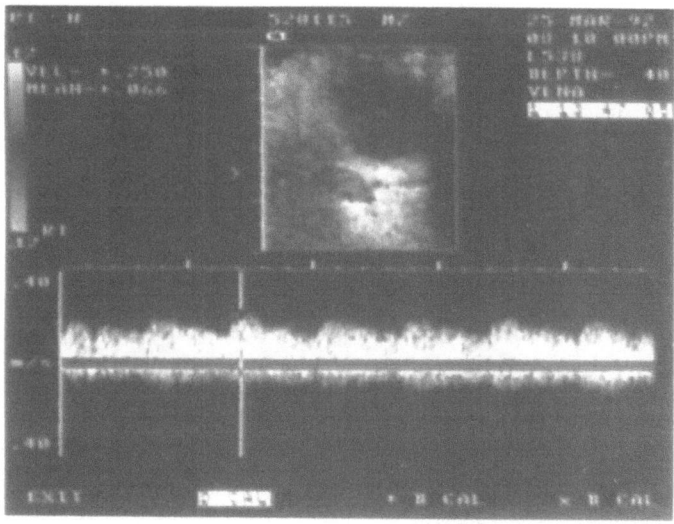

Figure 1. Color-coded Doppler imaging of the superior ophthalmic vein in carotid-cavernous fistula. The direction of the flow is from the apex of the orbit to the anterior. The Doppler spectrum is typical of arterial circulation.

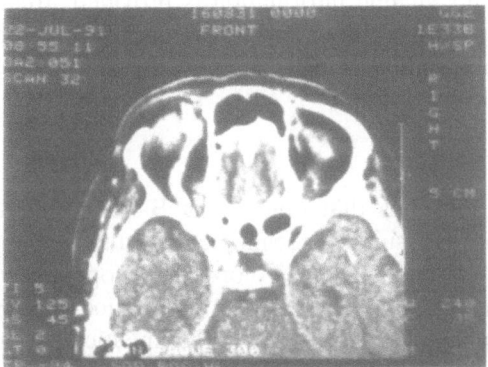

Figure 2. CT-scan of a patient with carotid-cavernous fistula. After contrast filling, the dilated superior ophthalmic vein is well visible in the left orbit.

the extraocular muscles, enlargement of the optic nerve and intracranial malformations can also be displayed. Figure 2 shows the CT-scan of a patient where a dilated superior ophthalmic vein is clearly visible in the left orbit.

With *digital subtraction angiography*, the filling of different pathological veins in the early arterial phase can be demonstrated both in the orbit and also in the brain. In the very early arterial phase, the filling of the shunt

214

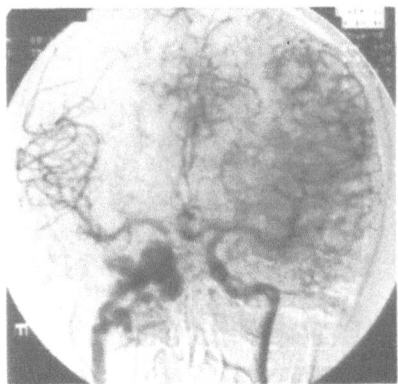

Figure 3. Digital subtraction angiography of the contralateral internal carotid artery of a patient with a carotid-cavernous fistula on the right side. Filling of the aneurysm-like malformation in the sinus cavernous on the right side is exactly visible.

vessel can be observed; later, the aneurysm-like enlargement of veins after the fistula is clearly visible (cf. Fig. 3).

The advantages of digital subtraction angiography include: accurate mapping of orbital and intracranial vessels; the exact site of the fistula can be verified; haemodynamic information is provided; treatment planning is facilitated; and the possibility can be revealed of interventional radiologic treatment by embolization or balloon implantation [3].

Conclusion

Our experience indicates that ophthalmic B-scan echography, as a quick screening method, is a suitable technique for establishment of the diagnosis of carotid-cavernous sinus fistula. Color-coded Doppler imaging is appropriate to confirm the final diagnosis. Digital subtraction angiography is required only for the planning or performance of therapeutic or surgical intervention.

References

[1] E. Balázs, L. Rózsa and S. Szabó. A carotideo-cavernous fistulakat koveto véráramlás-változások. Szemészet 1992;129:159–162.
[2] O. Berges. Doppler flow imaging of the orbital veins. Acta Ophthalmol Supplement 1992;204,70:55–58.
[3] G.M. Debrun. Treatment of carotid cavernous fistulas, and cavernous and paraophthalmic aneurysms. In: J. L. Smith (ed.): Neuro-ophthalmology Now. Springer 1986, pp. 211–225.
[4] S.J. Erickson, L.E. Hendrix and B.M. Masaro *et al*. Color Doppler flow imaging of normal and abnormal orbit radiology 1989;173:511–516.
[5] P.M. Flaharty, W.E. Lieb, R.C. Sergott *et al*. Color Doppler imaging. A new noninvasive technique to diagnose and monitor carotid cavernous sinus fistulas. Arch Ophthalmol. 1991;109:522–526.

215

[6] R Guthoff and J Jorgensen Long term follow-up in patients with spontaneous AV-fistulas affecting the orbit Orbit 1987,6 229–235

[7] R Guthoff Ultrasound in ophthalmologic diagnosis A practical guide Thieme, Stuttgart, 1991

[8] P S Kotval, I Weitzner and M S Tenner Diagnosis of carotid-cavernous fistula by periorbital color Doppler imaging and pulsed Doppler volume flow analysis J Ultrasound Med 1990,9 101

[9] W E Lieb, D A Merton, J A Shields et al Colour Doppler imaging in the demonstration of an orbital varix Br J Ophthalmol 1990,74 305–308

[10] J MacNeill The diagnosis of intracranial A V malformation with orbita involvement by 'standardized echography' Orbit 1987,6 217–222

[11] N R Miller Walsh and Hoyt's clinical neuro-ophthalmology Chapter 57 Carotid-cavernous sinus fistulas Williams and Wilkins, Baltimore, 1991

[12] J Németh, T Forster and L Heiner Carotideo-cavernosus fistula diagnózisa ultrahanggal A Magyar Szemorvos Társaság Vándorgyulése nemzetkozi részvétellel Szeged, 1989

[13] J Németh, Z Morvay, Z Horóczi and E Nagy A színkódolt Doppler ultrahang vizsgálat szemészeti alkalmazása Szemészet 1992,129 34–37

[14] J Németh, M Végh, Z Horóczi and I Suveges A szemgolyó és az orbita vizsgálata nemszemészeti ultrahang készulékekkel Orvosi Hetilap 1992,133 2563–2565

[15] K C Ossoinig Standardized Echography Basic Principles, Clinical Applications, and Results In R D Dallow (ed) Ophthalmic ultrasonography comparative techniques Little, Brown and Co , Boston, 1979, pp 127–210

[16] C D Phelps, H S Thompson and K C Ossoinig The diagnosis and prognosis of atypical carotid-cavernous fistula (red-eye shunt syndrome) Am J Ophthalmol 1982,93 423–436

Dr J Németh
1st Department of Ophthalmology
Semmelweis Medical University
Tomo u 25–29
H-1083 Budapest
Hungary

4.6. Color Doppler Imaging of Orbital Blood Flow in Dysthyroid Ophthalmopathy

YOSHIKO NAKASE, TOSHI HIGASHIDE, KEIJI YOSHIKAWA and
YOUICHI INOUE
(*Tokyo, Japan*)

Abstract. 39 orbits of 20 patients with dysthyroid ophthalmopathy and 22 orbits of 11 healthy control subjects were studied by color Doppler imaging. The authors found that blood in the superior ophthalmic vein flowed in the postero-anterior direction in 6 of the dysthyroid orbits. The superior ophthalmic vein blood flow in the postero-anterior direction was seen more frequently in the orbits in which apical orbital crowding, i.e. compression of the optic nerve by enlarged extraocular muscles, was observed on CT than in orbits without evidence of apical orbital crowding. Blood flow in the postero-anterior direction in the superior ophthalmic vein was seen also more frequently in orbits with dysthyroid optic neuropathy than in orbits without dysthyroid optic neuropathy. Color Doppler imaging has been shown to be a useful noninvasive tool for both the analysis of the venous stasis in the orbit and management of dysthyroid ophthalmopathy, especially with respect to assessing the risk of developing optic neuropathy.

Key words: Color Doppler flow imaging, dysthyroidism, Graves' disease, orbitopathy, ophthalmic vein.

Introduction

Among eye changes associated with Graves' disease, optic neuropathy is a serious complication which results in visual impairment. Orbital CT scan studies of dysthyroid optic neuropathy patients have revealed enlarged extraocular muscles, which cause a demonstrable compression of the optic nerve at the orbital apex [1, 2]. It has also been suggested that relative to individuals without optic neuropathy, dysthyroid ophthalmopathy patients with optic neuropathy have more severe venous stasis in the orbit due to increased intra-orbital pressure [2, 3]. We used color Doppler imaging which allows us to visualize a quasi-real time image of the retrobulbar structure with color-coded vascular images. We could determine the condition of the superior ophthalmic vein with this new technique to understand the

J.M. Thijssen, H.C. Fledelius and S. Tane (eds.), Ultrasonography in Ophthalmology 14, 216–224.
© *1995 Kluwer Academic Publishers, Dordrecht.*

relationship between venous stasis and apical compression in the orbit and its role in the pathophysiology of dysthyroid optic neuropathy.

Material and Methods

39 orbits of 20 patients with dysthyroid ophthalmopathy were studied. The average age of the patients was 45.4 years (range, 17 to 68 years). 9 patients were male and 11 patients were female. All of the patients had Graves' disease and were under treatment to maintain a euthyroid state.

Axial and coronal CT were evaluated based on the criteria described in our previous report [4]. Enlargement of extraocular muscles was noted on CT in 33 orbits. Enlargement of the inferior, medial, superior and lateral recti was seen in 11 orbits. Enlargement of the inferior, medial and superior recti was seen in 11 orbits. Enlargement of the inferior and superior recti was seen in 3 orbits. Enlargement of the inferior and medial recti occurred in 1 orbit and the inferior rectus alone was enlarged in 7 orbits. 6 orbits were free from any extraocular muscle enlargement.

CT scans showed apical orbital crowding, i.e. compression of the optic nerve by enlarged extraocular muscles at the orbital apex, in 14 orbits.

According to the Inoue classification system, 9 eyes were diagnosed as having moderate to severe dysthyroid optic neuropathy based on the presence of decreased visual acuity, abnormal visual field and/or redness of the optic disc [5]. Visual acuity varied from 20/800 to 20/20. Visual fields were evaluated by Octopus 201. Visual field loss was noted in 9 eyes.

Our control group consisted of 22 healthy subjects with an average age of 41.8 years (range, 20 to 58 years). 5 subjects were male and 6 subjects were female.

Color Doppler imaging was performed using an EUB 565A (Hitachi) with a 7.5 MHz linear array transducer. Each subject was asked to lie supine for 5 minutes prior to the examination. The transducer was applied with a coupling gel to the subject's closed eye lids. Horizontal and vertical scans through the eye and the orbit were performed. Different angles were used if necessary, to ensure that the probe was along the axis of the vessel.

Results

Of the 39 orbits with dysthyroid ophthalmopathy, the superior ophthalmic vein was detectable in 26 (67%) and not detectable in 13 (33%). Of the 22 control orbits, the superior ophthalmic vein was detectable in 13 (59%) and not detectable in 9 (41%) (Table 1).

In dysthyroid ophthalmopathy orbits, the superior ophthalmic vein was detectable in 13 (93%) of the 14 orbits in which apical orbital crowding was observed on CT, but in only 13 (52%) of 25 orbits without evidence of apical orbital crowding (Table 2) ($p < 0.05$). Apical orbital crowding was seen in 8 of 9 optic neuropathy orbits. The superior ophthalmic vein was detectable

Table 1 Detectability of the superior ophthalmic vein in color Doppler imaging

	SOV Detectability		
	(+)	(−)	Total
Dysthyroid ophthalmopathy	26 (67%)	13 (33%)	39 (100%)
Control	13 (59%)	9 (41%)	22 (100%)

SOV = the superior ophthalmic vein   ns

Table 2 Detectability of the superior ophthalmic vein in color Doppler imaging and apical orbital crowding on CT

	SOV Detectability		
	(+)	(−)	Total
Dysthyroid ophthalmopathy			
Apical crowding (+)	13 (93%)	1 (7%)	14 (100%)
*			
Apical crowding (−)	13 (52%)	12 (48%)	25 (100%)

* P < 0.05

in 8 (89%) of 9 optic neuropathy orbits and in 18 (60%) of 30 nonneuropathy orbits (Table 3).

In Color Doppler imaging, blood flow in the superior ophthalmic vein is usually blue indicating a flow away from the transducer. In contrast to the arterial spectrum in the ophthalmic artery and its branches, Doppler spectrum in the superior ophthalmic vein showed a continuous, linear wave or minimally pulsatile wave influenced by the cardiac cycle (Fig. 1). In some cases, we detected blood flow in the superior ophthalmic vein toward the

Table 3. Relationship between detectability of the superior ophthalmic vein in color Doppler imaging dysthyroid optic neuropathy.

	SOV Detectability		
	(+)	(−)	Total
Dysthyroid ophthalmopathy			
Optic neuropathy (+)	8 (89%)	1 (11%)	9 (100%)
Optic neuropathy (−)	18 (60%)	12 (40%)	30 (100%)

ns = not significant.

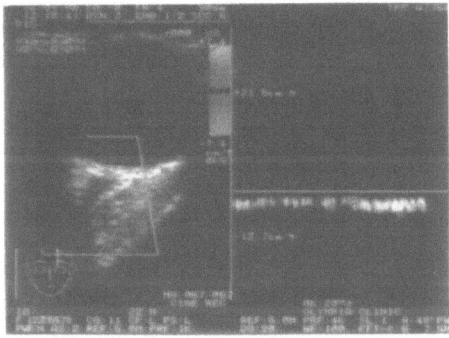

Figure 1. Antero-posterior blood flow in the superior ophthalmic vein in a healthy subject (vertical section). Blood flow is coded in blue. Doppler spectrum shows a minimally pulsatile wave.

transducer, coded in red with a positive continuous wave (Fig. 2). We use the words "the flow in the postero-anterior direction" when referring to the the blood flow in the superior ophthalmic vein toward the transducer.

The superior ophthalmic vein blood flow in the postero-anterior direction was seen in 6 (15%) of 39 dysthyroid ophthalmopathy orbits but in none (0%) of the 22 control orbits (Table 4).

In dysthyroid ophthalmopathy orbits, the blood flow in the superior ophthalmic vein was in the postero-anterior direction in 5 (36%) of 14 orbits with apical orbital crowding as compared to only 1 (4%) of the 25 orbits without apical orbital crowding ($p < 0.05$) (Table 5). The reversed blood

220

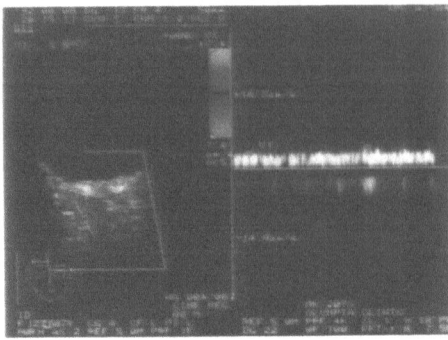

Figure 2. Postero-anterior blood flow in the superior ophthalmic vein in a dysthyroid optic neuropathy patient (horizontal section). Reversed blood flow is coded in red. Doppler spectrum shows continuous wave.

Table 4. Direction of blood flow in the superior ophthalmic vein in color Doppler imaging.

	SOV Blood flow		
	postero-anterior	antero-posterior	not detected
Dysthyroid ophthalmopathy	6 (15%)	20 (52%)	13 (33%)
Control	0 (0%)	13 (59%)	9 (41%)

ns

flow in the superior ophthalmic vein was also seen in 4 (44%) of 9 orbits with optic neuropathy as opposed to 2 (7%) of 30 orbits without optic neuropathy ($p < 0.05$) (Table 6).

Apical orbital crowding on CT is one of the most important findings with regard to the diagnosis of dysthyroid optic neuropathy. To evaluate the diagnostic value of color Doppler imaging, the sensitivity and specificity of diagnosis based on the superior ophthalmic vein blood flow in the postero-anterior direction in color Doppler imaging was compared to that based on apical orbital crowding on CT. Apical orbital crowding on CT yielded a sensitivity of 89% and a specificity of 80% in our series of examinations. The postero-anterior flow in the superior ophthalmic vein in color Doppler imaging had a low level of sensitivity of 44% but a specificity as an indicator

Table 5. Relationship between the direction of blood flow in the superior ophthalmic vein in color Doppler imaging and apical orbital crowding on CT.

	SOV Blood flow		
	postero-anterior	antero-posterior	not detected
Dysthyroid ophthalmopathy			
Apical crowding (+)	5 (36 %)	8 (57 %)	1 (7 %)
	*		
Apical crowding (−)	1 (4 %)	12 (48 %)	12 (48 %)

* P < 0.05

Table 6. Relationship between the direction of blood flow in the superior ophthalmic vein in color Doppler imaging and optic neuropathy.

	SOV Blood flow		
	postero-anterior	antero-posterior	not detected
Dysthyroid ophthalmopathy			
Optic neuropathy (+)	4 (44 %)	4 (44 %)	1 (11 %)
	*		
Optic neuropathy (−)	2 (7 %)	16 (53 %)	12 (40 %)

* P < 0.05

Table 7. Sensitivity and specificity of reversed blood flow in the superior ophthalmic vein in color Doppler imaging and apical orbital crowding on CT.

	Postero-anterior SOV blood flow	Apical crowding
Sensitivity (No. positive) of neuropathy orbits	44 % (4 / 9)	89 % (8 / 9)
Specificity (No. negative) of nonneuropathy orbits	93 % (28/30)	80 % (24/30)

of dysthyroid optic neuropathy of 93%, i.e, even higher than that of apical orbital crowding on CT (Table 7).

Discussion

The present study demonstrated that color Doppler imaging can provide information on venous stasis in orbits with dysthyroid ophthalmopathy. Blood flow in the superior ophthalmic vein was visualized by color Doppler imaging. A reverse flow in the superior ophthalmic vein was demonstrated in orbits with dysthyroid ophthalmopathy orbits. This has not been demonstrated using any technique other than color Doppler imaging [6].

No difference in the detectability of the superior ophthalmic vein by color Doppler imaging was found between dysthyroid ophthalmopathy orbits and control orbits. Among orbits with dysthyroid ophthalmopathy orbits, however, the detectability of the superior ophthalmic vein was higher in those orbits in which apical orbital crowding was observed on CT than in orbits without evidence of apical orbital crowding. The detectability of the superior ophthalmic vein also tended to be higher, though not significantly, in orbits with optic neuropathy than in those without optic neuropathy. Apical compression by enlarged extraocular muscles causes optic neuropathy and impedes orbital venous flow. Venous stasis in the orbit made it much easier than normal to detect the superior ophthalmic vein in color Doppler imaging.

The superior ophthalmic vein enters the muscle cone near the tendon of the superior oblique muscle and extends backwards and laterally. It exits the muscle cone along the superior border of the origin of the lateral rectus muscle. The superior ophthalmic vein is severely constricted at its posterior end near the point where it turns downward to enter the cavernous sinus [7]. The blood flow in the superior ophthalmic vein is normally toward the cavernous sinus [6, 8].

We found the blood flow in the superior ophthalmic vein toward the transducer in 6 dysthyroid ophthalmopathy orbits in our series of examinations. A reverse flow was not seen in any of the control orbits. Of the 6 orbits in which the superior ophthalmic vein blood flow was in the postero-anterior direction, 5 were found to have apical orbital crowding on CT. The postero-anterior blood flow in the superior ophthalmic vein was seen more frequently in orbits with apical orbital crowding than in those without apical orbital crowding. Reversed blood flow in the superior ophthalmic vein was also more frequently found in orbits with optic neuropathy than in those without optic neuropathy.

Compression of the optic nerve by enlarged extraocular muscles is seen at the orbital apex, where the superior ophthalmic vein is severely constricted. Orbital veins have no valves [7]. The direction of orbital venous flow can be reversed by apical compression, especially when the venous stasis due to apical compression is severe as is common in the orbits with optic neuropathy.

Whether the venous stasis in the orbit has some effect on the development of dysthyroid optic neuropathy or is merely the result of apical compression is a question in need of further investigation.

Since dysthyroid optic neuropathy is a sight-threatening complication and its onset is very often insidious, it is important to evaluate the usefulness of venous stasis analysis in dysthyroid ophthalmopathy orbits by color Doppler imaging as a means of assessing the risk of developing optic neuropathy. Compared to apical orbital crowding on CT, reversed blood flow in the superior ophthalmic vein had a low level of sensitivity of 44% probably because of the large range of variation normally seen in orbital veins, especially taking into account the possibility of anastomosis between extra-and intraorbital veins through the inferior orbital fissure [9]. But a specificity of reversed blood flow in the superior ophthalmic vein as an indicator of dythyroid optic neuropathy was higher than that of apical orbital crowding on CT.

We believe color Doppler imaging is a useful noninvasive tool for both the analysis of the venous stasis in the orbit and the management of dysthyroid ophthalmopathy. Those patients who are found to have reversed blood flow in the superior ophthalmic vein should be carefully examined for signs of dysthyroid optic neuropathy, a serious and frequently insidious complication of Graves' disease.

The authors do not have any commercial or propriety interest in the instruments and devices used in this study.

References

[1] J.S. Kennerdell and A.E. Rosenbaum et al. Apical optic nerve compression of dysthyroid optic neuropathy on computed tomography. Arch. Ophthalmol.1981;99:807–809.
[2] J.M. Neigel and J. Rootman et al. Dysthyroid optic neuropathy. The crowded orbital apex syndrome. Ophthalmology 1988;95:1515–1521.

224

[3] K Yoshikawa and T Higashide *et al* Fluorescein angiographic findings in optic discs with dysthyroid optic neuropathy Orbit 1991,10 89–96

[4] K Yoshikawa and T Higashide *et al* Role of rectus muscle enlargement in clinical profile of dysthyroid ophthalmopathy Jpn J Ophthalmol 1991,35 175–181

[5] Y Inoue and T Inoue Clinical studies on dysthyroid ophthalmopathy in Japanese Report 2 Classification of dysthyroid ophthalmopathy Acta Soc Ophthalmol Jpn 1971,75 2057–2062

[6] O Berges Colour Doppler flow imaging of orbital veins Acta Ophthalmol Suppl 1992,204 55–58

[7] K Murakami and G Murakami *et al* Gross anatomical study of veins in the orbit Acta Soc Ophthalmol Jpn 1991,95 31–38

[8] J Brismar Orbital phlebography I Anatomy of superior ophthalmic vein and its tributaries Acta Radiologica Diagnosis 1974,15 481–496

[9] J Brismar Orbital phlebography III Topography of intraorbital veins Acta Radiologica Diagnosis 1974,15 577–594

Eye Division of Olympia
Medical Clinic
6-35-3 Jingunae, Shibuyaku
Tokyo 150
Japan

4.7. New Echographic Findings in Orbital Vascular Diseases

N. ROSA, G. CENNAMO and A. LA RANA
(Naples, Italy)

Abstract. Calcifications and ossifications in orbital tumors are quite rare. Vascular orbital diseases sometimes show calcification. These findings can be very important in the differential diagnosis of orbital tumors, as they are consistent with the presence of benign vascular orbital disease. Calcifications can be found with CT scan, plain X ray, echography. While MRI is not useful, standardized echography is the most sensitive test in finding this kind of lesions showing small and very reflective areas followed by a shadow, related to the presence of phleboliths. Moreover in this paper the effects of a contrast agent in the evaluation of an orbital tumor is discussed.

Key words: Echography, color Doppler imaging, orbit, varix, calcification, contrast agent.

Introduction

Among the orbital lesions, the vascular diseases are quite frequent [1]. Most of the time, the differential diagnosis with Standardized Echography [2] is quite easy, but sometimes can be challenging.

For these reasons, we describe 5 clinical cases of orbital vascular disease where an additional echographic sign has been detected. The presence of this sign can be very useful in reaching a correct differential diagnosis.

Moreover, another clinical case where the use of a contrast agent was very useful to show the internal vascularity will be described.

Clinical Cases

Case I. A 71 y.o. white male was referred to our echographic service for a L.E. exophthalmos. In his clinical history there was a surgery to his left superior lid for an epithelioma.

J M Thyssen, H C Fledelius and S Tane (eds), Ultrasonography in Ophthalmology 14, 225–229
© *1995 Kluwer Academic Publishers, Dordrecht*

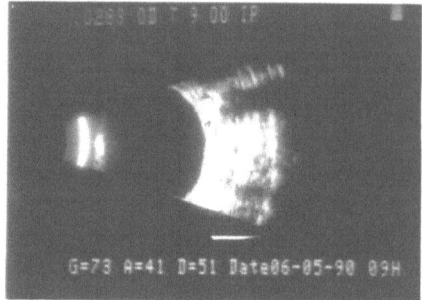

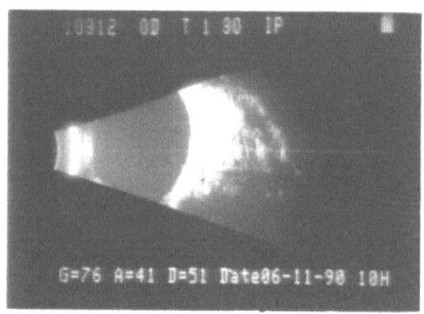

Figure 1. Contact B Scan in patient number 1 showing 2 roundish, very reflective areas followed by a shadow.

Figure 2. Contact B Scan in patient number 2 showing a roundish, very reflective area followed by a shadow.

The patient underwent an echographic examination of both orbits, according to the technique of Standardized Echography [2].

This examination detected in the left orbit an infiltrative lesion invading the left frontal sinus with the characteristics of a periorbital malignancy. But the examination disclosed also another lesion in the fellow orbit with the characteristics of vascular malformation, and with some very highly reflective, foreign body like, signals, probably due to calcifications (Fig. 1).

The same lesions where then detected with CT scan and MRI, even if the latter test obviously was not able to show the calcifications. The patient underwent a surgery in the suspicion of bilateral malignancy localization, and a varix like malformation was found.

Case II. A 22 y.o. white female was referred to our echographic service for R.E. exophthalmos and headache. The echographic examination detected an intraconal lesion typical for a lymphangioma, with the presence of calcification (Fig. 2). The patient underwent a surgery and the histology report was hemangiolymphangioma with phleboliths.

Case III. A 69 y.o. white male presented in the last years a progressive right eye exophthalmos. The echographic examination showed a retrobulbar mass with the characteristics of a trombosed varix with calcification (Fig. 3). During the surgery a large mass originating from the superior ophthalmic vein was found. The pathology report was cavernous hemangioma with phleboliths.

Case IV. A 72 y.o. white female presented a right eye exophthalmos. The echographic examination showed a trombosed varix with phleboliths (Fig. 4). No surgery was performed.

Case V. A 13 y.o. white child with a right eye exophthalmos. The echo-

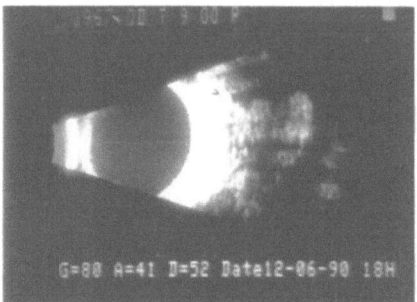

Figure 3. Contact B Scan in patient number 3 showing 2 roundish, very reflective areas followed by a shadow.

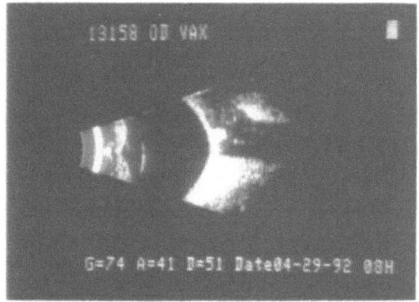

Figure 4. Contact B Scan in patient number 4 showing a very high reflective area followed by a shadow close to the optic nerve.

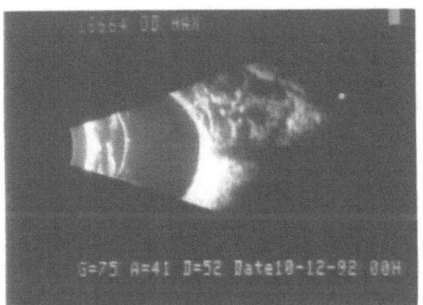

Figure 5. Contact B scan showing a mass lesion with large internal spaces.

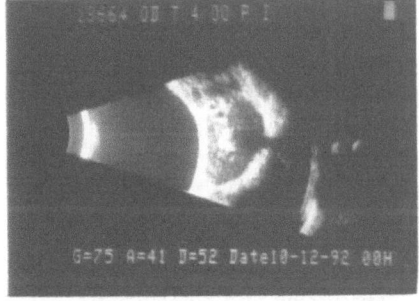

Figure 6. Contact B Scan showing a very highly reflective area inside a large vascular space in patient number V.

graphic examination revealed a lesion with the characteristics of a lymphangioma and the presence of phlebolithe (Figs. 5, 6). The patient underwent surgery and a phlebolithe was found in the mass lesion. The pathologic report was: lymphangioma.

Case VI. A 70 y.o. white female was referred to our echographic service for the evaluation of her left eye exophthalmos. The echographic examination showed the characteristics of a metastatic carcinoma. The patient underwent a further examination with echo-Doppler using a contrast agent. The results showed the presence of a marked blood flow after the injection of this agent (Fig. 7).

228

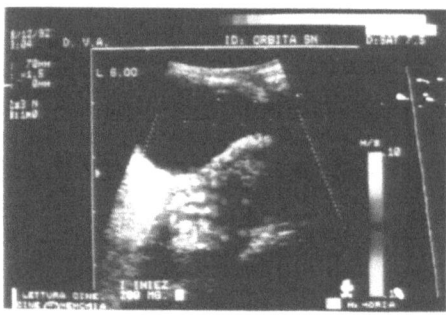

Figure 7. The lesion of Case VI after injection of the contrast agent. A very high blood flow can be detected.

Table 1. Metastatic orbital carcinoma characteristics

STRUCTURE	Irregular
REFLECTIVITY	High (V shape)
SOUND ATTENUATION	Minimal
BORDERS	Infiltrative
SHAPE	Irregular
LOCATION	Superior Orbit
BLOOD FLOW	No
MOBILITY	No
CONSISTENCY	Hard

Discussion and Conclusions

Standardized echography can be very important in the differential diagnosis of orbital lesions, with the evaluation of topographic, quantitative and kinetic criteria [3]. In this way most of the orbital lesions are identified with a high degree of precision. Some echographic findings, such as calcifications, can add information and a more precise diagnosis can be performed [4].

To find the calcifications inside an orbital lesion, as in our 5 clinical cases, can be very important in the differential diagnosis of orbital tumors, as they are consistent with the presence of phleboliths. Phleboliths are small, rounded calcifications that are the result of organizing thrombi, which are diagnostic for vascular malformations [5].

These calcifications can be found by CT Scan, plain X Ray, and echography. While MRI is not useful, standardized echography is the most sensitive test in finding this kind of disease showing small and very reflective areas followed by a shadow, related to the presence of phleboliths.

The diagnosis of a metastatic carcinoma in the orbit can be performed by standardized echography following the criteria in Table 1.

In particular no vascularity can be detected in these lesions. Doppler examination confirm this finding showing no significant signs of blood flow. The intravenous injection of a contrast agent (SH 508A by Schering), that is able to bypass the pulmonary circle, gives an enhancement of the echosignals from the blood flow and allows to show the real blood flow inside this lesion.

The possibility to better evaluate with a contrast agent, the internal vascularity, could be very useful in the differential diagnosis of bulbar and orbital lesions.

References

[1] J. Henderson. Orbital Tumors. N.Y. Thieme Stratton Inc. 1980;451, 471.
[2] K.C. Ossoinig. Standardized echography: basic principles, clinical applications and results. Int. Ophth. Clin. 1979;19:4.
[3] G. Cennamo. Ecodiagnostica orbitaria. In: La Semeiologia strumentale in oftalmologia di G. Bertoni Ed. Tip. Bari 1987.
[4] N. Rosa, G. Cennamo, L. De Palma, F. Tranfa. Fleboliti orbitari: studio ecografico. Clin. Ocul. N.4 1991, 300–304.
[5] I.S. Jones and F.A. Jakobiec. Diseases of the orbit. Harper and Row Publ. Inc., 1979.
[6] R. Schlief. Ultrasound contrast agents. Current opinion in radiology 1991;3:198–207.

Eye Department
University Federico II
Naples
Italy

4.8. Standardized A-scan Evaluation of the Ophthalmic Artery-Optic Nerve Sheath Complex

C. TAMBURELLI, A. CAPOBIANCO, C. ANILE and A. MANGIOLA

(Rome, Italy)

Abstract. The authors report a new echographic sign characterized by rapid oscillation of echo spikes, displayable, usually, on the nasal side of the optic nerve. This finding is detectable only with the standardized A-scan unit. The source of the rapid oscillations is most likely due to the pulsation of the ophthalmic artery walls. Optic nerve sheaths may also pulsate (especially if subarachnoid fluid fills perioptic spaces) by transmission of the pulsation of the ophthalmic artery. In normals, the pulsation decreases with aging. In Graves' disease there is always a reduced pulsation; on the contrary, it is increased in patients with Idiopathic Intracanial Hypertension.

Key words: A-mode echography, vascularity sign, pulsation index, Graves' disease, hypertension.

Introduction

Standardized A-scan evaluation of the contents of the orbit permits precise assessment of the dimensions and morphology of the optic nerve, its sheaths, the extraocular muscles as well as of the adipose tissue of the orbit (Ossoinig 1979, Tamburrelli *et al.* 1990).

In normal persons, both arterial as well as venous structures may occasionally be visualized by B-scan (for example the vertical venous branches of the superior ophthalmic vein). In pathological conditions such as caroticocavernous fistulae, orbital varicosities or vascular malformations, B-scan allows correct delineation of the course of some of the major branches and standardized A-scan permits evaluation of the characteristics of blood flow besides correct measurement of vessel dimensions (Ossoinig 1981, Ossoinig *et al.* 1984, Phelps *et al.* 1982).

The introduction of new instruments which allow simultaneous B-scan assessment and Doppler evaluation of the orbital vascular flow (Lieb *et al.* 1989) together with the possibility of outlining flow areas by means of colour introduction on B-scan images with visualization of anterograde and retro-

J.M. Thijssen, H.C. Fledelius and S. Tane (eds.), *Ultrasonography in Ophthalmology 14*, 230–235.

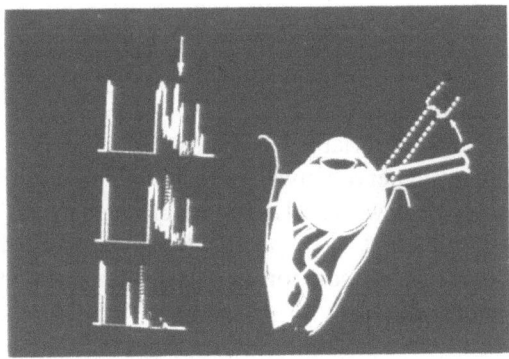

Figure 1. Relevant acoustic anatomy, cf. text.

grade flow (with respect to the probe scan zone) have brought about new developments of promising clinical value.

To our knowledge, no article regarding A-scan evaluation of the pulsations of the ophtalmic artery or of other orbital vessels has been published in the literature.

The purpose of the present study is to point out the finding of a pulsation as an echographic sign noticeable both in normal subjects and in pathological conditions and to report the results obtained concerning the pulsation characteristics we have noticed in normal persons as well as in patients with pathological conditions. The ultrasonographic spikes which present such a pulsation at standardized A-scan of the orbit are due to the ophtalmic artery pulse and/or to its possible repercussions on the optic nerve sheath. The origin of this observation is referable to these structures since the pulsating ultrasonic spikes are noticed in the area crossed by the ophthalmic artery and the medial sheaths of the optic nerve.

Methods and Material

We used the Mini A (Biophysic Medical) when performing standardized A-scan of the ophthalmic artery/optic nerve complex.

This instrument permits high frequency imaging (2000/sec) and hence allows kinetic evaluation of the registered movements with no appreciable latencies. This evaluation may be considered similar to that obtained with the old Kretzthecnik Unit/Analogic instruments. This apparatus is hence particularly adapt for the representation of the rapid arterious pulses.

It was possible to show, at examination of the medial side of the optic nerve, the spontaneous pulsation of the single or less often the bifid spike. This spike very often corresponds to the spike of the arachnoid sheath of thc nasal side of the optic nerve. In some cases, however, it is situated between the sheath of the optic nerve and that of the medial rectus muscle

(Fig. 1). The pulsation of this spike consists of rapid vertical oscillations which are clearly distinguishable from the surrounding immobile spikes. These oscillations are not accompanied by horizontal displacements along the abscissa of the monitor.

The site of pulsation is variable but is most often localized at the intermediate portion of the optic nerve between the orbital apex and bulbar insertion.

The pulsation may however also be visible at a more anterior site just behind the optic bulb and even on the temporal side of the optic nerve sheath. This oscillation is more or less easily localized depending on the subject being examined.

The amplitude of the oscillation is also variable. Sometimes it is very low, with a vertical displacement below 0.5 mm, but it may also be rather high with a vertical displacement above 2 mm. The rate of variation of the spike amplitude is also variable, depending probably on the cardiac frequency.

On the basis of these characteristics, we have formulated an intensity scale which allows us to obtain an ultrasonic index of pulsation for each subject. The criterion utilized takes two parameters into consideration: the first is the ease with which pulsation is observed, the second is the amplitude of oscillation of the spike.

We could not take the velocity of oscillation into consideration since we could not record the ultrasonic pictures.

The ease of observation includes four levels:
0 pulse observation is impossible
1 observation is difficult
2 immediate observation
3 evident observation

The amplitude of pulsation also includes four levels:
0 absent
1 just visible (up to 0.5 mm)
2 evident (0.5–1 mm)
3 very wide (up to 2 mm and above)

We have examined 34 normal persons and 52 subjects with different pathologies chosen in such a manner that we could consider any alterations of ophthalmic artery pulsation or of the optic nerve and/or its sheath. 28 patients with Graves ophthalmopathy (Werner class II–III) and 24 patients with idiopathic endocranial hypertension were included.

The 34 normal subjects represented our control group and enabled us to evaluate pulsation characteristics according to the following parameters: age, minimum, maximum and differential arterial blood pressure, diameter of the optic nerve (in some cases echo-colour Doppler was employed).

The mean age of the control group was 57 years (range 12–88).

Results

The mean calculated value chosen as 'echographic index of pulsation' for all the subjects of the control group was 1.602 (range 0–3; s.d. 0.88).

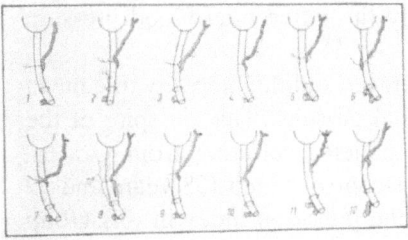 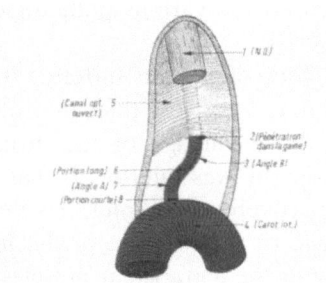

Figure 2 Liquor in the subarachnoidal space

We have evaluated the relationship between the pulsation index and age for the control group. A negative correlation was found (correlation coefficient = −0.47). The correlation of the calculated pulsation index to the diastolic arterial blood pressure was −0.019; to the systolic arterial blood pressure it was −0.22; the differential pressure was −0.303.

The correlation of the pulsation index as related to the diameter of the optic nerve was +0.54.

The values obtained in the group of patients with various pathologies were the following: in case of Graves' ophthalmopathy, the mean age was 38 years (range 17–51), the mean pulsation index was 1.24 (range 0–3; s.d.0.93); the correlation coefficient between the pulsation index and the diameter of the optic nerve was +0.121.

For the group of patients suffering from benign intracranial hypertension, the mean age was 45 years (range 11–65), the mean pulsation index was 1.88 (range 1–3; s.d. 0.59), the correlation coefficient between the pulsation index and the diameter of the optic nerve was −0.185.

Discussion and Conclusions

The ultrasonographic pulsation which we have come across is localized at the ophthalmic artery where it crosses above the optic nerve to pass nasally to it. However given the close relationship of these two structures, it is possible that the vessel's pulsation is transmitted to the sheath of the optic nerve especially if liquor (even in minimal amounts) is present in the sub-arachnoid spaces (Fig. 2).

The fact that the pulsation is sonographically less evident in older patients is due to the lesser expansion of the vessels due to arteriosclerotic processes which diminish the elasticity of these structures. In fact the correlation coefficient between age and sonographic index of pulsation is definitively negative (−0.47). There was no significant correlation with the systolic, diastolic and differential blood pressure in either group of patients (in the group of patients suffering from the various pathologies only the differential blood pressure was evaluated).

In the group of patients suffering from Graves' ophthalmopathy, the mean pulsation index was less than that of normal persons. This, in spite of the fact that the mean age of the group of patients suffering from Graves' ophthalmopathy was inferior to that of the control group (38 years and 57 years respectively). The inferior value of the pulsation index in this group may be due to the increase in the intraorbital pressure resulting from the thickening of the extraocular muscles and of the adipose tissue of the orbit. This condition explains both the decreased expansibility (increased impedance) of the arteries as well as the presence of less liquor in the subarachnoid perioptic spaces.

On the other hand the pulsation index in patients suffering from idiopathic intracranial hypertension is superior to that of normal subjects and especially to that of patients suffering from Graves' ophthalmopathy (1.88). In these patients the optic nerve sheaths are expanded by the abundant liquor present in the subarachnoid spaces. Hence, the pulsation of the ophthalmic artery may be transmitted to the liquor surrounding the optic nerve in the subarachnoid space. For this reason, the pulsation is most evident in patients suffering from idiopathic endocranial hypertension. We believe that it is improbable that the pulsation originates in the cranium to be transmitted through the optic canal and ultrasonographically visualized as displacement and oscillations of the nerve sheaths.

We conclude that the pulsation is due to the rapid displacements of the ophthalmic artery walls as the arterial pressure varies between diastolic and systolic values. Using A-scan echography, we can detect even minimal displacements of large to medium acoustic interfaces. For this reason, if liquor is present in the subarachnoid perioptic spaces, this technique enables us to visualize both the displacements of the arterial walls as well as those of the arachnoidal and dural sheaths caused by the arterial pulse.

A further confirmation of our results may be obtained by comparing orbital studies using standardized ultrasonography and colour Doppler flow imaging.

References

Lieb Jr , W , Cohen. S M , Mitchell, D , Merton, D and Shields, J Darstellung von intraokularen und orbitalen Gefaessen mittels Angiodynografie Paper presented at 87th Meeting German Ophthalmologic Society, Heidelberg, 1989

Ossoinig, K C Standardized echography basic principles, clinical application and results Int Ophthal Clin 1979,19(4) 127

Ossoinig K C Echographic differentiation of vascular tumors in the orbit In Ophthalmic Echography Proc SIDUO VIII, Docum Ophthal Proc Series 1981, 29 283

Ossoinig, K C , Frieling, E , Tamburrelli, C and Warner, L Superior ophthalmic vein thrombosis an echographic diagnosis In Ophthalmic Echography Proc SIDUO X, Docum Ophthal Proc Series 1984,48 527–537

Phelps, C.D., Thompson, H.S. and Ossoinig, K.C. The diagnosis and prognosis of atypical carotid-cavernous fistula (red eyed shunt syndrome). Am. J. Ophthal. 1982;93:423.

Tamburrelli, C., Anile, C., Mangiola, A., Falsini, B. and Palma, P. CFS dynamic parameters and changes of optic nerve diameters measured by standardized echography. In Ophthalmic Echography. Proc. SIDUO XIII, Docum. Ophthal. Proc. Series. 1990;55:101–109.

Department of Ophthalmology
Catholic University of Rome
Largo F. Vito 1
I-00168 Roma
Italy

4.9. Ultrasonographic Measurements of Extraocular Muscle Thickness in Normal Eyes and Eyes with Orbital Disorders Causing Extraocular Muscle Thickening

AKIRA KOMATSU and SADANAO TANE

(Kawasaki, Japan)

Abstract. The thickness of the extraocular muscles was determined by ultrasonography using St. Marianna's high-powered ultrasonic diagnostic equipment (ZD-252). The mean thickness of the extraocular muscles was 3.5 mm for the medial rectus muscle. 3.4 mm for the lateral rectus muscle, 3.3 mm for the superior rectus muscle, and 3.4 mm for the inferior rectus muscle in 240 eyes of Japanese normal adults. The thickness ranged from 4.1 to 4.3 mm in 34 eyes with dysthyroid ophthalmopathy, showing significantly thicker muscles than that in normal persons. As a result of ultrasonography of the extraocular muscles in patients with orbital myositis and inflammatory pseudotumor, the thickness of the extraocular muscles of the affected eye was significantly greater than that of the healthy eye. Ultrasonography of the extraocular muscle was considered to be useful for early diagnosis and observation of the course of dysthyroid ophthalmopathy, as well as certain other orbital disorders, and for evaluating therapeutic effects.

Key words: Biometry, A-mode echography, extraocular muscle thickness, Graves' disease

Introduction

Measurement of thickened extraocular muscles in orbital disorders such as exophthalmos in hyperthyroidism, orbital inflammatory pseudotumor and orbital myositis is clinically useful because the procedure provides information for early diagnosis and determination of morbid condition and for evaluation of therapeutic efficacy.

Ultrasonic measurements of extraocular muscle thickness was performed on normal subjects and patients with certain orbital disorders, such as exophthalmos in hyperthyroidism, as an aid to elucidating the morbid condition of the extraocular muscles in orbital disorders. The clinical significance of these measurements is discussed.

J.M. Thijssen, H.C. Fledelius and S. Tane (eds.), Ultrasonography in Ophthalmology 14, 236–246.
© 1995 *Kluwer Academic Publishers, Dordrecht.*

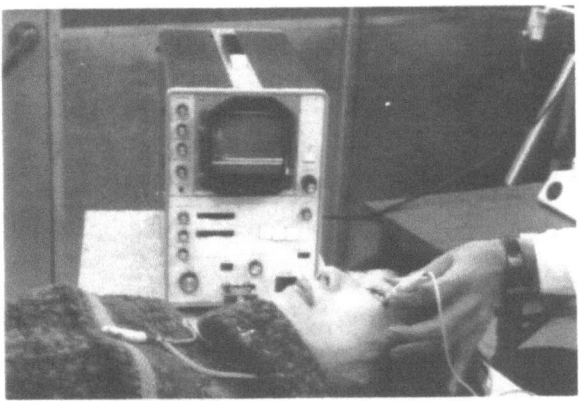

Figure 1. Measurement of extraocular muscle thickness using A-scan ultrasonogram.

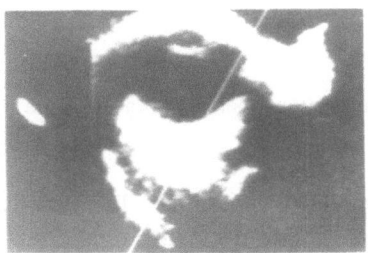
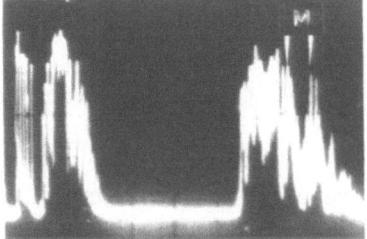

Figure 2. Left: A-scan and B-scan ultrasonogram. Right: A-scan ultrasonogram, M is the defect pattern in the orbital ultrasonogram representing a cross section of the extraocular muscle.

Methods and Material

St. Marianna's high-powered ultrasonic diagnostic equipment ZD-252 was used for ultrasonography, and PZT type focussed probes (5–10 MHz) were used. According to Ossoinig's method, A-mode images of the extraocular muscles were measured (Fig. 1). Figure 2 shows B-mode ultrasonogram, composite figures of A-mode images by a scan converter, and wave forms of the extraocular muscles obtained by the A-mode method. The width displayed by M was calculated as the values determined by ultrasonography of the extraocular muscles.

As a preliminary experiment, ultrasonography and actual anatomical measurement of the extraocular muscles were carried out on orbital specimens from 10 cadaver orbits, and the accuracy of ultrasonography was confirmed (Fig. 3).

Then, the thickness of the extraocular muscles was determined by ultrasonography to sex and age, on 320 eyes of 160 normal persons aged 5 to 80

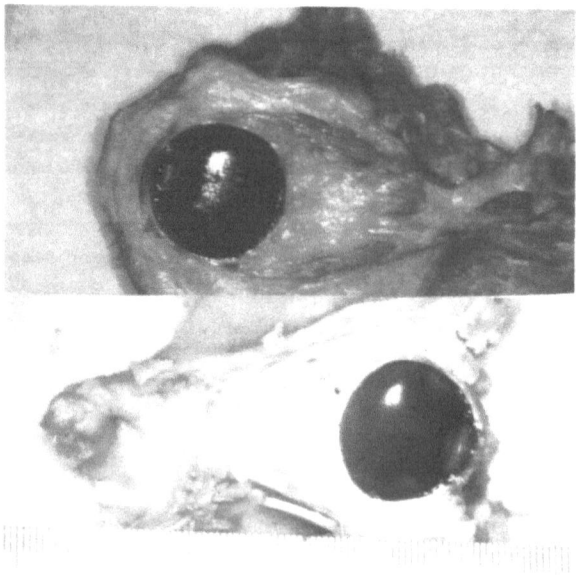

Figure 3. The horizontal section (top) and the sagittal section (bottom) in cadaver orbit

years. The measurement of extraocular muscle thickness in a living body, and the thickness value in a normal subject were thus decided. To determine the thickness of the extraocular muscles in a morbid eye, the thickness was measured ultrasonographically in 34 eyes of 17 patients with exophthalmos in hyperthyroidism. Eight eyes of 4 patients with orbital myositis and 10 eyes of 5 patients with orbital inflammatory pseudotumor, whose ages ranged from 18 to 68 years.

Results

1. *Measurement Results in Normal Eyes.* In our experiment, there was no significant difference between the thickness values determined by ultrasonography of the extraocular muscles and actual anatomical values, at a 5% level (Tables 1.1 and 1.2).

Table 2 shows the results of ultrasonography of four rectus muscles of 20 eyes of 10 normal subjects, taken from among 160 normal subjects (320 eyes) who had been divided according to age group and sex. There was no significant difference or right-left difference among the four rectus muscles.

Table 3.1 shows the mean thickness of the extraocular muscles according to sex in normal persons of all age groups. There was no significant sex difference. Table 3.2 shows the mean thickness of the extraocular muscles of adults. The mean thickness of the medial rectus muscle was 3.5 mm, that of the lateral rectus muscle 3.4 mm, that of the superior rectus muscle

Table 1.1. The comparative values between thickness of extraocular muscles measured with A-scan echography and actual measurement in the post-mortem orbit

No.	Age	Sex	Medial rectus		Lateral rectus		Superior rectus		Inferior rectus	
			Actual m.	A-scan	Actual m.	A-scan	Actual m.	A-scan	Actual m.	A-scan
1	56	f	3.4	3.4	3.5	3.1	3.4	3.5	4.2	4.0
2	77	m	3.4	3.5	3.2	3.1	4.0	3.5	3.6	3.1
3	59	m	3.2	3.2	3.3	3.1	3.5	3.1	3.5	3.0
4	75	f	3.1	3.2	3.2	3.2	3.3	3.4	3.2	3.3
5	60	f	3.2	2.8	3.6	3.2	2.9	2.8	3.2	2.7
6	46	m	3.4	3.1	3.1	2.8	3.0	3.1	3.3	3.1
7	66	m	3.5	3.6	3.0	3.2	–	–	–	–
8	60	f	2.8	2.8	2.7	2.8	–	–	–	–
9	68	f	3.0	3.5	3.2	3.7	–	–	–	–
10	69	m	3.0	2.8	3.2	3.7	–	–	–	–

Table 1.2. Average of extraocular muscle thickness in cadaver orbit and test

Muscle	Medical rectus		Lateral rectus		Superior rectus		Inferior rectus	
	Actual m.	A-scan	Actual m.	A-scan	Actual m.	A-scan	Actual m.	A-scan
Mean	3.2	3.2	3.2	3.2	3.4	3.2	3.5	3.2
S.D.	±0.21	±0.29	±0.24	±0.29	±0.36	±0.26	±0.34	±0.40
Max	3.5	3.6	3.6	3.7	4.0	3.5	4.2	4.0
Min	2.8	2.8	2.7	2.8	2.9	2.8	3.2	2.7
Range	0.7	0.8	0.9	0.9	1.1	0.7	1.0	1.3
Test	$t = 2.020$ $t(0.05) = 2.262$ N.S.		$t = 2.156$ $t(0.05) = 2.262$ N.S.		$t = 2.122$ $t(0.05) = 2.571$ N.S.		$t = 1.993$ $t(0.05) = 2.571$ N.S.	

241

Table 2. Thickness of extraocular muscles in normal human eyes as measured with A-scan echographic biometry [N(each age group) = 20 eyes, right and left combined)]

	Year Sex	1–10	11–20	21–30	31–40	41–50	51–60	61–70	71–80
Medial rectus muscle	m	2.9 ± 0.18	3.3 ± 0.16	3.5 ± 0.17	3.5 ± 0.09	3.5 ± 0.15	3.5 ± 0.13	3.3 ± 0.22	3.5 ± 0.22
	f	2.9 ± 0.10	3.3 ± 0.22	3.4 ± 0.19	3.6 ± 0.11	3.5 ± 0.11	3.5 ± 0.14	3.5 ± 0.11	3.4 ± 0.10
Lateral rectus muscle	m	2.9 ± 0.15	3.3 ± 0.21	3.5 ± 0.23	3.5 ± 0.10	3.4 ± 0.13	3.5 ± 0.15	3.3 ± 0.26	3.4 ± 0.20
	f	2.8 ± 0.11	3.3 ± 0.21	3.4 ± 0.17	3.4 ± 0.12	3.5 ± 0.07	3.4 ± 0.11	3.4 ± 0.17	3.3 ± 0.11
Superior rectus muscle	m	2.9 ± 0.16	3.3 ± 0.18	3.3 ± 0.15	3.4 ± 0.13	3.4 ± 0.22	3.3 ± 0.15	3.2 ± 0.24	3.3 ± 0.13
	f	2.8 ± 0.10	3.3 ± 0.14	3.3 ± 0.11	3.4 ± 0.13	3.4 ± 0.10	3.4 ± 0.08	3.3 ± 0.10	3.3 ± 0.08
Inferior rectus muscle	m	2.9 ± 0.13	3.3 ± 0.16	3.3 ± 0.16	3.4 ± 0.12	3.4 ± 0.23	3.3 ± 0.15	3.2 ± 0.18	3.3 ± 0.15
	f	2.8 ± 0.12	3.3 ± 0.14	3.4 ± 0.11	3.5 ± 0.09	3.4 ± 0.10	3.3 ± 0.13	3.3 ± 0.14	3.2 ± 0.07

Table 3.1. Average thickness of extraocular muscles in normal human eyes as measured with A-scan echographic biometry (right and left combined). Average of 5–79 years (male) and 7–80 years (female)

	Sex	N	Mean value (mm)	Maximum value (mm)	Maximum difference OD-OS (mm)
Medial rectus	male	160	3.4 ± 0.20	4.3	0.5
muscle	female	160	3.4 ± 0.20	4.1	0.4
Lateral rectus	male	160	3.4 ± 0.19	4.1	0.6
muscle	female	160	3.3 ± 0.20	4.2	0.8
Superior rectus	male	160	3.3 ± 0.28	4.1	1.2
muscle	female	160	3.3 ± 0.18	4.2	1.3
Inferior rectus	male	160	3.3 ± 0.24	3.9	0.9
muscle	female	160	3.3 ± 0.20	4.0	1.4
Average degree of protrusion (Hertel) R, L 12.8 mm					

Table 3.2. Average of adults (In 21 ~ 80 years old male and female combined)

	N	Mean value (mm)	Maximum value (mm)	Maximum difference OD-OS (mm)
Medial rectus muscle	240	3.5 ± 0.24	4.3	0.5
Lateral rectus muscle	240	3.4 ± 0.26	4.2	0.8
Superior rectus muscle	240	3.3 ± 0.35	4.2	1.3
Inferior rectus muscle	240	3.4 ± 0.28	4.0	1.4

Average degree of protrusion (Hertel) R, L 13.1 mm

3.3 mm, and that of the inferior rectus muscle 3.4 mm. The mean degree of exophthalmos was 13.1 mm.

2. Measurement Results in Eyes with Exophthalmos. The mean ultrasonographically determined value for extraocular muscles was 4.1–4.3 mm in 34 eyes with dysthyroid ophthalmopathy, being significantly thicker than the extraocular muscles of normal subjects (Tables 4 and 5). When the eye with exophthalmos was regarded as the first eye and the healthy eye as the second eye, the thickness values for the extraocular muscles of patients with orbital myositis ranged from 3.8 to 5.1 mm in the first eye, which was significantly greater than that of the second eye. In patients with inflammatory pseudo-tumor, the thickness values ranged from 3.7 to 3.9 mm in the first eye, again significantly greater than in the second eye (Tables 6 and 7).

Discussion

The method of ultrasonographic determination of the thickness of the extraocular muscles and the values thus obtained have been reported by Ossoinig *et al.* [1–3], and McNutt *et al.* [4]. According to their reports on 102 eyes of healthy western subjects, the medical rectus muscle was 4.2 mm,

Table 4. Thickness of extraocular muscles in Dysthyroid ophthalmopathy as measured with A-scan echography

Case	Age	Sex	Hertel		Medial		Lateral		Superior		Inferior	
			R	L	R	L	R	L	R	L	R	L
1	56	f	24	24	4.4	4.5	4.6	4.6	4.4	4.5	4.7	4.6
2	48	m	16	16	3.9	4.1	4.1	3.8	3.6	3.9	3.8	3.6
3	49	f	16	17	3.9	4.2	3.9	4.1	4.2	4.0	3.9	3.9
4	42	f	18	18	4.6	4.5	4.5	4.7	4.7	4.6	4.9	4.8
5	39	f	19	18	3.8	3.9	3.6	3.7	3.8	3.9	3.8	3.7
6	32	f	17	18	3.8	3.9	3.8	3.9	3.8	3.7	3.6	3.7
7	33	f	17	19	3.8	3.9	4.1	3.8	4.1	4.2	4.3	4.0
8	39	f	22	20	4.6	4.7	4.8	4.7	4.8	4.8	4.4	4.4
9	49	f	20	20	4.1	4.2	4.1	4.3	4.1	4.8	4.3	4.2
10	18	f	18	18	3.9	4.0	3.8	3.8	3.9	3.7	3.8	3.9
11	36	m	19	18	3.9	3.8	3.7	3.6	3.8	3.6	3.6	3.6
12	56	f	24	24	4.5	4.7	4.2	4.2	4.6	4.6	4.4	4.2
13	47	f .	18	18	4.7	4.5	4.3	4.3	4.5	4.6	4.2	4.4
14	37	f	16	16	3.8	3.8	3.6	3.5	4.1	4.0	3.8	3.7
15	46	f	17	18	4.3	4.3	4.0	4.1	4.1	4.2	4.0	3.9
16	53	f	22	24	5.4	5.5	5.2	5.0	5.6	5.7	5.1	5.1
17	68	f	22	20	4.2	4.0	4.0	3.9	4.3	4.1	3.9	4.0

Table 5. Average of extraocular muscle thickness in Dysthyroid ophthalmopathy (right and left eye combined)

	N	Mean value (mm)	Maximum value (mm)	Maximum difference OD-OS (mm)
Medial rectus muscle	34	4.3 ± 0.43	5.5	0.3
Lateral rectus muscle	34	4.1 ± 0.42	5.2	0.3
Superior rectus muscle	34	4.3 ± 0.49	5.7	0.7
Inferior rectus muscle	34	4.2 ± 0.48	5.3	0.4

Average degree of protrusion (Hertel) R, L 19 mm

lateral rectus muscle 4.3 mm, superior rectus muscle 3.8 mm and inferior rectus muscle 3.6 mm, in thickness.

As a result of our present study on 240 eyes of normal Japanese subjects by ultrasonography, the medial rectus muscle was 3.5 mm, lateral rectus muscle 3.4 mm, superior rectus muscle 3.3 mm and inferior rectus muscle 3.4 mm, in thickness, showing that the thickness of the extraocular muscles of Japanese people is slightly less than that of Western people.

In our experimental set-up, the thickness of the extraocular muscles was determined by the A-mode method after observation by the B-mode method. It was difficult to determine the thickness by the A-mode contact method because of considerably increased absorption due to formalin fixation of the cadaver orbit. The angle of the ultrasonic transducer was changed on an

Table 6. Thickness of extraocular muscles in myositis and pseudotumor as measured with A-scan echography

① Myositis

Case	Age	Sex	Hertel		Medial		Lateral		Superior		Inferior	
			R	L	R	L	R	L	R	L	R	L
1	60	f	15	18	3.4	4.1	3.3	3.8	3.3	3.8	3.2	3.8
2	54	m	16	12	6.9	3.4	3.8	3.5	3.7	3.3	3.5	3.4
3	43	f	17	14	4.0	3.6	3.8	3.5	3.8	3.7	3.6	3.6
4	41	f	18	13	5.2	3.5	4.9	3.6	4.0	3.5	4.8	3.5

② Pseudotumor

Case	Age	Sex	Hertel		Medial		Lateral		Superior		Inferior	
			R	L	R	L	R	L	R	L	R	L
1	18	f	17	14	3.8	3.3	3.6	3.4	3.8	3.3	3.8	3.3
2	56	f	14	17	3.6	4.2	3.8	4.1	3.4	3.8	3.3	4.1
3	32	f	15	19	3.6	3.8	3.6	3.8	3.4	3.6	3.4	3.8
4	18	m	18	13	3.8	3.4	3.8	3.5	3.6	3.4	3.6	3.3
5	28	f	17	14	3.8	3.6	3.7	3.4	3.7	3.4	3.8	3.4

Table 7. Average of extraocular muscle thickness in Myositis and Pseudotumor.

① Myositis

	Exophthalmic eye		Fellow eye	
	N	Mean ± SD	N	Mean ± SD
Medial rectus muscle	4	5.1 ± 1.17	4	3.5 ± 0.10
Lateral rectus muscle	4	3.9 ± 0.13	4	3.5 ± 0.11
Superior rectus muscle	4	3.8 ± 0.11	4	3.4 ± 0.17
Inferior rectus muscle	4	3.9 ± 0.52	4	3.4 ± 0.15

Average degree of protrusion (Hertel)
Exopthalmic eye: 17 mm, Fellow eye: 13 mm.

② Pseudotumor

	Exophthalmic eye		Fellow eye	
	N	Mean ± SD	N	Mean ± SD
Medial rectus muscle	5	3.9 ± 0.18	5	3.5 ± 0.13
Lateral rectus muscle	5	3.8 ± 0.17	5	3.5 ± 0.15
Superior rectus muscle	5	3.7 ± 0.11	5	3.5 ± 0.10
Inferior rectus muscle	5	3.8 ± 0.16	5	3.3 ± 0.10

Average degree of protrusion (Hertel)
Exophthalmic eye: 18 mm, Fellow eye: 14 mm.

extension line of the sclera of the contralateral meridian of the extraocular muscles tested. When the echo spikes corresponding to the extraocular muscles showed the maximum width and surface signal, at which the bilateral heights of echo spikes were the same, the distance between the spikes was regarded as the thickness of the extraocular muscles, and was determined as such. The superior and inferior rectus muscles and oblique muscles were examined from their courses and crossing sites in the cadaver orbit. There seemed to be no problem because the sites expected for ultrasonography of the superior and inferior rectus muscles were distant from the crossing sites. This has been confirmed by Duke-Elder [5] and Sobotta [6]. The superior and inferior oblique muscles were excluded from the present study because of the potential difficulty of applying echo beams vertically to the fascia. Although the levator muscle showed a course similar to that of the superior rectus muscle, both of these muscles could be differentiated by estimating echo wave forms because they were isolated with the fascia. Thus, the thickness of the superior rectus muscle could also be determined.

The group of patients with dysthyroid ophthalmopathy included those in whom hyperthyroidism was definitely diagnosed according to criteria based on internal medicine, who belonged to class 1-3 of Werner's classification and who showed a degree of exophthalmos of 15 mm or more. Although the degree of exophthalmos has been believed not to be correlated with thickening of the extraocular muscles, there was a correlation of 0.461, at a significance level of 5%. As reported by Coleman [7–8], Shammas [9], Werner [10], hyperthyroidism of Werner's classification 0-2 should be differentiated from orbital myositis and inflammatory pseudotumor.

References

[1] K. McNutt and K. Ossoinig. Echographic measurement of extraocular muscles, ultrasound in medicine, Vol. 3A. (Proceedings of the 1st WFUMB) Plenum Press, New York, 1976;927.
[2] K. Ossoinig. Die Ultraschalldiagnostik der Orbita. Klin Monatsbl. Augenheilk. 1966;149:817.
[3] K. Ossoinig. Echography of the eye, orbit, and periorbital region. (Orbit roentogenology, edited by P.G. Ager), John Wiley & Sons, New York, 1977.
[4] L.C. McNutt. Echographic measurement of extraocular muscles applied in Graves' orbitopathy, Proceeding of XXIII Concilium Ophthalmologicum Kyoto 1978. (ACTA), 1842, Excerpta Medica, Amsterdam, 1979.
[5] S. Duke-Elder. System of ophthalmology. Vol. II, 414. Henry Kimpton, London, 1976.
[6] Becher Sobotta. Atlas der Anatomie des Menschen Band 3. Urban & Schwarzenbeg, Munchen–Berlin–Wien, 1973.
[7] D.J. Coleman and J.R.L. Franzen. High resolution B-scan ultrasonography of the orbit. Arch. Ophthalmol. 1972;88:358.
[8] D.J. Coleman and R.L. Pallow. Orbital ultrasonography. (Diseases of the orbit, edited by I.S. Jones and F.A. Iackobiec), Harper & Row, Hagerstown, 1979.
[9] H.J.F. Shammas, D.S. Minckler and C. Ogden. Ultrasound in early thyroid orbitopathy. Arch. Ophthalmol. 1980;98:277.

[10] S C Werner, D J Coleman and L A Franzen Ultrasonographic evidence of a consistent orbital involvement in Graves' disease N Engl J Med 1974,290 1447–1450

Department of Ophthalmology
St Marianna University, School of Medicine
2-16-1 Sugao
Miyamaeku
Kawasaki
216 Japan

4.10. The Merit of Electronic Linear Scan Ultrasonic Tomography of the Orbit

KAZUO EMI, MOTO KATAOKA and YUKITAKA UJI

(*Mie, Japan*)

Abstract. In this paper the electronic linear-scanning ultrasonography is compared to the mechanical sector scanning method in optic nerve and orbital lesions. Mechanical sector scanners display the optic nerve as if it were wedge-shaped. The posterior enlargement of the diameter is an acoustic artefact. On the contrary, electronic linear scanners show the optic nerve straight as it is. For evaluating orbital tumors, it is important to see the optic nerve accurately, for the purpose of the tumor site determination. Therefore, the electronic linear scanner is considered to be superior to the mechanical sector scanner. This statement is supported by four case reports.

Key words: B-mode echography, linear array, mechanical sector scanner, orbit.

Introduction

The difference of the video images is related to the scanning method. A linear scanner projects parallel beams over a scan width, which is identical to the lateral size of the array. Mechanical sector scanners cannot project the beams parallel to the optic nerve but divergently. For this reason, mechanical sector scanners produce an image distortion, resulting in the posterior enlargement of the optic nerve and orbital image.

A linear scanner does not have such an artefact (Figs. 1 and 2).

Methods

Tomey B-scan IS-500 has the following properties of the transducer: 1, center frequency 7.5 MHz; 2, focal length 22 mm; 3, depth of focus 20 mm; 4, 30 frames/s; 5, 30 mm $*$ 6 mm (width and length of the transducer); 6, beam width is 0.6 mm at the focus.

Nidek Echoscan US-2500 has these properties of transducer as follows: 1, center frequency 10 MHz; 2, focal length 20 mm; 3, depth of focus 20 mm;

J.M. Thijssen, H.C. Fledelius and S. Tane (eds.), Ultrasonography in Ophthalmology 14, 247–252.

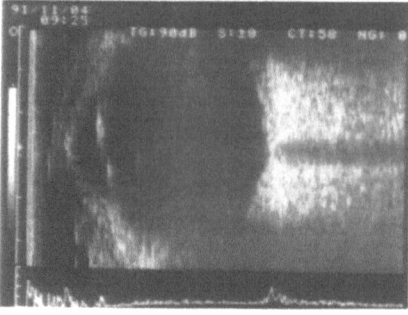

Figure 1. Image of electronic phase array scanner.

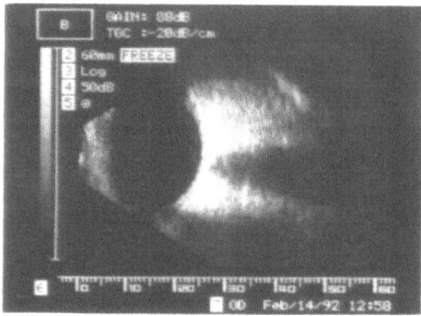

Figure 2. Image of mechanical sector scanner.

4, 10 frames/s; 5, diameter of the transducer 5 mm; 6, beam width is 0.6 mm at the focus.

Case Reports

Case 1

The first case was a 55-year-old female with non-Hodgkin, B-cell follicular type malignant lymphoma. Both her eyes had gradually extruded in spite of chemotherapy. Hertel was 15 mm right and 19 mm left. The visual acuity decreased to 0.1 right and 0.4 left. Critical fusion frequency was 22 right and 35 left. Computed tomography showed extraocular muscle swellings due to venous stasis (Fig. 3). Acoustically, there was superior orbital vein dilation of both eyes because of tumor mass invasion to the cavernous sinus (Fig. 4). As the cause of the exophthalmos, it was considered that venous return was obstructed by the invaded mass at the cavernous sinus. The patient was treated by irradiation with a dose of 30 Gy in fifteen fractions over a period of three weeks. After that, exophthalmos was diminished to 15 mm right and

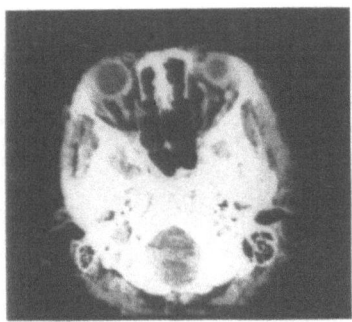

Figure 3 Horizontal CT showed extraocular muscle swellings, case 1

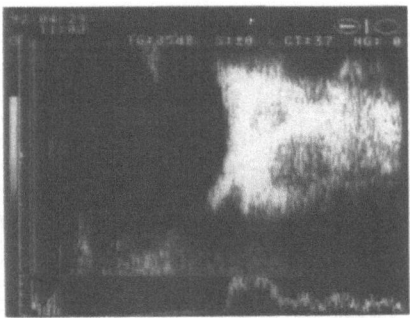

Figure 4 Echo shows right superior orbital vein dilation, case 1

16 mm left. The visual acuity recovered to 0.7 right and 0.8 left. Critical fusion frequency was unchanged.

Case 2

The second case was a 61-year-old male with proptosis of the right eye. Hertel was 18 mm right and 11 mm left. He was suffering from T-cell diffuse type non Hodgkin malignant lymphoma which arose from the right ethomoidal sinus (Fig. 5). Acoustically, the medial wall of the right orbita was destroyed by the tumor (Fig. 6). Tumor invaded close to the optic nerve (Fig. 7). The tumor diminished by irradiation with a dose of 40 Gy.

Case 3

The third case was a 35-year-old female who had an inflammatory pseudotumor of the left orbita. Her left eye had gradually protruded for three months. The visual acuity was both (1.2). Hertel was 12 mm right and 16 mm left. Computed tomography and magnetic resonance imaging showed mass lesion at the medial portion in the muscle cone of the left orbita (Fig. 8).

250

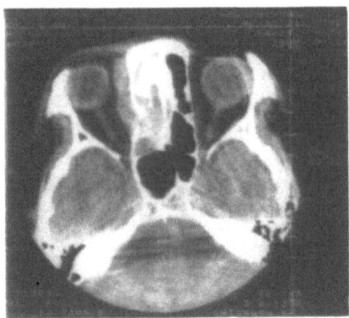

Figure 5 Horizontal CT of the ethomoidal tumor invading into the orbita, case 2

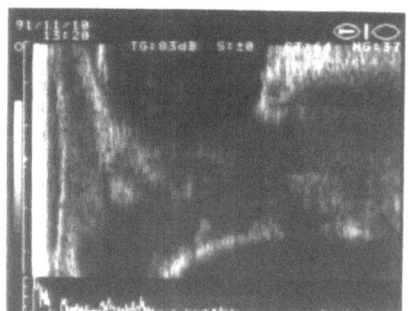 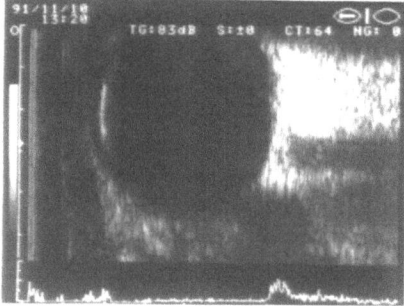

Figures 6 and 7 Acoustically the tumor destroyed the medial wall of right orbita (Fig 6) and invaded close to the optic nerve (Fig 7), case 2

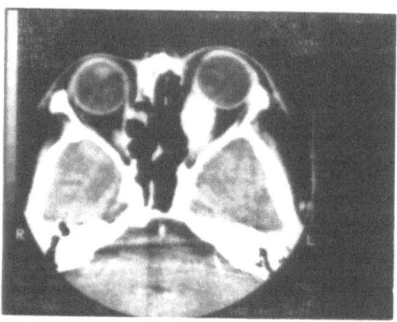

Figure 8 CT showed mass lesion behind the left eye, case 3

Acoustically, there was a mass lesion adjacent to the optic nerve just posterior to the globe (Fig. 9). An open biopsy was performed. Histologically, there was inflammatory involvement of connective tissue and lymphocytes, and plasma cell infiltration. Systemic corticosteroid was administered intraven-

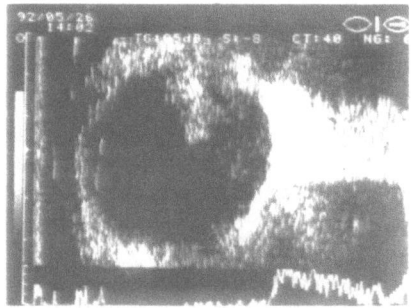

Figure 9 B-scan ultrasonogram shows mass lesion adjacent to the globe, case 3

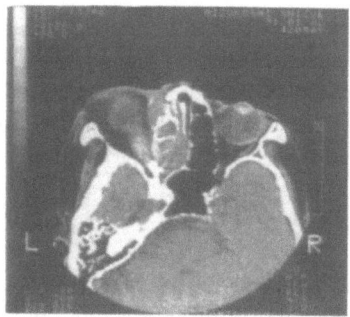

Figure 10 The maxillary tumor also invades the ethmoidal sinus, case 4

ously. But the tumor did not diminish at all. Irradiation therapy for this condition is controversial. This time irradiation therapy was not performed.

Case 4
The fourth case was an 85-year-old female who had a left maxillary carcinoma invading into the orbit. MRI indicates the invading tumor from maxillary sinus to orbita. CT shows the tumor invading to left orbita and ethmoidal sinus (Fig. 10) Electronic linear scanner can display the invading tumor from the floor of the orbita (Fig. 11), while mechanical sector scanner cannot detect it (Fig. 12). Chemotherapy and irradiation were performed. Tumor was markedly diminished.

Conclusion

In this presentation we emphasized the merit of the electronic linear-scanning echography in orbital examination. Electronic linear scanner shows the optic nerve straight as it is. When we examine orbital tumors, it is important that we can see the optic nerve accurately for the aim of orientation. I think the

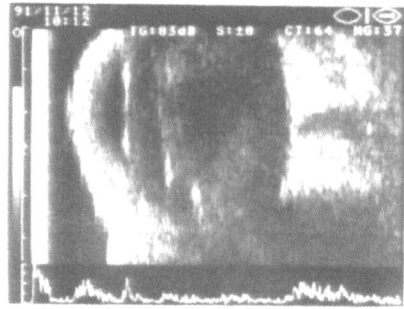 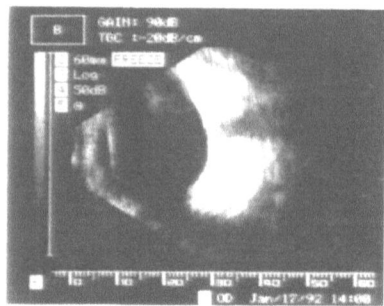

Figures 11 and 12. Electronic linear scanner (Fig. 11) displays the tumor more clearly than the mechanical sector scanner (Fig. 12), case 4.

electronic linear scanner is superior to the mechanical sector one in orbital examination. When we evaluate the B-mode color Doppler imaging of ophthalmic artery or orbital vein in near future, I think it is more important than ever.

References

Lünborg, H.G. and Trier, H.G. The accuracy of ultrasonic and other methods in orbital diagnosis demonstrated on selected pathological cases. In Proceedings of the 10th SIDUO Congress, Florida, USA, November 7–10, 1984. Martinus Nijhoff/Dr. W. Junk Publishers, Dordrecht, 1987, pp. 453–461.

Lieb, W. and Rochels, R. Echographic pattern of an orbital myxoma and schwannoma. In Proceedings of the 11th SIDUO Congress, Capri, Italy, 1986. Kluwer Academic Publishers. Dordrecht, 1988, pp. 270–275.

Dr. Kazuo Emi
Mie Prefectural
Shiohama General Hospital
Mie, Japan

4.11. Orbital Veins at the B-Scan Image

V. MAZZEO, P. PERRI, L. RAVALLI, R. SCORRANO, P. MONARI
and S. NADERI

(*Ferrara, Italy*)

Abstract. Normal antero-posterior superior and inferior orbital veins are rarely seen during orbital examination. Sometimes, it is possible instead to show on the screen the vertical veins.

When a pathologic event takes place, i.e. low and high pressure A-V fistulas, the superior orbital vein enlarges and in particular cases, vortex veins or inferior orbital veins are also clearly visible.

Key words: B-mode echography, orbit, arterio-venous fistula, orbital vein.

Introduction

The ophthalmic superior and inferior veins (OSV, OIV) are the main venous vascular channels in the orbit. The OSV originates anteriorly near the root of the nose and it extends posteriorly and laterally to reach the superior orbital fissure to end into the cavernous sinus. The IOV originates from the venous net that occupies the anterior inferior aspect of the orbit, it also extends posteriorly to end, alone or joined with the OSV, into the cavernous sinus.

Many other venous channels are also present in the orbit: some of them drain the blood from all the orbital structures (muscular branches, lacrimal, angular and ethmoidal veins, vortex veins) and some other connecting the OSV with the OIV. Among these anastomotic vessels, the commonest is the medial vertical vein (MVV) that has a roughly vertical course and is situated between the medial rectus muscle and the optic nerve in the anterior aspect of the orbit.

The MVV is the only vein that can be revealed by echography in half of the normal patients; one must look for it very attentively on the B-scan at reduced sensitivity in the space between the medial rectus and the optic nerve [6, 10, 12].

Normal OSV are not visible on echography. This feature can be explained

J.M. Thijssen, H.C. Fledelius and S. Tane (eds.), Ultrasonography in Ophthalmology 14, 253–257

by their anterior-posterior courses practically parallel to the examining sound beam [1, 8].

When the venous pressure increases, due to an obstruction of any reason of flow towards the cavernous sinus, the venous channels enlarge and become echographically visible.

Arterio-venous fistulas (A-VF) are the commonest cause of orbital venous pressure increase.

They are due to the rupture of the carotid artery itself or of very thin meningeal arteries of the cavernous sinus wall originating from the carotid into the cavernous sinus itself.

A-VF can be traumatic or spontaneous with high or low pressure.

Traumatic A-VF is generally due to the rupture of the carotid itself into the cavernous sinus because of a very severe cranial trauma associated or not with a base fracture.

Carotid-cavernous fistulas due to a perforating injury are much more rare. The traumatic forms are generally with high pressure, while spontaneous fistulas are more often with low pressure.

The rupture of the carotid or of a little meningeal vessel into the cavernous sinus increases the pressure and determines an orbital stasis or even an inverted venous flow.

In high-pressure cases an arterialization of the OSV occurs.

High-pressure A-VF are characterized by: pulsating proptosis, bruit, conjunctival and retinal vessel acute congestion, choroidal oedema, and sometimes ophthalmoplegia.

Low-pressure A-VF are instead characterized by subtler clinical features with insidious onset.

The signs are: unilateral and non pulsatile proptosis, conjunctival and retinal venous conjection, ocular hypertension, optic disk oedema, choroidal detachment, sixth cranial, or less frequently third cranial nerves palsies.

The bruit is not always present [3].

Echography

The pathognomonic A-scan pattern is characterized by the enlarged OSV that appears as a clear-cut defect in the orbital echopattern.

Boundary echoes are maximal and internal echoes are low reflective and show very fast spontaneous movements due to the very high blood flow into the dilated and arterialized vein [5]; less clear-cut defects may be encountered otherwise in the orbit that are due to the enlargement of other orbital veins, like MVV or OIV.

On the B-scan we can more easily follow the course of the dilated OSV visible as a channel with parallel or slightly diverging borders towards the apex.

This channel bends with its convexity towards the centre of the orbit on its anterior-posterior course (Fig. 1).

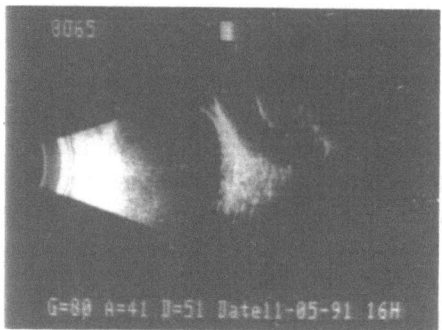

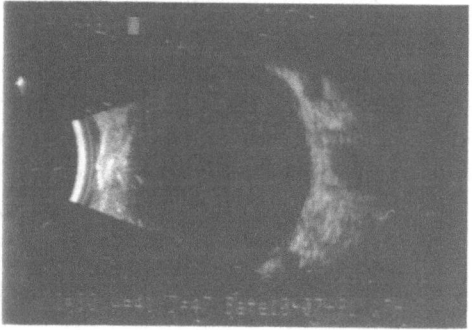

Figure 1 Arterio-venous fistula The oph-thalmic superior vein appears highly dilated It shows no internal echoes and well defined borders

Figure 2 Arterio-venous fistula Two vortex veins appears as empty round spaces just behind the eye wall

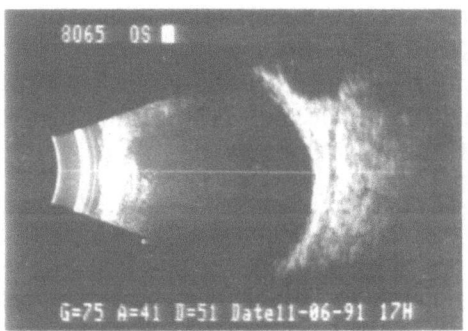

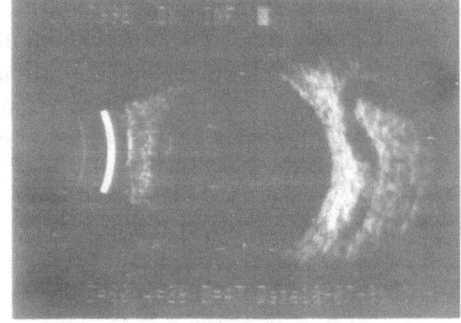

Figure 3 Arterio-venous fistula The enlarged medial vertical vein or its anastomosis with the superior ophthalmic vein

Figure 4 Arterio-venous fistula The inferior ophthalmic vein appears enlarged and very tortuous

In coronal section the vein appears like a really well defined round cavity. The 'cystic' behaviour of this is often characterized by posterior reinforcement echoes [7, 8].

Internal echogenicity may go from no echoes to medium reflectivity depending on the blood flow level into the vein.

The vein enlargement can displace the optic nerve. The vortex vein just ouside the eye wall can be as visible (Fig. 2) as the vertical vein with origin from the dilated OSV (Fig. 3). The OIV is more rarely visible: it appears like a highly banding channel going posteriorly under the optic nerve (Fig. 4). Its internal echogenicity seems higher than that of the OSV.

In some cases anterior ethmoidal veins may be revealed as multiple cavernous little spaces in the anterior medial part of the orbit [2, 6, 11]. They show a low medium reflectivity underlined by the pulsatility of the dilated vessel as a sign of arterialization.

Pulsatility would be present when tissue pressure overcomes the diastolic pressure in the vessel, furthermore it would be used in the differential diagnosis with vein enlargement not due to A-VF, like in OSV thrombosis.

Venous stasis also produces an extraocular muscles thickening, their internal reflectivity is increased; the optic nerve may be enlarged either because it is compressed by the enlarged muscles or because there is the venous stasis of the optic nerve sheets [11].

Some A-V fistulas may cause a choroidal detachment associated to ocular hypertension.

Whatever cause compresses, infiltrates or obstructs the cavernous sinus, or the OSV, it will cause a venous stasis and so the enlargement of the veins before the obstruction.

The most common cause of this obstruction is OSV thrombosis. This illness shows some differences compared with the OSV engorgement due to an A-VF [6]; in the first conditions the enlargement of the OSV is mild, very often it is more visible anteriorly, while the posterior thrombotic part is hardly visible and shows a high internal reflectivity.

In the anterior dilated portion of the vein spontaneous movements are practically absent on kinetic echography, while the MVV is always visible and enlarged due to its function of alternative drainage.

References

[1] M.J. Dadd, H.L. Hughes and G. Kossoff. Ultrasonic examination of the orbital vasculature. J. Cl. U. 1978;6:36–40.

[2] R. Guthoff. Ultrasound in ophthalmologic diagnosis. Georg Thieme Verlag, 1991.

[3] W. Hauff and P. Till. Echography in carotid-cavernous fistulas Ophthalmic Ultrasonography. Proceedings of the 9th S.I.D.U.O. Congress. J.S. Hillman and M.M. Le May (eds.), Dr W. Junk Publishers, 1984;399–405.

[4] V. Mazzeo, G. Galli, D. Signori and P. Perri. Spontaneous choroidal detachment and 'red eyed shunt syndrome'. Two clinical entities with the same cause? International Ophthalmology 1985;8:129–138.

[5] K.C. Ossoinig. A-scan echography and orbital disease. Orbital disorders. G.H. Bleeker et al. (eds.), Mod. Probl. Ophthal. 14, Karger, 1975;203–235.

[6] K.C. Ossoinig, E. Frieling, C. Tamburrelli and L. W. Arner. Superior ophthalmic vein thrombosis, an echographic diagnosis. Ophthalmic echography. Proceedings of the 10th S.I.D.U.O. Congress. K.C. Ossoinig (ed.), Martinus Nijhoff–Dr W. Junk Publishers, 1987;527–537.

[7] J. Poujol and M. Le Roy. Echographic appearance of orbital veins. Orbit 1983;2:79–81.

[8] L. Ravalli. Diagnostica ecografica. Ecografia del l'apparato oculare. V. Mazzeo (ed.), Fogliazza, 1987;279–327.

[9] J. Rootman and D.A. Graebs. Vascular lesion. Diseases of the orbit. J. Rootman (ed.), J.B. Lippincott Company, 1988;525–568.

[10] N. Rosa, G. Cennamo and A. Zitelli, La vena verticale mediale: un interessante reporto ecografico. Clin. Oc. e Pat. Ocul. XI. 1990;366–368.

[11] R.H. Spector. Echographic diagnosis of dural carotid cavernous sinus fistulas. Am. J. Ophthalmol. 1991;111:77–83.

[12] C. Tamburrelli, F. Focosi, G. Lazetera and E. Buratto. Rami verticali della vena oftalmica superiore: valutazione ecografica. Clin. Oc. e Pat. Ocul. 1990;XI:369–372.

University Eye Clinic
Ferrara, Italy

4.12. Orbital Teratoma
Presentation of a Case

EDUARDO MORAGREGA

(Coyoacan, Mexico)

Abstract. A case is presented of a newborn with a large orbital teratoma. The results of echographic examination and of the resection of the tumor with a two year follow-up are discussed.

Key words: Teratoma, orbit, echography, resection.

A teratoma is by defination a congenital tumor that consists of tissues from more than one of the three germinal layers: ectoderm, endoderm, or mesoderm. The tumor is considered a choristoma. Ninety percent of teratoids consist of only ectodermal and mesodermal tissue, whereas 10 percent consist of only mesodermal and endodermal tissue. The tumor typically causes marked unilateral proptosis and upward displacement of the globe due to the rapid growth after birth in a full term infant. In teratoma, at birth the proptotic globe tends to protrude through the palpebral fissure.

Females with teratoma outnumber males by a ratio of 2:1. The tumor may represent an abortive attempt at formation of the human body since a complete embryo has been found implanted in the orbit. Typically, the bony orbit has expanded without erosion so that its volume is doubled or tripled. Nasal and malar deformities result. The tumor may transilluminate due to its cystic components, including endoderm forming a primitive gut and surface ectoderm forming a dermoid cyst. The former structure may produce copious mucus. The tumor is irreducible. Ependymal cells and even choroid plexus may also be present. Malignant teratomas may occur.

The present case is a newborn with orbital teratoma in which the eyeball protruded through the palpebral fissure, producing an ulceration of the cornea (Fig. 1). The ultrasonography reported an axial length of 18.0 mm, with big cystic areas surrounding the eyeball, and dense tissue within the cyst giving high reflectivity (Fig. 2). The mass was not compressible and optic nerve and extraocular muscles were very difficult to demonstrate. Three days after birth we performed the resection of the tumor, making a peritomy and

J M Thijssen, H C Fledelius and S Tane (eds), Ultrasonography in Ophthalmology 14, 258–260

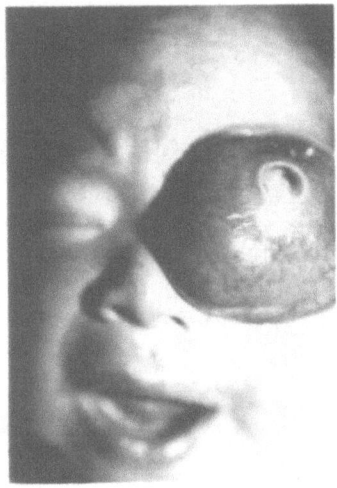

Figure 1 Clinical appearance of the great proptosis in O S

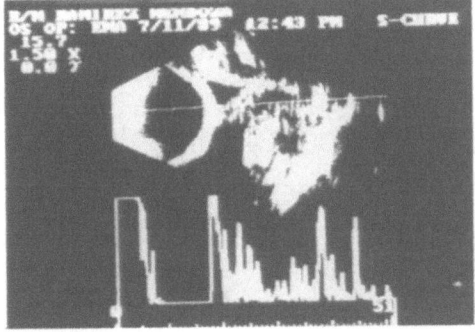

Figure 2 Echogram showing big cystic areas

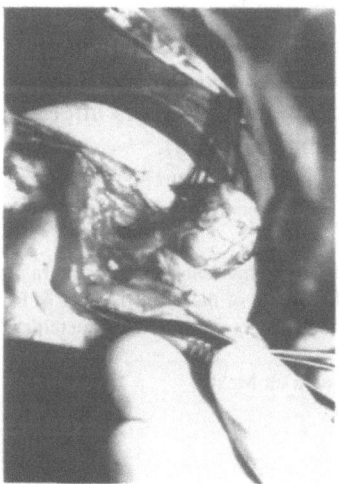

Figure 3 Surgery dissecting the cyst

following the extraocular muscles all the way from their insertion in the sclera, to the orbital apex, dissecting the cyst and leaving the eyeball, muscles and optic nerve in the fat-empty orbit (Fig. 3).

The histopathology reported a cyst formation with epithelium from the upper respiratory tract, intestine, and neuroectoderm with rosette formation.

260

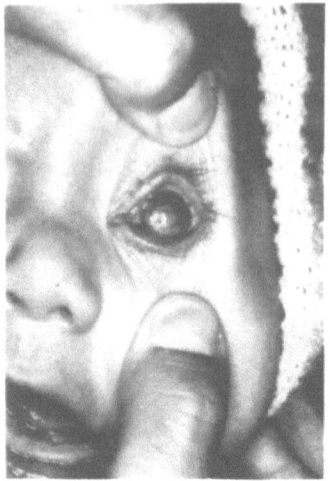

Figure 4. 8 days post-op.

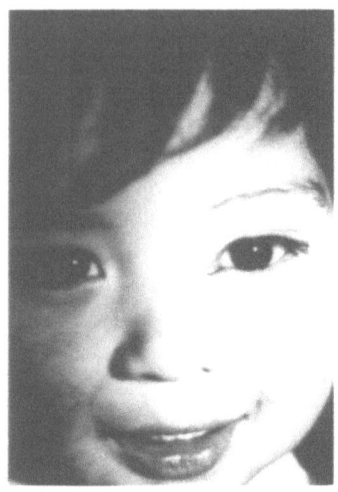

Figure 5. One year after surgery with prothesis O.S

There was also some lacrimal gland tissue. All these tissues were surrounded by conjunctival tissue with cartilage and smooth muscle.

The patient had a bad visual outcome with no light perception, and a total corneal leucoma, but with excellent cosmetic appearance (Fig. 4). A cosmetic scleral prosthesis was made and two years after surgery the difference between the eyelids was minimal (Fig. 5).

References

Herreman, R. and Gomez Leal, A. Oftalmologia. Edit. Interamericana 1989, pp. 41–42.
Snow, Ira and Jakobiec, Fred. Disease of the orbit. Harper & Row 1979, pp 135–136.
Villanueva, Gil. Introducción a la oftalmología. Edit Senefelder 1978, p 211

Asociacion para Evitar la Ceguera en Mexico
Vicente Garcia Torres No. 46
Col. El Rosedal
Coyoacan
C.P. 04030 Mexico, D.F.

Index

Documenta Ophthalmologica Proceedings Series

1. J. François (eds.): *Symposium on Light-Coagulation.* Argon Laser and Xenon Arc (Ghent, Belgium, 1972). 1973   ISBN 90-6193-141-X
2. J.T. Pearlman (ed.): *10th ISCERG Symposium* (Los Angeles, Calif., USA, 1972). 1973   ISBN 90-6193-142-8
3. H.E. Henkes (ed.): *Photography, Electro-Ophthalmology and Echo-Ophthal-mology in Ophthalmic Practice.* 1973   ISBN 90-6193-143-6
4. E. Dodt & J.T. Pearlman (eds.): *11th ISCERG Symposium* (Bad Nauheim, Germany, 1973). 1974   ISBN 90-6193-144-4
5. W.J. Holmes (ed.): *Public Health Ophthalmology.* Papers Presented at the Conference on the Prevention of Impaired Vision and Blindness (Paris, France, 1974). 1975   ISBN 90-6193-145-2
6. A. Th. M. van Balen (ed.): *First International Symposium on Artificial Len-simplantation* (Utrecht, The Netherlands, 1974). 1975   ISBN 90-6193-146-0
7. A.F. Deutman (ed.): [Symposium on] *New Developments in Ophthalmology.* (Nijmegen, The Netherlands, 1975) 1976   ISBN 90-6193-147-9
8. O. Hockwin (ed.): *Progress of Lens Biochemistry Research.* In Honour of Prof. Dr. med. J. Nordmann. 1976   ISBN 90-6193-148-7
9. J.J. de Laey (ed.): *International Symposium on Fluorescein Angiography* (Ghent, Belgium, 1976). 1976   ISBN 90-6193-149-5
10. R. Alfieri & P. Solé (eds.): *12th ISCERG Symposium* (Clermont-Ferrand, France, 1974). 1976   ISBN 90-6193-150-9
11. E. Auerbach (ed.): *Experimental and Clinical Amblyopia. 13th ISCERG Symposium* (Kibbutz Ginossar, Israel, 1975). 1977   ISBN 90-6193-151-7
12. E.L. Greve (ed.): *Symposium on Medical Therapy in Glaucoma* (Amsterdam, The Netherlands, 1976) 1977   ISBN 90-6193-152-5
13. T. Lawwill (ed.): *ERG, VER and Psychophysics. 14th ISCERG Symposium* (Louisville, USA, 1976). 1977   ISBN 90-6193-153-3
14. E.L. Greve (ed.): *2nd International Visual Field Symposium* (Tübingen, Germany, 1976). 1977   ISBN 90-6391-154-1
15. J. François & A. De Rouck (eds.), J.T. Pearlman and J. Kelsey (co-eds.): *Electrodiagnosis, Toxic Agents and Vision. 15th ISCEV Symposium* (Ghent, Belgium, 1977). 1978   ISBN 90-6193-155-X
16. H.-J Merté (ed.): *Genesis of Glaucoma.* Contributions of the Wessely Symposium in Munich (October 1974) with final Considerations by H. Goldmann. 1978   ISBN 90-6193-156-8
17. A.F. Deutmann & J.R.M. Cruysberg (eds.): *5th International Congress on Neurogenetics and Neuro- Ophthalmology* (Nijmegen, The Netherlands, 1977). 1978   ISBN 90-6193-159-2
18. O. Hockwin & W.B. Rathbun (eds.): *Progress in Anterior Eye Segment. Research and Practice.* In Honour of Prof. J.E. Harris. 1979
          ISBN 90-6193-158-4
19. E.L. Greve (ed.): *3rd International Visual Field Symposium* (Tokyo, Japan, 1978). 1979   ISBN 90-6193-160-6
20. J. François, S.I. Brown & M. Itoi (eds.): *Proceedings of the Symposium of the International Society for Corneal Research* (Kyoto, Japan, 1978). 1979
          ISBN 90-6193-157-6

Documenta Ophthalmologica Proceedings Series

Documenta Ophthalmologica Proceedings Series

38. J.S. Hillman & M.M. Le May (eds.): *Ophthalmic Ultrasonography*. Proceedings of the 9th SIDUO Congress (Leeds, UK, 1982). 1984   ISBN 90-6193-734-5
39. G. Verriest (ed.): *Colour Vision Deficiencies VII*. Proceedings of the 7th Symposium of the International Research Group on Colour Vision Deficiencies (Geneva, Switzerland, 1983). 1984   ISBN 90-6193-735-3
40. J.R. Heckenlively (ed.), G.H.M. van Lith & T.Lawwill (ass. eds): *Pattern Electroretinogram, Circulatory Disturbances of the Visual System and Pattern-Evoked Responses*. 21st ISCEV Symposium (Budapest, Hungary, 1983). 1984   ISBN 90-6193-503-2
41. E.C. Campos (ed.): *Sensory Evaluation of Strabismus and Amblyopia in a Natural Environment*. In Honour of Prof. Bruno Bagolini. 1984
    ISBN 90-6193-508-3
42. A. Heijl & E.L. Greve (eds.): *6th International Visual Field Symposium* (Santa Margherita Ligure, Italy, 1984). 1985   ISBN 90-6193-524-5
43. E.L. Greve, W. Leydhecker & C. Raitta (eds.): *2nd European Glaucoma Symposium* (Hyvinkää, Finland, 1984). 1985   ISBN 90-6193-526-1
44. P.C. Maudgal & L. Missotten (eds.): *Herpetic Eye Diseases*. Proceedings of an International Symposium (Leuven, Belgium, 1984). 1985
    ISBN 90-6193-527-X
45. B. Jay (ed.): *Detection and Measurement of Visual Impairment in Pre-Verbal Children*. Proceedings of a Workshop (London, UK, 1985). 1986
    ISBN 0-89838-789-2
46. G. Verriest (ed.): *Colour Vision Deficiencies VIII*. Proceedings of the 8th Symposium of the International Research Group on Colour Vision Deficiencies (Avignon, France, 1985). 1987   ISBN 0-89838-801-5
47. P.L. Emiliani (ed.): *Development of Electronic Aids for the Visually Impaired*. Proceedings of a Workshop on the Rehabilitation of the Visually Impaired (Florence, Italy, 1984). 1986   ISBN 0-89838-805-8
48. K.C. Ossoinig (ed.): *Ophthalmic Echography*. Proceedings of the 10th SIDUO Congress (St. Petersburg Beach, Florida, USA, 1984). 1987
    ISBN 0-89838-873-2
49. E.L. Greve & A. Heijl (eds.): *7th International Visual Field Symposium* (Amsterdam, The Netherlands, 1986). 1987   ISBN 0-89838-882-1
50. D. BenEzra, S.J. Ryan, B.M. Glaser & R.P. Murphy (eds.): *Ocular Circulation and Neovascularization*. Proceedings of the First International Symposium (Jeruzalem, Israel, 1986). 1987   ISBN 0-89838-892-9
51. J.M. Thijssen, J.S. Hillman, P.E. Gallenga & G. Cennamo (eds.): *Ultrasonography in Ophthalmology 11*. Proceedings of the 11th SIDUO Congress (Capri, Italy, 1986). 1988   ISBN 0-89838-378-1
52. B. Drum & G. Verriest (eds.): *Colour Vision Deficiencies IX*. Proceedings of the 9th Symposium of the International Research Group on Colour Vision Deficiencies (Annapolis, Md., USA, 1987). 1989   ISBN 0-89838-403-6

Documenta Ophthalmologica Proceedings Series

53. R. Sampaolesi (ed.): *Ultrasonography in Ophthalmology 12.* Proceedings of the 12th SIDUO Congress (Iguazú Falls, Argentina, 1988). 1990
ISBN 0-7923-0765-8

54. B. Drum, J.D. Moreland & A. Serra (eds.): *Colour Vision Deficiencies X.* Proceedings of the 10th Symposium of the International Research Group on Colour Vision Deficiencies (Cagliari, Italy, 1989). 1991   ISBN 0-7923-0948-0

55. P. Till (ed.): *Ophthalmic Echography 13.* Proceedings of the 13th SIDUO Congress (Vienna, Austria, 1990). 1993   ISBN 0-7923-1808-0

56. B. Drum (ed.): *Colour Vision Deficiencies XI.* Proceedings of the 11th Symposium of the International Research Group on Colour Vision Deficiencies (Sydney, Australia, 1991). 1993   ISBN 0-7923-1864-1

57. B. Drum (ed.): *Colour Vision Deficiencies XII.* Proceedings of the 12th Symposium of the International Research Group on Colour Vision Deficiencies (Tübingen, Germany, 1993). 1995   ISBN 0-7923-2889-2

58. J.M. Thijssen, H.C. Fledelius & S. Tane (eds.): *Ultrasonography in Ophthalmology 14.* Proceedings of the 14th SIDUO Congress (Tokyo, Japan, 1992). 1995
ISBN 0-7923-3475-2

KLUWER ACADEMIC PUBLISHERS – DORDRECHT / BOSTON / LONDON